ABC of Pediatric Surgical Imaging

Savvas Andronikou • Angus Alexander
Tracy Kilborn • Alastair J. W. Millar
Alan Daneman (Eds.)

ABC of Pediatric Surgical Imaging

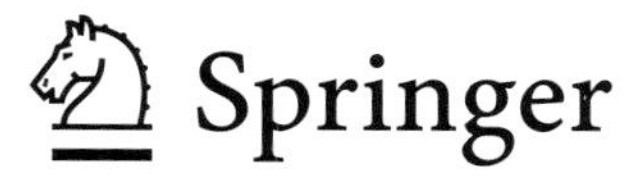

Springer

Dr. Savvas Andronikou
University of Cape Town
Dept. Radiology
Observatory
South Africa
docsav@mweb.co.za

Dr. Angus Alexander
The Hospital for Sick Children
555 University Avenue, Toronto
ON M5G 1X8, Canada
angus.ceiri@gmail.com

Dr. Tracy Kilborn
Red Cross Children's Hospital
Dept. Radiology
Klipfontein Road
Rondebosch, Cape Town 7700
South Africa
tracykilborn@gmail.com

Prof. Alastair J. W. Millar
University of Cape Town
Red Cross War Memorial Children's Hospital
Rondebosch, Cape Town 7700
South Africa
alastair.millar@uct.ac.za

Dr. Alan Daneman
University of Toronto
Hospital for Sick Children
Dept. Diagnostic Imaging
555 University Ave.
Toronto ON M5G 1X8
Canada
alan.daneman@sickkids.ca

ISBN: 978-3-540-89384-4 e-ISBN: 978-3-540-89385-1

DOI: 10.1007/978-3-540-89385-1

Springer Heidelberg Dordrecht London New York

Library of Congress Control Number: 2009929163

Cover design: eStudioCalamar Figueres/Berlin

Printed on acid-free paper

Springer is part of Springer Science+Business Media (www.springer.com)

Introduction

This handbook is intended for doctors working in this field. It belongs to the pocket of a student, house officer, resident, medical officer or generalist consultant, who will first see the patient.

The clinician needs to suspect at least one disease process as a starting point, because the book is ordered alphabetically according to diagnoses. From this point there are both surgical and imaging differential diagnoses listed. These can also be looked at within the book.

For the clinician there is a dedicated page to assist with clinical symptoms and signs, alternative diagnoses and urgency of the radiological investigation, based on important information that is needed from imaging.

With regard to imaging, there is a list of primary, follow-on and alternative investigations appropriate for the suspected diagnosis. There are lists of imaging features with supporting images, tips and radiological differential diagnoses.

The alphabetic organization makes for a jump to the next suspected diagnosis with ease to find something more suitable for the current patient's needs.

The editors are experts in their field, with extensive practical experience and clarity into the complexity of problems encountered daily. They are also up to date on new imaging techniques and apply what they teach in clinical practice. They cannot be responsible for any errors in diagnosis, however, as clinical medicine still requires meticulous history and examination, as well as subjective opinion, which remains a product of knowledge, experience and even luck. Medicine is constantly changing and medical opinion changes over time and due to an increasing body of knowledge. The user of this book should keep this in mind. The editors hope that this book will be used to help the clinician make better decisions and help sick children.

South Africa Savvas Andronikou

Acknowledgements

Dr. Arthur Maydell – For assistance with images and digital post processing
Mrs. Annette Hinze – For believing in the project and her patience
Mrs. Annalie Rich – For her unwavering support and assistance
Dr. Kieran McHugh – For immediate assistance with images
Dr. Douglas Jamieson – For immediate assistance with images
Dr. Irene Borzani – For immediate assistance with images
Dr. Ian Cowan – For immediate assistance with images

Contents

Contributors

Surgeons

A. Alexander
The Hospital for Sick Children,
555 University Avenue, Toronto,
ON M5G 1X8, Canada
angus.ceiri@gmail.com

J. Alves
Tygerberg Academic Hospital,
Faculty of Medicine,
University of Stellenbosch, PO Box 19063,
Tygerberg 7505, South Africa
jalves@mtnloaded.co.za

M. Arnold
Department of Paediatric Surgery,
Tygerberg Academic Hospital,
Faculty of Medicine,
University of Stellenbosch, PO Box 19063,
Tygerberg 7505, South Africa
Mariondonald@mweb.co.za

O. Basson
Department of Otorhinolaryngology,
Red Cross War Memorial Children's
Hospital, Klipfontein Road, Rondebosch,
Cape Town 7700, South Africa
Ola_basson@hotmail.com

A. Brooks
Red Cross War Memorial Children's
Hospital, Klipfontein Road, Rondebosch,
Cape Town 7700, South Africa
andre.brooks@uct.ac.za

S. Cox
Department of Paediatric Surgery,
Red Cross War Memorial Children's
Hospital, Klipfontein Road, Rondebosch,
Cape Town 7700, South Africa
sharon.cox@uct.ac.za

A. Darani
Department of Paediatric Surgery, Hôpital
des Enfants, Geneva University Hospital,
6 Rue Willy-Donzé, 1211 Geneva 14,
Switzerland
Adarani@worldcom.ch

C. Davies
Department of Pediatrics, The Hospital
for Sick Children, 555 University Avenue,
Toronto, ON M5G 1X8, Canada
angus.ceiri@gmail.com

J. Karpelowsky
Department of Paediatric Surgery,
Red Cross War Memorial Children's
Hospital, Klipfontein Road, Rondebosch,
Cape Town 7700, South Africa
jonathan.karpelowski@uct.ac.za

J. Lazarus
Department of Paediatric Surgery,
Red Cross War Memorial Children's
Hospital, Klipfontein Road, Rondebosch,
Cape Town 7700, South Africa
may1968@geocities.com

J. Loveland
Department of Paediatric Surgery, Baragwanath Hospital, University of the Witwatersrand, PO Bertsham, Johannesberg 2013, South Africa
Loveland@wol.co.za

S.W. Moore
Department of Paediatric Surgery, Tygerberg Academic Hospital, Faculty of Medicine, University of Stellenbosch, PO Box 19063, Tygerberg 7505, South Africa
swm@sun.ac.za

A. Numanoglu
Department of Paediatric Surgery, Red Cross War Memorial Children's Hospital, Klipfontein Road, Rondebosch, Cape Town 7700, South Africa
Alp.Numanoglu@uct.ac.za

H. Peens-Hough
Department Paediatrics, Red Cross War Memorial Children's Hospital, Klipfontein Road, Rondebosch, Cape Town 7700, South Africa
hyla.peenshough@gmail.com

A. Potgieter
Department of Plastic and Reconstructive Surgery, University of Witwatersrand, Chris Hani Baragwanath Hospital for Sick Children, PO Bertsham, Johannesberg 2013, South Africa
antonpot@global.co.za

D. Sidler
Department of Paediatric Surgery, Tygerberg Academic Hospital, Faculty of Medicine, University of Stellenbosch, PO Box 19063, Tygerberg 7505, South Africa
ds2@sun.ac.za

I.F. Simango
Eastern Cape Paediatric Surgical Services, East London Hospital Complex, Private Bag X9047, East London 5200, South Africa
ifsimango@yahoo.com

A.B. van As
Department of Paediatric Surgery, Red Cross War Memorial Children's Hospital, Klipfontein Road, Rondebosch, Cape Town 7700, South Africa
sebastian.vanas@uct.ac.za

J.C.H. Wilde
Paediatric Surgical Center, Academic Medical Center, PO Box 22660, 1100 DD Amsterdam, The Netherlands
j.c.wilde@amc.uva.nl

Radiologists

Christelle Ackermann
Radio-diagnosis Department, Stellenbosch University, Medical Faculty Building, 5th floor, Parow, Cape Town, South Africa, ca@sun.ac.za

Asif Bagadia
Radio-diagnosis Department, Stellenbosch University, Medical Faculty Building, 5th floor, Parow, Cape Town, South Africa, asif@sun.ac.za

Andrew Brandt
Radio-diagnosis Department, Stellenbosch University, Medical Faculty Building, 5th floor, Parow, Cape Town, South Africa, andrewdbrandt@yahoo.com

Shaheen Cader
Groote Schuur Hospital, Anzio Road, Observatory, Cape Town, South Africa, shaheen.cader@gmail.com

Gerrit Dekker
Radio-diagnosis Department, Stellenbosch University, Medical Faculty Building, 5th floor, Parow, Cape Town, South Africa, gerritdekker@mweb.co.za

Hassan Douis
University Hospitals Birmingham, NHS Foundation Trust Selly Oak Hospital, Raddlebarn Rd, Birmingham B29 6JD, UK, douis.hassan@gmx.de

Anne-Mari du Plessis
Radio-diagnosis Department, Stellenbosch University, Medical Faculty Building, 5th floor, Parow, Cape Town, South Africa, docams@iafrica.com

Jaco du Plessis
Radio-diagnosis Department, Stellenbosch University, Medical Faculty Building, 5th floor, Parow, Cape Town, South Africa, drjjdup@hotmail.com

Reena George
Cowichan District Hospital, Duncan, British Columbia, Canada, deepujosephgeorge@gmail.com

Petrus J. Greyling
Radio-diagnosis Department, Stellenbosch University, Medical Faculty Building, 5th floor, Parow, Cape Town, South Africa, jacothea@telkomsa.net

Murray Hayes
Radio-diagnosis Department, Stellenbosch University, Medical Faculty Building, 5th floor, Parow, Cape Town, South Africa, murrayhayes@hotmail.com

Linda Tebogo Hlabangana
Faculty of Health Sciences, University of the Witwatersrand, 7 York Road, Parktown, Gauteng 2193, South Africa, bogoness@yahoo.com

Bryan Darryl Khoury
Groote Schuur Hospital, Anzio Road, Observatory, Cape Town, South Africa, bryan@dhcare.org

Tracy Kilborn
Department of Radiology, Red Cross War Memorial Children's Hospital, Klipfontein Road, Rondebosch, Cape Town 7700, South Africa, tracykilborn@gmail.com

Hassan M.A. Lameen
Radio-diagnosis Department, Stellenbosch University, Medical Faculty Building, 5th floor, Parow, Cape Town, South Africa, h_alameen1@yahoo.com

Jan Lotz
Radio-diagnosis Department, Stellenbosch University, Medical Faculty Building, 5th floor, Parow, Cape Town, South Africa, Lotz@sun.ac.za

Ayanda Mapukata
Radio-diagnosis Department, Stellenbosch University, Medical Faculty Building, 5th floor, Parow, Cape Town, South Africa, mapu@discoverymail.co.za

Arthur T. Maydell
Radio-diagnosis Department, Stellenbosch University, Medical Faculty Building, 5th floor, Parow, Cape Town, South Africa, atmaydell@hotmail.com

Jaishree Naidoo
Department of Radiology, Red Cross War Memorial Children's Hospital, Klipfontein Road, Rondebosch, Cape Town 7700, South Africa, jaishreenaidoo@hotmail.com

Stefan Jerzy Przybojewski
1835 Westmount Road NW, Hillhurst, Calgary, Alberta, Canada, drstefanp@hotmail.com

Salomine H. Theron
PO Box 5729, Helderberg 7135, South Africa, salomine@adept.co.za

Dirk Johannes van der Merwe
Radio-diagnosis Department, Stellenbosch University, Medical Faculty Building, 5th floor, Parow, Cape Town, South Africa, dirkenanje@yahoo.ca

Pieter Janse van Rensburg
Division Radiodiagnosis, Department of Medical Imaging and Clinical Oncology, Faculty of Health Sciences, University of Stellenbosch, PO Box 19063, Tygerberg 7505, South Africa, p.xray@yahoo.com

Leon Janse van Rensburg
Department of Radiology and Diagnostics, University of the Western Cape, Tygerberg 7535, South Africa, leonj@xray.co.za

Hofmeyr Viljoen
Radio-diagnosis Department, Stellenbosch University, Medical Faculty Building, 5th floor, Parow, Cape Town, South Africa, hviljoen74@yahoo.com

Helga von Bezing
Radio-diagnosis Department, Stellenbosch University, Medical Faculty Building, 5th floor, Parow, Cape Town, South Africa, helgavonbezing@gmail.com

Nicky Wieselthaler
Department of Radiology, Red Cross War Memorial Children's Hospital, Klipfontein Road, Rondebosch, Cape Town 7700, South Africa, ruznix@wol.co.za

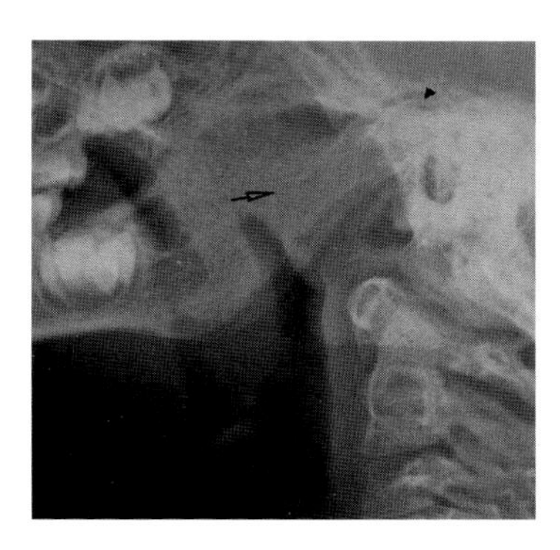

"Soft-tissue" lateral view of the post-nasal space demonstrates the adenoidal soft-tissue pad (*arrow*) encroaching on the nasopharyngeal air space. As a clue, look for soft tissue immediately inferior to the pituitary fossa (*arrowhead*) and internal auditory canal

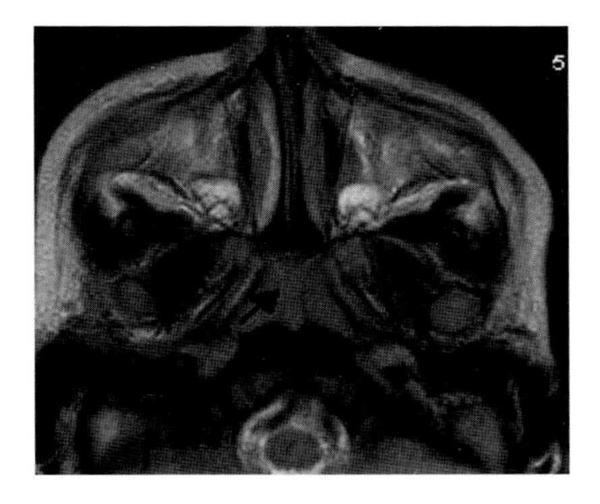

Axial T2 MRI demonstrates the lymphoid tissue in the nasopharynx as homogenous high-signal soft tissue posteriorly (*arrow*)

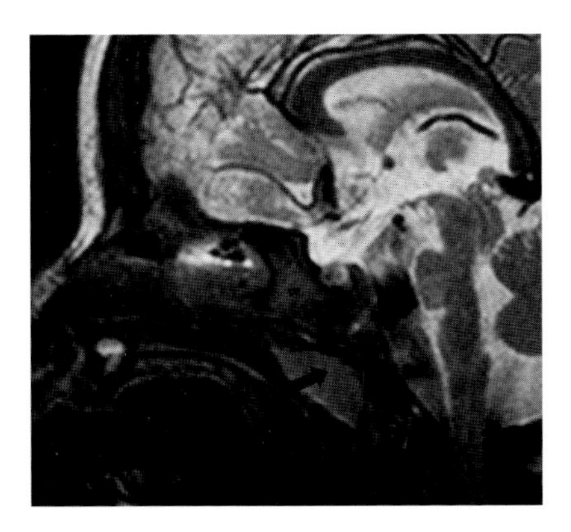

Sagittal T2 demonstrates the adenoidal soft tissue as a high-signal soft-tissue mass (*arrow*) inferior to the pituitary fossa/sphenoid bone (*arrow head*) and clivus

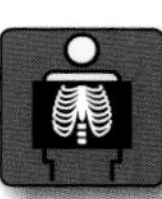

Imaging Options

- Primary: Lateral "soft-tissue" radiograph
- Secondary: Dynamic MRI (for obstructive sleep apnea)

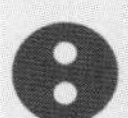

Imaging Findings

- Thick soft tissue in posterior nasopharynx.
- Considered enlarged when adenoids narrow the nasopharynx, or when >12 mm.

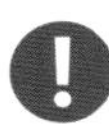

Tips

Lateral Radiograph

- Adenoids rarely seen radiographically <6 months.
- Rapid growth during infancy.
- Peak size between 2–10 years.
- Decrease in size during the second decade.
- Beginners find adenoids by looking inferior to pituitary fossa or sphenoid bone/sinus.

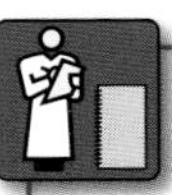

Radiological Differential Diagnosis

- Juvenile angiofibroma
- Lymphoma
- Rhabdomyosarcoma
- Encephalocoele
- Neuroblastoma
- Traumatic haematoma
- Nasopharyngeal teratoma

Adrenal Masses (Other than Neuroblastoma)

Surgeon: D. Sidler
Radiologist: R. George

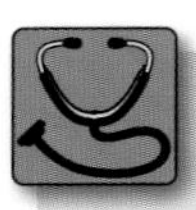

Clinical Insights

- Adrenal masses in childhood may be benign or malignant, intra- or extra-adrenal.
- They may be found incidentally or may be hormonally active and present with:
  - Hypertension
  - Metabolic crises (watery diarrhoea, hypokalaemia)
  - Endocrinopathies (pheochromocytoma)
- Neuroblastoma accounts for greater than 90% of paediatric adrenal cancers.
- The primary therapy for most adrenal lesions is surgical excision.
- Laparoscopy has become the surgical approach of choice with localized disease.
- Surgery is indicated if:
  - A malignancy is suspected.
  - The tumour is hormonally/metabolically active.

Warning

- Pre-operative and intra-operative control of hypertension in a child with a pheochromocytoma is crucial to prevent an intra-operative crisis.

Controversy

- It has been recommended that all paediatric adrenal masses should be resected because of the high proportion of malignant lesions.

Urgency

- ❑ Emergency
- ❑ Urgent
- ☑ Elective

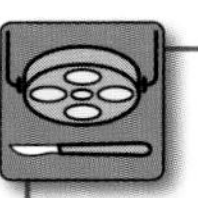

What the Surgeon Needs to Know

- Is the tumour clearly originating from the adrenal gland?
- What is the size of the lesion? (Larger lesions suggest malignancy.)
- Is the CT attenuation less than 10 HU?
- Is there an evidence of a primary lesion suggesting the mass is a metastasis?

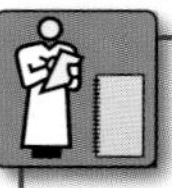

Clinical Differential Diagnosis

- Neuroblastoma, pheochromocytoma, adrenocortical tumours
- Traumatic haemorrhage
- Cysts and pseudocysts

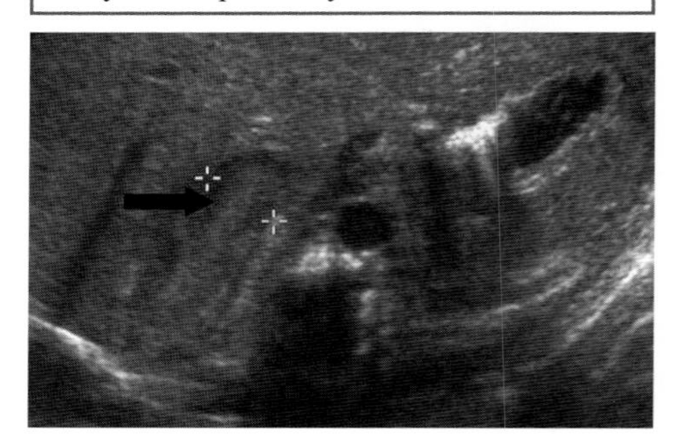

US transverse – Hyperechoic acute adrenal haematoma (*arrow*) of the right adrenal gland in a neonate [Image courtesy Dr. Kieran McHugh]

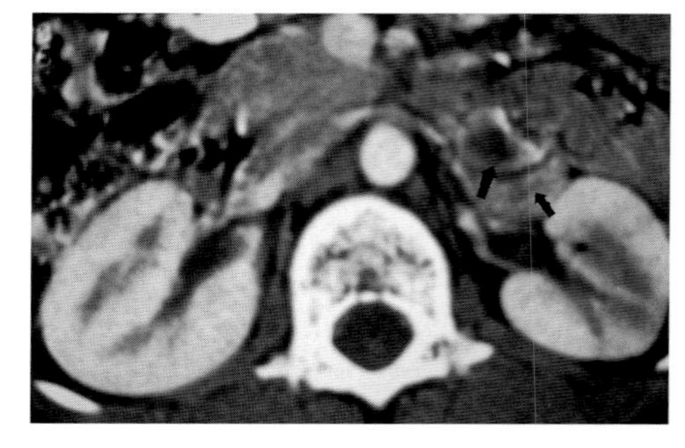

Contrasted CT – Heterogeneously enhancing pheochromocytoma of the left adrenal (*arrows*)

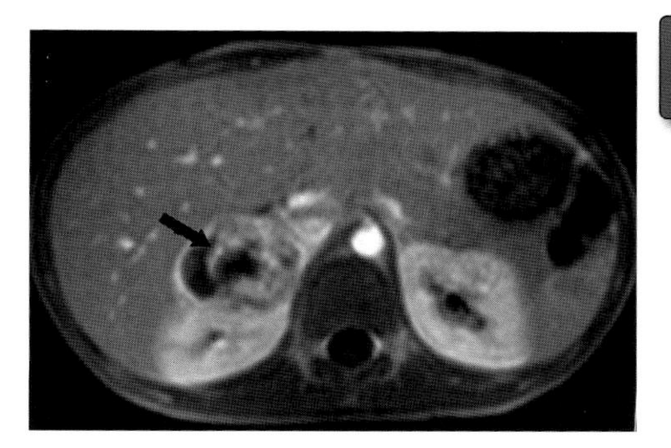

Post-contrast T1 axial MRI – Mixed signal intensity mass in the right adrenal (*arrow*) representing a malignant pheochromocytoma

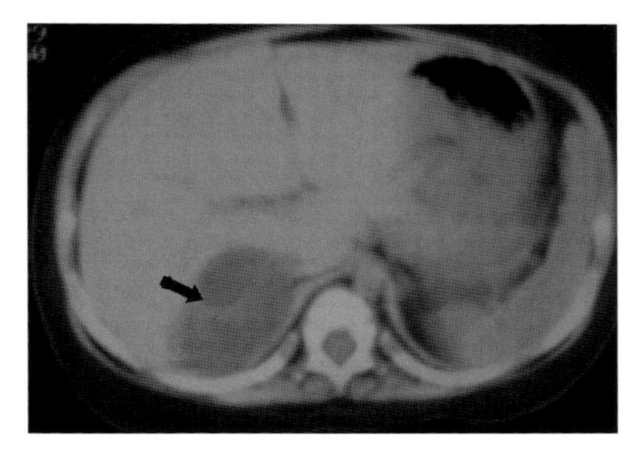

CT low-density adenoma in the right adrenal (*arrow*) of a child with Cushing's disease

Tips

- Normal neonatal adrenal glands are very well seen on US and appear "enlarged" with clearly discernible cortex and medulla.
- Neonatal adrenal haemorrhage – serial ultrasound for reduction in size.

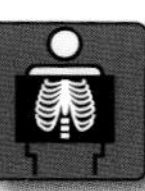

Imaging Options

- Primary: US
- Back-up: MRI/CT/Nuc med

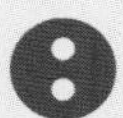

Imaging Findings

Neonatal Adrenal Haemorrhage

US

- Echogenic solid lesion – Initial 1–2 days.
- Anechoic mass as the blood liquefies and then echogenic as it clots.
- Triangular calcification with reduction in the size of mass in weeks to months.
- Mass is avascular and may be bilateral.

Pheochromocytoma

I 131 MIBG

- Initial modality for localization
- 5% bilateral, multiple and malignant

CT/MRI

- Hypervascular mass on CT
- Hyperintense on T2-weighted MRI

Adrenal Adenoma/Carcinoma

CT

- Adenoma – Well-defined soft-tissue mass 0–20 HU on CT. Invariably associated with endocrine dysfunction.
- Carcinoma – Solid invasive mass, calcification 30%
- Imaging cannot always differentiate adenoma and carcinoma; this requires histology.

Adrenal Myelolipoma

- Rare, incidental, small or large mass with intratumoural fat

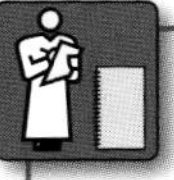

Radiological Differential Diagnosis

- Neuroblastoma

Anorectal Malformation

Surgeon: A. Numanoglu
Radiologist: R. George

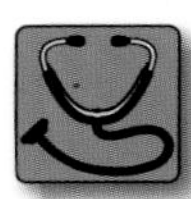

Clinical Insights

- Degree of malformation is a spectrum, from anal stenosis to extrophy and cloaca.
- Vestibular anus is the most common lesion in females.
- Recto-urethral fistula is the commonest abnormality in males.
- The VACTREL syndrome and associated abnormalities need to be excluded.
- Management is based on the relationship of the most distal bowel anomaly to the pelvic-floor muscle–sphincter complex and the genito-urinary tract.

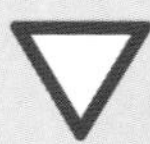

Warning

- Anatomy can be complex, and a surgeon should be present during the imaging procedure for operative planning.

Controversy

- An invertogram performed 24 h after birth is designed to detect those infants who have no clinical fistula and who have a rectal stump below the coccyx. It is thought that they can safely undergo a primary surgical correction.

Urgency

- ☐ Emergency
- ☐ Urgent
- ☑ Elective

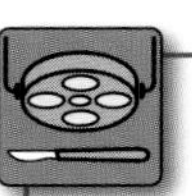

What the Surgeon Needs to Know

At Birth

- Are there associated defects?
  - Vertebral/spinal cord, sacrum
  - Cardiac
  - Tracheo-oesophageal
  - Renal
  - Limb
- The "level" of the anomaly in relation to the muscle–sphincter complex

Elective

- Where does the fistula open into the genito-urinary tract?
- In those with colostomy, is the length of bowel distal to mucus fistula adequate for pull-through?

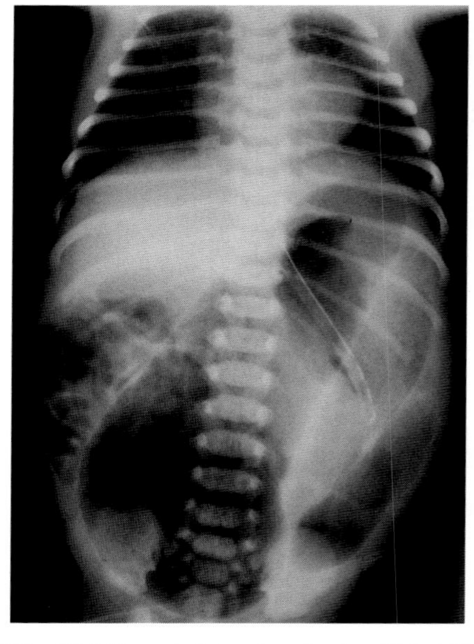

AXR – Distal bowel obstruction due to a high ARM. Also note the elevated cardiac apex due to Fallot's tetrology (VACTREL)

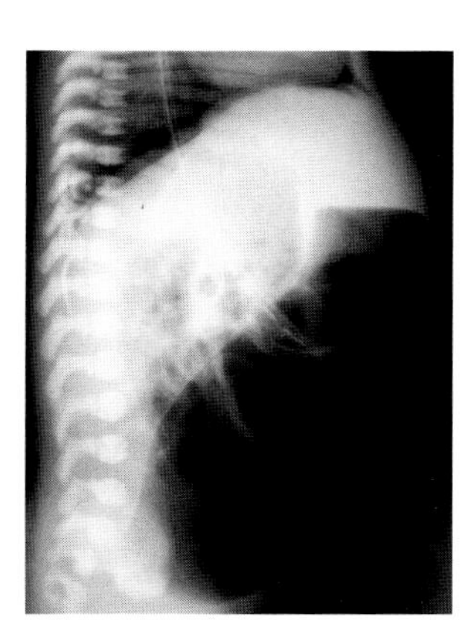

Lateral shoot-through – Sacral hypogenesis indicating a high ARM

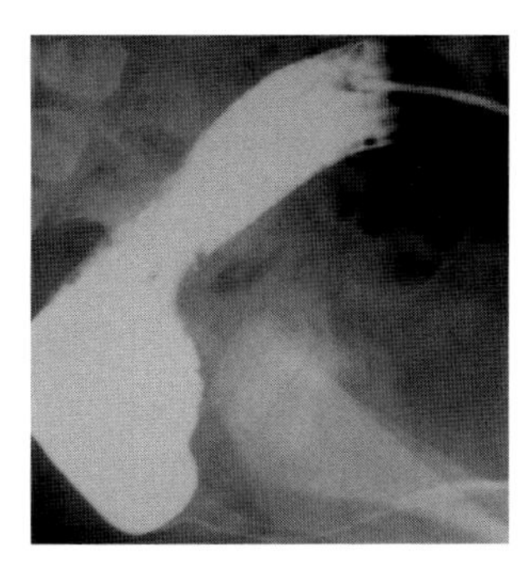

Distal loopogram – High anorectal malformation and fistula with the posterior urethra in a male

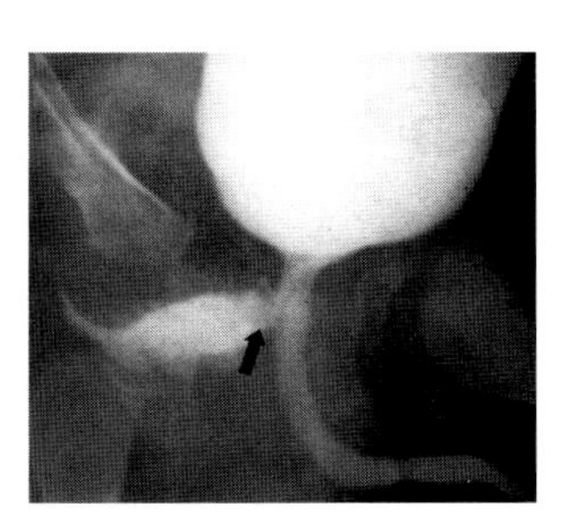

MCUG – Shows the fistula of the posterior urethra with rectum (*arrow*)

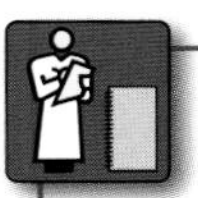

Radiological Differential Diagnosis

All causes of distal obstruction, but physical examination should rule these out.

- Hirschsprung's disease
- Meconium plug syndrome
- Distal bowel obstruction
- Small left colon syndrome

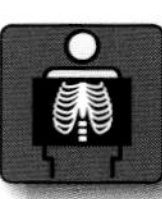

Imaging Options

- Primary: AXR/lateral shoot through
- Back-up: US/fluoroscopy – distal loopogram (via mucus fistula)
- Follow on: MRI

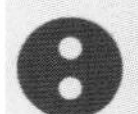

Imaging Findings

AXR

- Distal obstruction.
- Sacrum may be deficient, and vertebral anomalies constitute VACTREL.
- ±Meconium/air in bladder (males) due to fistula (colo-vesical/prostatic/urethral).

US

- Transperineal for distance from distal pouch to skin
- Routine KUB for renal anomalies
- Spinal US routine for tethered cord

Fluoroscopy – distal loopogram

- Via mucus fistula for distal pouch and demonstration of fistula prior to closure
- MCUG to demonstrate VUR

MRI

- Post-operative assessment of neo-rectum and pelvic muscles
- For diagnosing tethered cord in high ARM

Tips

- AXR and ultrasound unreliable to determine the exact level.
- Absent sacral elements indicate a "high" ARM.
- Fluoroscopy – True lateral with open collimators to include bladder and perineum.
- Fluoroscopy – a contrast marker at anal dimple helps to measure the distance from distal pouch to skin.

Appendicitis (Acute)

Surgeon: H. Peens-Hough
Radiologist: A. Bagadia

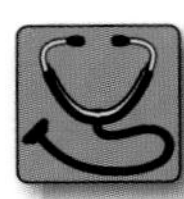

Clinical Insights

- Peak incidence: 4–15 years.
- Abdominal pain is typical, initially poorly localised to the umbilical region (visceral), and then migrates to the right iliac fossa (somatic) as the inflammatory process becomes transmural.
- An appendix mass may be a phlegmon or an abscess.
- The majority of appendixes are retro-caecal.

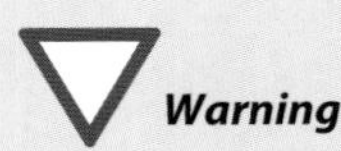

Warning

- Resuscitation and pain management are essential before imaging.

Controversies

- No imaging is required if the diagnosis is made clinically.
- Many institutions perform an ultrasound regardless of the diagnostic certainty.
- If the ultrasound diagnosis and grading can be performed it may allow for non-surgical treatment of early cases as these can be effectively treated with antibiotics.
- CT scanning is the most accurate imaging modality – When is it necessary?

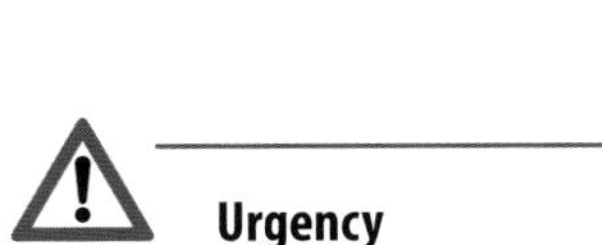

Urgency

- ❑ Emergency
- ☑ Urgent
- ❑ Elective

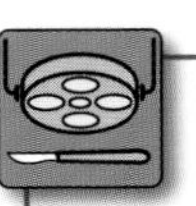

What the Surgeon Needs to Know

- Is the appendix inflamed and what is its position?
- If there is pus: Is it localised, regionally contained or lying free in the peritoneal cavity?
- Is there evidence of co-existing pathology?
- Is some other primary pathology mimicking appendicitis?

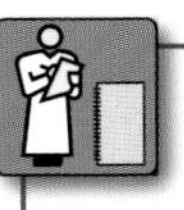

Clinical Differential Diagnosis

- Mesenteric adenitis
- Urinary tract infection
- Terminal ilieitis
- Meckel's diverticulum
- Ovarian pathology
- Pelvic inflammatory disease (older girls)
- Ectopic pregnancy (older girls)
- Renal calculus

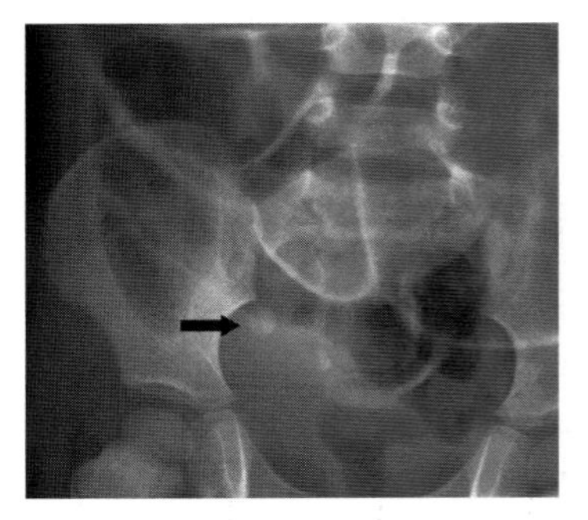

X-ray pelvis – The appendicolith in the right pelvis (*arrow*) is diagnostic in the right clinical setting. There is a relative paucity of bowel gas around it and massive gas distension suggesting ileus or obstruction

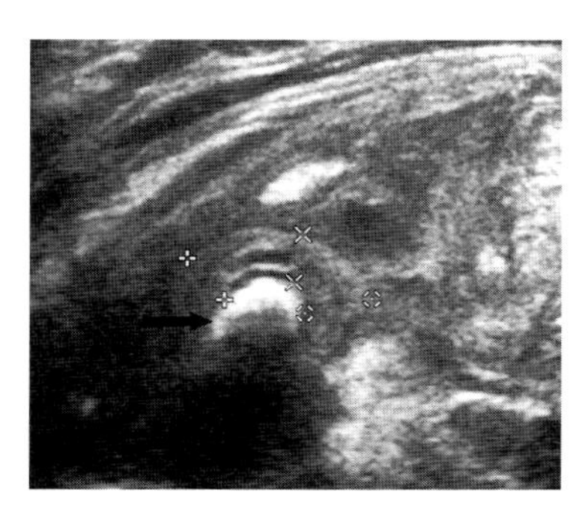

US transverse – Demonstrates an appendicolith (*arrow*) with an acoustic shadow diagnostic of appendicitis

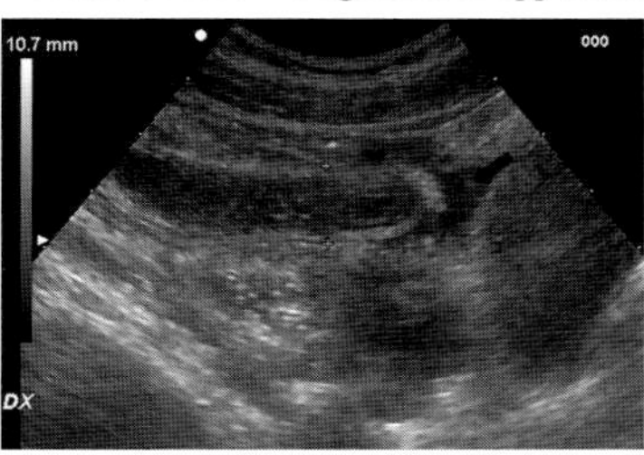

US longitudinal with curvilinear probe– Demonstrating a non-compressible, thickened appendix, measuring 10.7 mm (calipers) (normal: <6 mm) and demonstrating a pre-appendiceal fluid collection (*arrow*) [Image courtesy Dr. Irene Borzani]

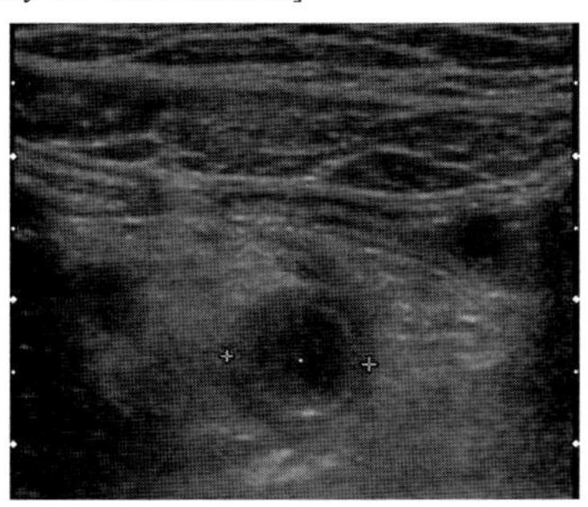

US transverse with linear probe – Demonstrates the non-compressible, thickened appendix (9.7 mm) (calipers) [Image courtesy Dr. Irene Borzani]

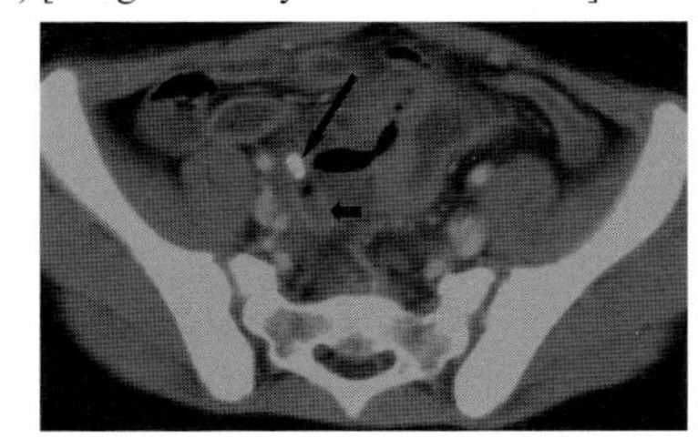

CT axial post-contrast – Demonstrating an appendicolith (*long arrow*) thickening of the appendix (*short arrow*), an associated fluid collection and features of local ileus. [Image courtesy Dr. Irene Borzani]

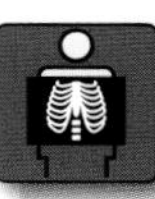

Imaging Options

- Primary: US
- Back-up: CT

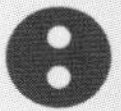

Imaging Findings

US

- Non-compressible, swollen, hypo-echoic appendix ≥ 6 mm
- Laminated wall with target appearance
- Sonographic "Mc Burney" tenderness
- Appendicolith – Echogenic with posterior acoustic shadowing
- Increased Doppler flow in inflamed appendicular region
- Focal/peri-appendiceal collection
- Free fluid in RIF or pelvis
- Echogenic mesentry due to oedema/ inflammation

CT

- Dilated hypodense appendix ≥ 6 mm with thick enhancing wall
- Appendicolith
- Periappendicular fat stranding
- Free fluid in RIF or pelvis
- Caecal apex changes
  - Focal mural thickening
  - Arrow head sign
  - Caecal bar
- Phlegmon, free fluid, air bubbles, abscess and ±adenopathy

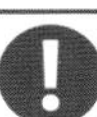

Tips

- CT: Contrast-enhanced CT with contrast distension of the caecum (controversial)
- CT better at detecting small abscesses and geography prior to intervention

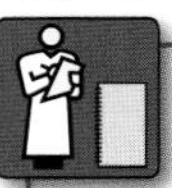

Radiological Differential Diagnosis

- Meckel's diverticulum
- Mesenteric lymphadenitis
- Crohn's/TB
- In girls: Ovarian cyst or torsion (adolescents – ruptured ectopic pregnancy)
- Omental infarction

Ascariasis (Worm Bolus Obstruction)

Surgeon: M. Arnold, J. Alves
Radiologist: J. du Plessis

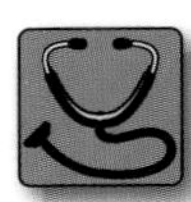

Clinical Insights

- Ascaris worms colonise 20–25% of world's population.
- May present with:
  - Vague abdominal complaints.
  - Evidence of malabsorption.
  - Bowel obstruction due to a worm bolus.
  - Biliary colic.
  - Cholangitis or pancreatitis.

Warnings

- A worm bolus may cause obstruction or volvulus.
- Worm bolus obstruction with fluid levels on X-ray usually indicates impending strangulation/necrosis.
- This clinical and radiological picture in the presence of a tender or peritonitic abdomen requires urgent surgical intervention.

Urgency

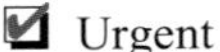

- ☐ Emergency
- ☑ Urgent
- ☐ Elective

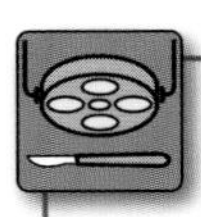

What the Surgeon Needs to Know

- Is there a worm infestation?
- Are the worms the likely cause of the symptoms?
- Are there worms in the biliary tree?

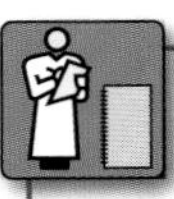

Clinical Differential Diagnosis

- Other causes of bowel and pancreatico-biliary duct obstruction.
- Sand ingestion (pica) may resemble worms on abdominal X-ray.

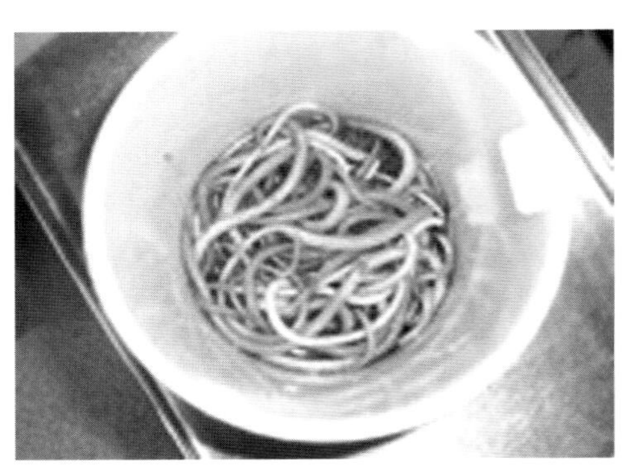

Ascaris worms "milked" from bowel during surgery for bolus obstruction

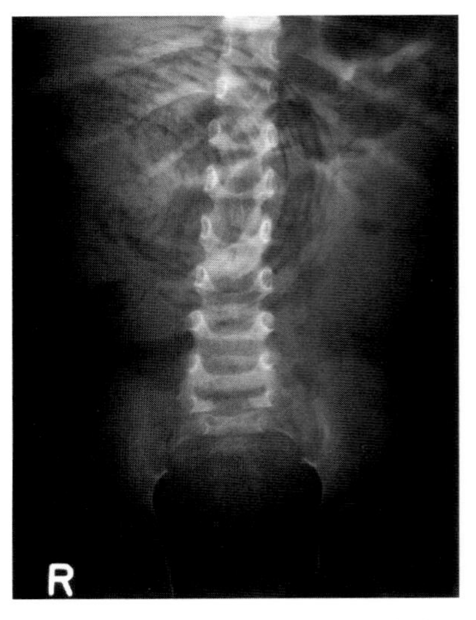

Plain abdominal film demonstrates a whorled appearance of the worms outlined by air

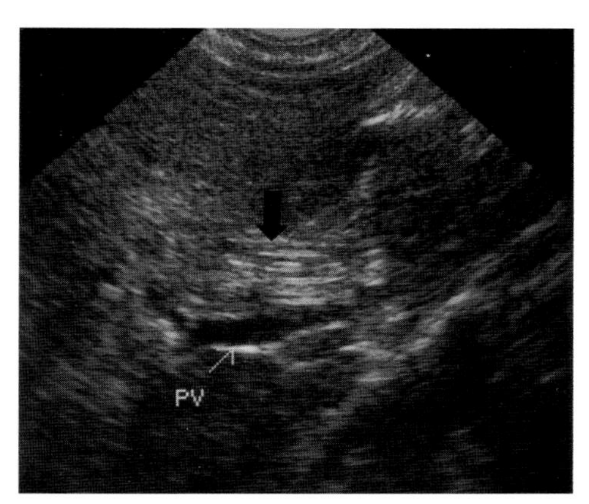

US of the billiary tree demonstrating linear structures in the common bile duct at the porta hepatis (*black arrow*) close to the portal vein (PV) representing ascaris worms [Courtesy Doug Jamieson]

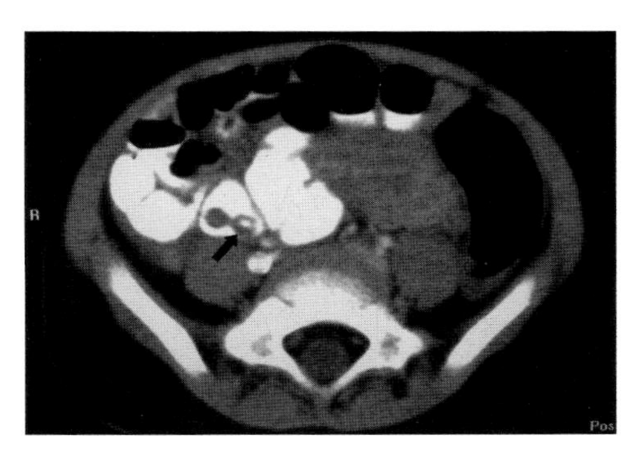

CT scan demonstrates the parasite as a filling defects in cross section with contrast within the parasites intestine (*arrow*)

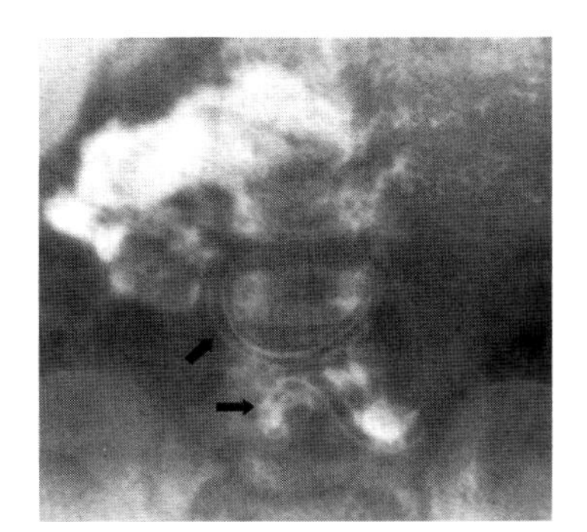

Contrast fluoroscopy demonstrates contrast-filled enteric canal within parasites (*arrows*)

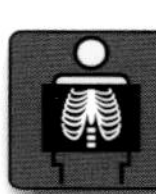

Imaging Options

- Primary: AXR
- Back-up: US, CT, contrast fluoroscopy

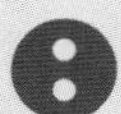

Imaging Findings

AXR

- Partial or complete bowel obstruction with distended bowel loops
- Whorled appearance
- Free intraperitoneal air if perforation of bowel

US

- "Spaghetti-like" structures in small bowel and/or billiary tree (gall bladder)

CT/Contrast Fluoroscopy

- Tubular filling defects in contrast-filled bowel
- Barium-filled enteric canal outlined within ascaris

Tips

- They look like worms!

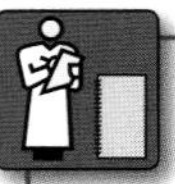

Radiological Differential Diagnosis

- As for bowel obstruction

Biliary Atresia

Surgeon: A. Alexander
Radiologist: L. Tebogo Hlabangana

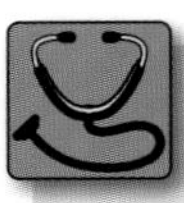

Clinical Insights

- Biliary atresia is a cholangio-destructive disease of the bile ducts of unknown aetiology.
- The most common, surgically treatable cause of cholestasis encountered during the newborn period.
- If untreated, the bile ducts obliterate leading to cholestasis, cirrhosis and liver failure.
- Type I involves obliteration of the common bile duct only (good prognosis but rare).
- Type II is atresia of the common hepatic duct.
- Type III (>90% of patients) involves atresia of the extra-hepatic ducts to the level of porta hepatis.
- Following Kasai portoenterostomy, 70% may clear jaundice, but complications include cholangitis (50%), portal hypertension (>60%) and progressive cirrhosis that requires transplantation.

Warnings

- Jaundice that is progressive or persisting beyond the first 2 weeks of life should always be investigated for an obstructive component.
- The success of portoenterostomy is reduced if the operation is delayed more than 60 days. Clinical investigations should be expedited.

Urgency

- ❑ Emergency
- ☑ Urgent
- ❑ Elective

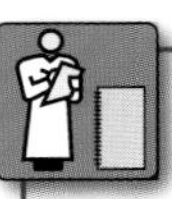

Clinical Differential Diagnosis

- Alagille syndrome
- Caroli disease
- Cholestasis
- Cystic fibrosis
- Neonatal hepatitis
- Alpha 1 antitrypsin deficiency
- Infections (toxoplasmosis, rubella, cytomegalovirus infection, herpes simplex virus infection, syphilis)
- Choledochal cyst

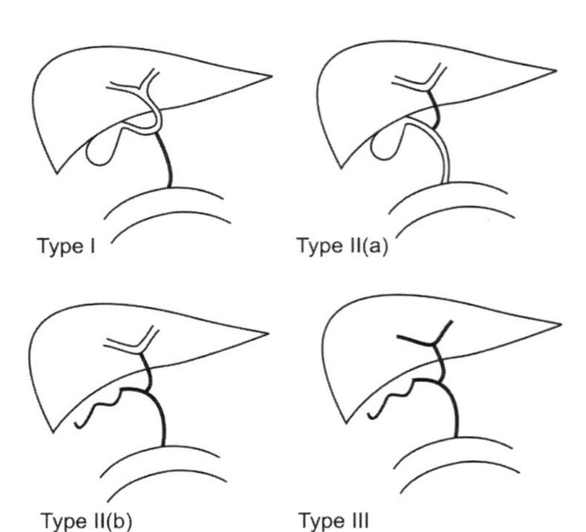

The four common types of biliary atresia

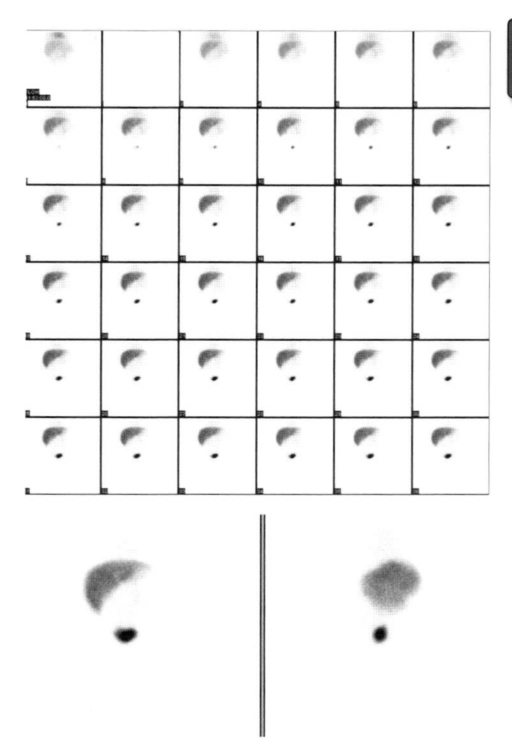

Nuc Med Tc99 DISIDA study showing hepatic uptake of radiopharmaceutical but lack of excretion into the biliary tree or bowel

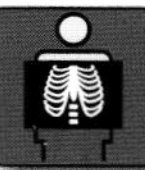

Imaging options

- Primary: US
- Followed on: Nuc Med

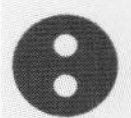

Imaging Findings

US

- Exclude other causes of jaundice (e.g. choledochal cyst).
- Liver echotexture is typically normal.
- A gallbladder may be present in 25% (absent GB is a positive sign).
- Extrahepatic bile ducts are not visible – replaced by a fibrotic remnant of the common duct – echogenic "triangular cord" sign.

Nuclear Hepatobiliary Scan

- Lack of excretion of radiotracer into the intestines on 24-h delay images is highly suggestive of biliary atresia (or other extrahepatic occlusion).
- Visualization of the gallbladder is not a helpful sign.

Tips

- Hepatobiliary scintigraphy is most accurate after 5 days of pretreatment with phenobarbital.

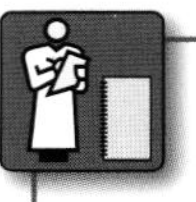

Radiological Differential Diagnosis

- Hepatitis
- Alagille syndrome
- Choledochal cyst

Bochdaleck Hernia (Congenital Diaphragmetic Hernia/CDH)

Surgeon: A. Alexander
Radiologist: J.W. Lotz

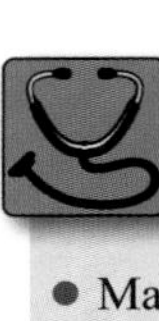

Clinical Insights

- Malformation of the primordial diaphragm (pleuroperitoneal folds).
- Eighty five percent occur on the left.
- Pulmonary hypoplasia may be part of the abnormality and is the major determinant of outcome.
- Associated congenital abnormalities:
  - Cardiac defects present in 63%
  - Neural tube defects
  - Uro-genital abnormalities
  - Chromosomal abnormalities (trisomy)
  - Pulmonary sequestrations
  - Anomalies of midgut rotation and fixation

Controversies

- Ante-natal diagnosis of an isolated defect cannot reliably predict the outcome and does not require a change in obstetric management.
- Surgical correction is delayed until cardio-respiratory status has been stabilized (trial of life).
- Permissive hypercapnoea and role of ECMO (extracorporeal membrane oxygenation).

Urgency

- ☐ Emergency
- ☐ Urgent
- ☑ Elective

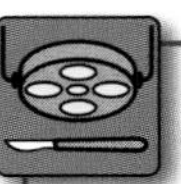

What the Surgeon Needs to Know

- Lung:head circumference ratio/fetal lung volume assessment on antenatal imaging.
- Has thoracic disease mimicking CDH been excluded?
- Presence of stomach or liver in the chest (indicators of poor prognosis).
- Are there any identifiable associated abnormalities?

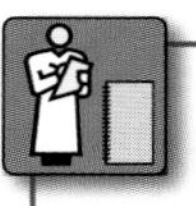

Clinical Differential Diagnosis

- Diaphragmatic: Eventration
- Pleural: Effusion, empyema
- Parenchymal: Consolidation, CCAM, sequestrations, bronchogenic cyst
- Mediastinal: Cystic hygroma, teratoma, neurogenic tumours

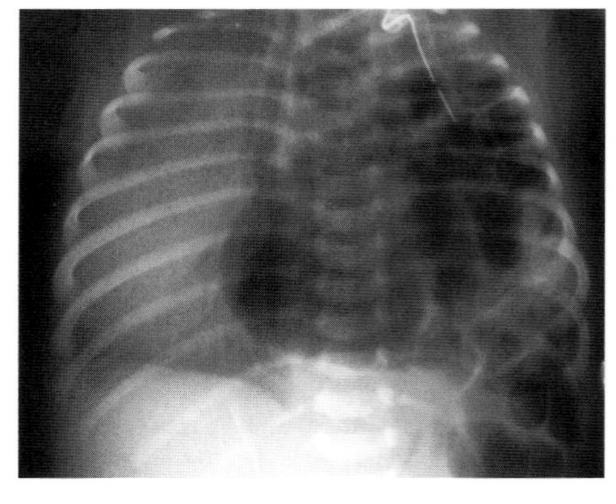

CXR – Bowel gas pattern within the left hemithorax continuous with bowel loops in the abdomen and displacement of the mediastinal structures to the right. Note that there is no significant aerated lung on the right. An intercostal drain has been inserted in error on the left

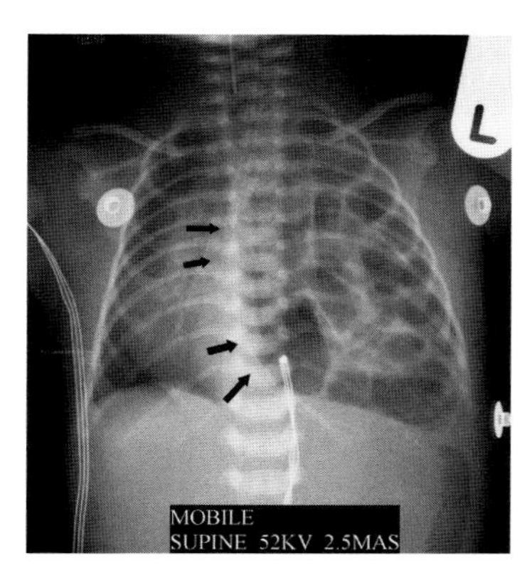

CXR – There are bowel loops in the left hemithorax displacing mediastinal structures to the right, including the nasogastric tube (*arrows*). Note the paucity of intra-abdominal bowel gas contributing to the diagnosis

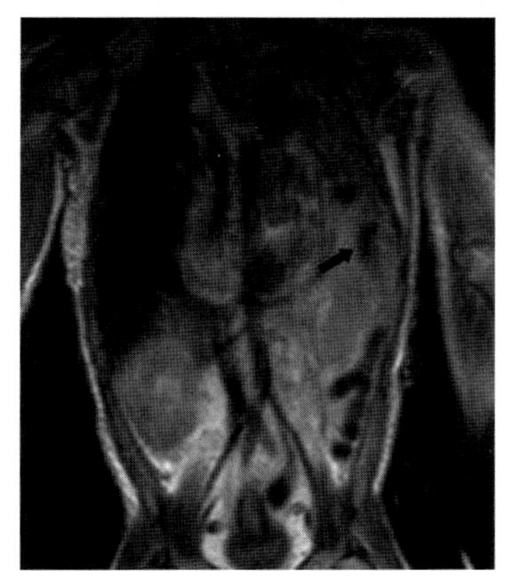

MRI coronal – In contrast to low-signal air-filled lung on the right, the left hemithorax shows some fluid-filled and some air-filled bowel loops (*arrow*) in continuity with abdominal bowel loops through a large diaphragmatic defect

Tips

- 5 "B"s: *B*ochdalek hernias are *b*ig and present at *b*irth with *b*owel in the *b*ack of the chest (in contrast to Morgagni, which present later, anteriorly and are small).
- Air-filled cysts often of the same diameter (CCAM cysts have different sizes and normal bowel gas in the abdomen).
- Associated with unilateral pulmonary hypoplasia (objective of treatment is to re-expand lung and allow growth).

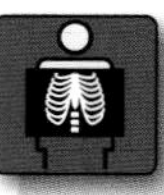

Imaging Options

Primary:	AXR, CXR, prenatal US
Follow-on:	US
Back-up:	CT, MRI
Not recommended:	Contrast meal (UGI)/ enema

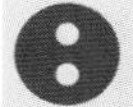

Imaging Findings

CXR/AXR

- More common left (L:R–5:1)
- Immediately after birth may be radiodense (no air in bowel)
- Air containing mass/air-filled cysts
- Less bowel loops in abdomen
- Abnormal position of support tubes (NGT, ETT, UVC)
- When right sided, contains liver and therefore radiodense
- Pulmonary hypoplasia – Low volume ipsi- and contra-lateral lung

US

- Demonstrates fluid-filled and peristalsing bowel loops in the chest
- Demonstrates paucity or lack of bowel loops in the abdomen and sometimes continuity with loops in the chest

CT

- Confirms bowel continuous from abdomen into chest
- Reconstructions may demonstrate defective diaphragm

MRI

- Bowel loops = high signal fluid content in the chest
- Liver = low signal in chest

UGI/Enema

- Enema confirms colon and UGI confirms stomach in chest

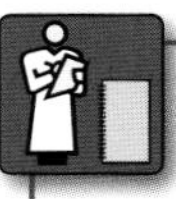

Imaging Differential Diagnosis

- CCAM
- Cavitating pneumonia
- Pneumatocoeles – Rare in neonates

Branchial Cleft Anomalies

Surgeon: J. Karpelowsky
Radiologist: L. Tebogo Hlabangana

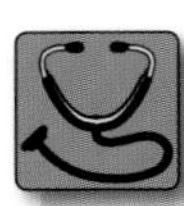

Clinical Insights

- Caused by a congenital anomaly of the branchial arches.
- Usually the second arch grows over the third and fourth arch. The branchial cleft is an ectoderm-lined cavity, which normally involutes. Persistence leads to an epithelium-lined cyst or sinus.
- Branchial cysts usually present later in life (6 years)
- May present as a recurrent infected abscess

Warnings

- May present as an abscess
- Very rarely may cause airway compromise

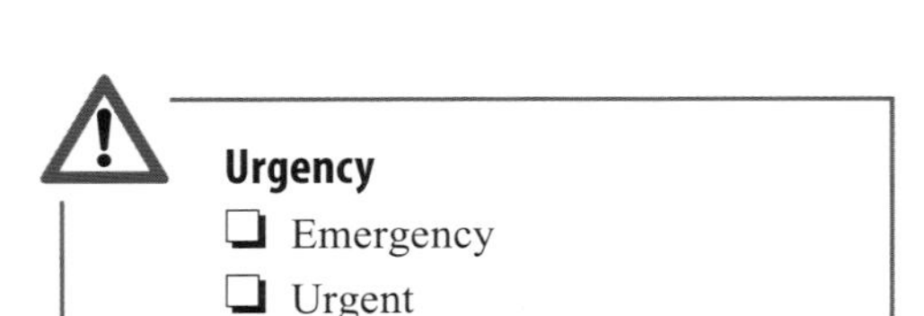

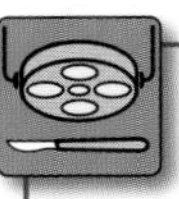

What the Surgeon Needs to Know

- Relationship to adjacent structures
- Whether it is solid or cystic

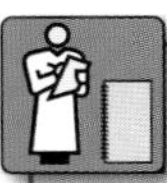

Clinical Differential Diagnosis

- Lymph node
- Dermoid cyst
- Parotid lesions
- Neoplasms
- Oesophageal duplication cysts
- Thymic cysts
- Laryngocoeles
- Cystic hygroma

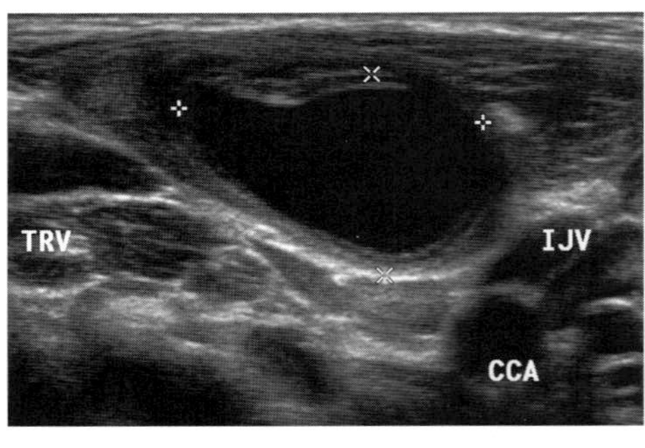

US – Demonstrates a cystic neck mass deep to the sternocleidomastoid and superficial but closely associated with the internal jugular vein (IJV) and common carotid artery (CCA) consistent with a second branchial cleft anomaly

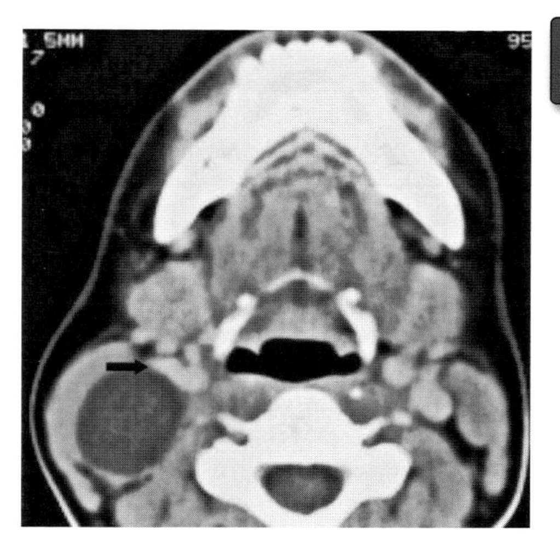

CT scan – Demonstrates an uncomplicated second branchial cleft cyst deep to the sternocleidomastoid muscle and closely associated with the carotid space (*arrow*)

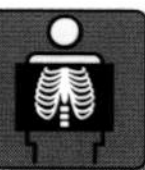

Imaging options

- Primary: US
- Secondary: CT/MRI
- Back-up: Fistulogram

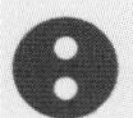

Imaging findings

US

- Hypo-echoic or anechoic cyst; may contain internal echoes if infected or haemorrhage

CT

- Well-defined hypodense cyst
- Peripheral enhancement if infected

MRI

- Typically T1 hypo-intense/T2 hyper-intense
- May have increase in T1 signal if proteinaceous content
- Peripheral enhancement if infected

Fisutlogram

- First branchial arch traverses parotid to external auditory canal
- Second branchial arch usually opens into tonsillar fossa
- Third branchial arch opens into pyriform sinus
- Fourth branchial arch opens into hypopharynx

Tips

- Anatomical boundaries of the cyst/fistula predict the type of anomaly.
- A child presenting with recurrent thyroid abscess should prompt a search for branchial cleft fistula.
- In second branchial cleft cysts, CT may demonstrate a "tail" extending from the cyst to the space between the internal jugular vein (IJV) and the common carotid artery (CCA)

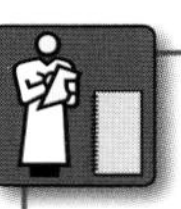

Radiological Differential Diagnosis

- Cystic hygroma
- Necrotic lymph nodes
- Abscess
- Cystic neoplasm of the parotid

Bronchogenic Cysts

Surgeon: A. Brooks
Radiologist: T. Kilborn

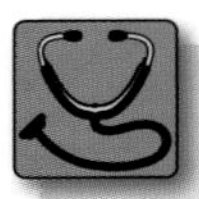

Clinical Insights

- Congenital cysts that result from an anomalous development of the ventral foregut and are along the tracheobronchial tree or within the lung parenchyma.
- When parenchymal in location the lower lobes are most commonly involved.
- They may communicate with the bronchial tree and if so usually present with signs of pulmonary sepsis and air–fluid levels.

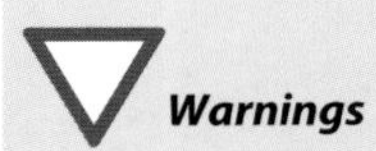

Warnings

- Cyst-related complications such as infection, rupture, bleeding and compression are common.
- There is also a risk of malignant degeneration.
- Other reported complications include airway-cyst fistula, ulceration and haemorrhage. Arrhythmias and superior vena cava syndrome may also develop.

Urgency

- ❑ Emergency
- ❑ Urgent
- ☑ Elective

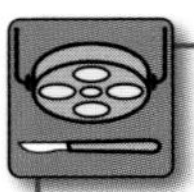

What the Surgeon Needs to Know

- Is this a bronchogenic cyst?
- What is its origin and location?
- Is there any evidence of complications that could be life threatening? Exclude airway and great vessel compression preoperatively.
- Is there a communication with the bronchial tree, oesophagus or stomach?

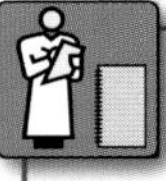

Clinical Differential diagnosis

- CCAM
- Pulmonary sequestration
- Empyema

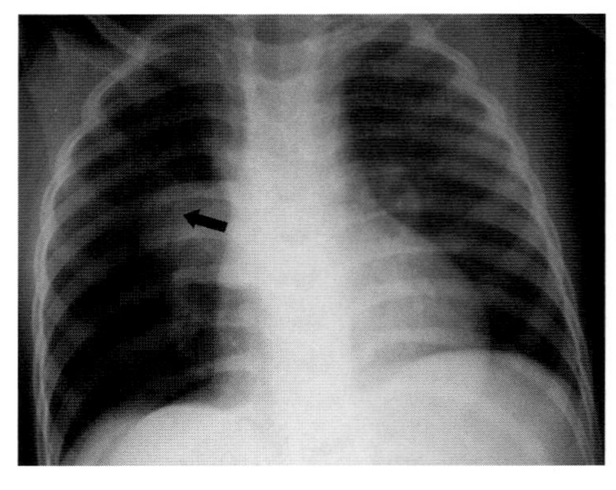

CXR demonstrates an oval soft-tissue density parahilar mass on the right (*arrow*) representing a bronchogenic cyst. This is causing air-trapping in the right lung because of compression of the main bronchus

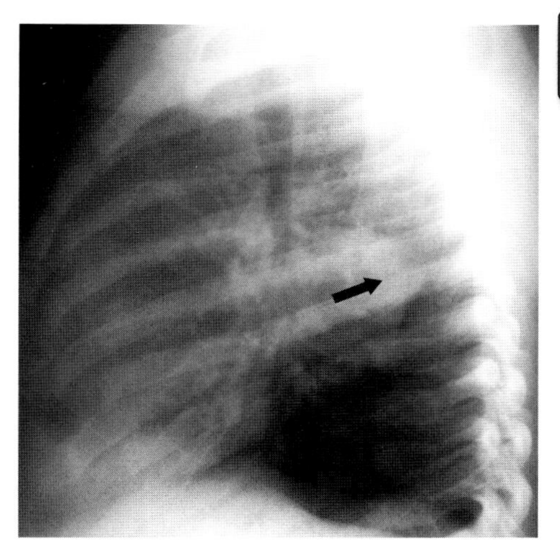

Lateral CXR confirms the parahilar soft-tissue density mass representing the bronchogenic cyst (*arrow*)

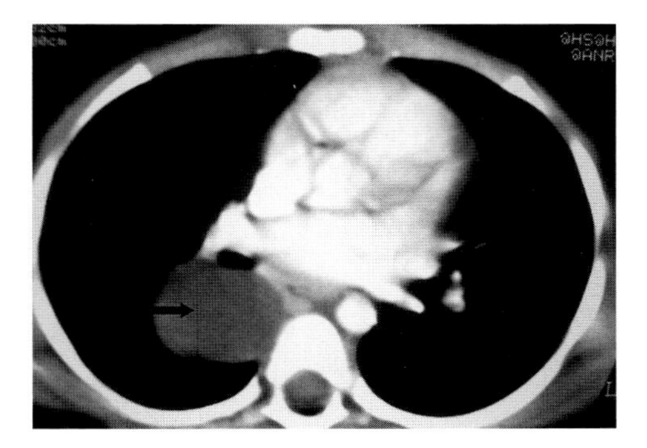

Axial CT post-contrast confirms the relatively posterior and right-sided mediastinal mass with low-density fluid content (*arrow*)

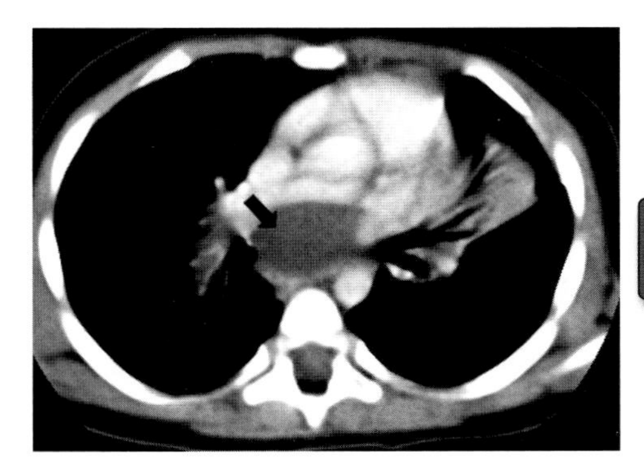

Axial CT post-contrast demonstrates a subcarinal, hypodense non-enhancing cyst (*arrow*) compressing the left main bronchus

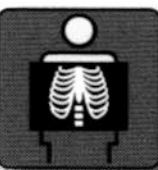

Imaging Options

- Primary: CXR
- Follow on: CT/MRI

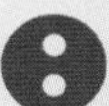

Imaging Findings

- Well-defined mass in middle mediastinum or lung parenchyma
- When in parenchyma involves the medial third of the lung
- Usually solitary with smooth borders

CXR

- Shows a soft tissue mass ± mass effect, hyperinflation, collapse

CT /MRI

- Cyst contents vary from water to proteinaceous fluid (usually hypodense on CT, T1 intermediate and T2 high signal on MRI).
- Non-enhancing and does not communicate with the airway.
- May sometimes contain air (infection may also result in an air content).

Tips

- MRI – use axial T1 and coronal T2/STIR

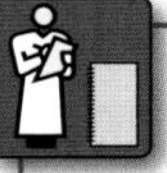

Radiological Differential Diagnosis

- Round pneumonia (does not cause mass effect and resolves)
- Lymphadenopathy
- Hydatid
- Pulmonary blastoma (rare)

Choledochal Cyst

Surgeon: S. Cox
Radiologist: A. M. du Plessis

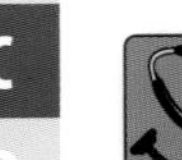

Clinical Insights

- Choledochal cysts are congenital anomalies, frequently (70%) associated with pancreatico-biliary mal-union, where the junction of the common bile duct with the pancreatic duct inserts abnormally proximal (1 cm) – "The long common channel."
- They present as cystic dilatations of the extra-hepatic and/or intra-hepatic bile ducts.
- Most will present in childhood with obstructive jaundice, pain, cholangitis or pancreatitis but increasingly are noted on antenatal ultrasound.
- The simplest classification is by Todani.

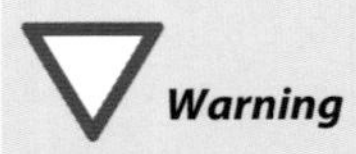

Warning

- Patients with pancreatitis or cholangitis should be resuscitated prior to imaging.

Urgency

- ❑ Emergency
- ❑ Urgent
- ☑ Elective

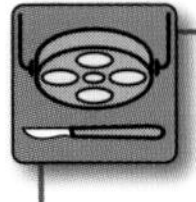

What the Surgeon Needs to Know

- Extent of biliary abnormality
- Anatomy of the pancreatic ducts
- Associated intra-hepatic ductal strictures, hepatolithiasis, hepatic abscesses or pancreatitis

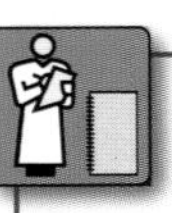

Clinical Differential Diagnosis

- Primary hepatic or pancreatic cyst
- Biliary atresia with associated cyst formation
- Choledocholithiasis
- Gall bladder duplication
- Cholangiocarcinoma

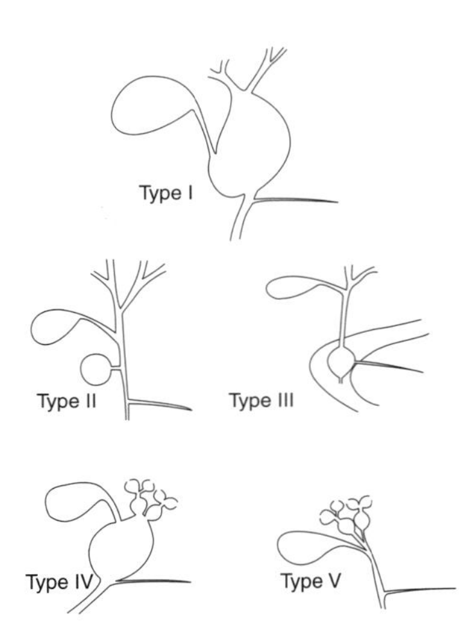

A simple classification of choledocal cysts by Todani

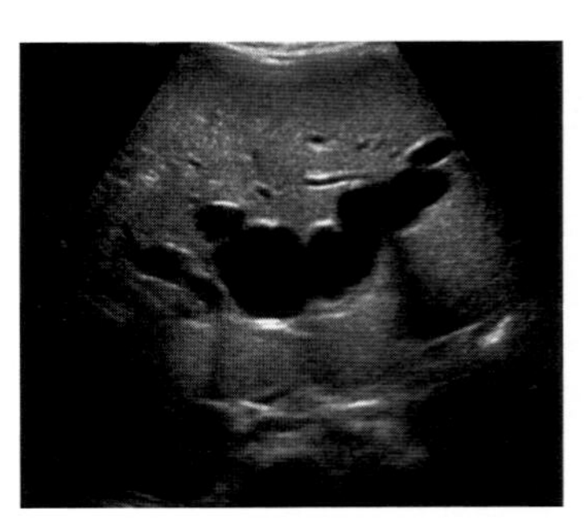

US – Demonstrates a lobulated cystic structure in the region of, but separate from the gallbladder (*arrow*) – representing both intra- and extra-hepatic cystic duct dilation

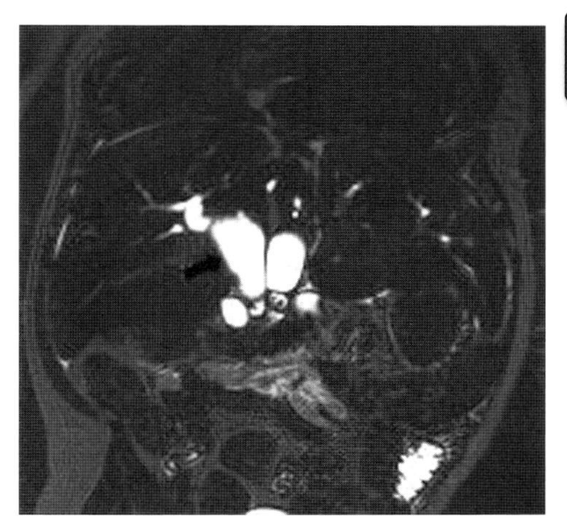

MRI – Heavily T2-weighted coronal demonstrates a cystic lesion occupying the porta hepatis, representing a choledochal cyst (*arrow*); some intra-hepatic bile duct dilation is present

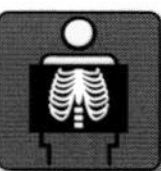

Imaging Options

- Primary: US
- Follow-on: Magnetic resonance cholangiopancreatography (MRCP)
- Back-up: CT, percutaneous transhepatic cholangiography (PTC)

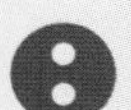

Imaging Findings

- Cystic/fusiform structure in porta hepatis, separate to gallbladder
- Intra- and extra-hepatic biliary dilatation

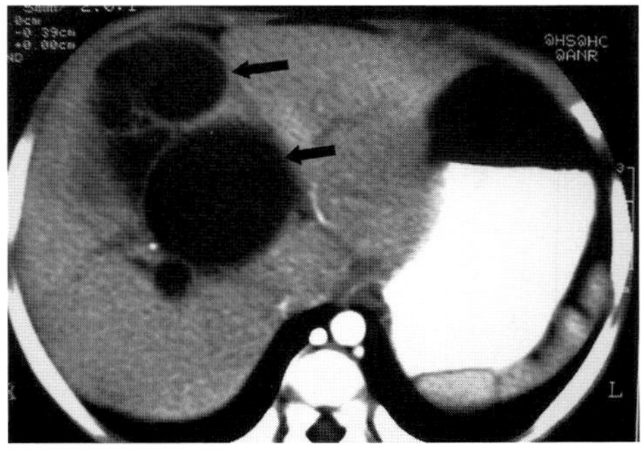

CT – Demonstrates an extra-hepatic "multiloculated" cystic lesion (*arrows*); no intra-hepatic bile duct dilatation is seen

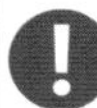

Tips

- MRCP/PTC – Confirms diagnosis, defines extent and visualises remaining biliary tract.
- MRCP is non-invasive, avoids radiation and provides the same information as PTC.
- Children under the age of 5 – Anaesthesia for successful MRCP.

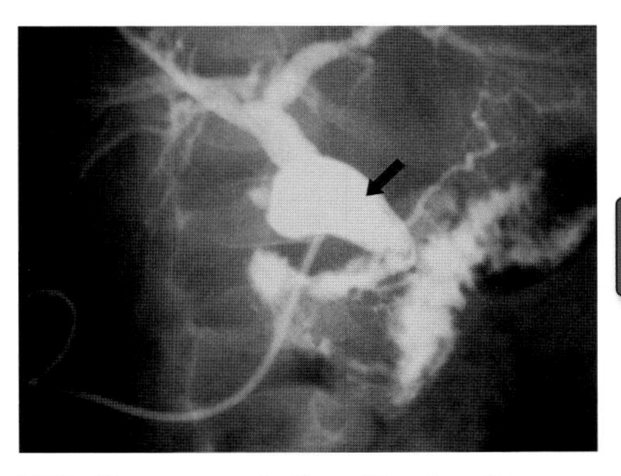

PTC – Demonstrates fusiform dilatation of the common bile duct (*arrow*), in keeping with a choledochal cyst

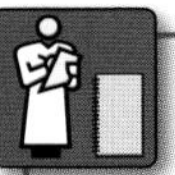

Radiological Differential Diagnosis

- Enteric duplication cyst
- Hydatid cyst (look for cyst-within-a-cyst appearance)
- Lymphatic malformation/mesenteric cyst
- Amoebic abscess

Congenital Cystic Adenomatoid Malformation (CCAM)

Surgeon: A. Brooks
Radiologist: C. Ackermann

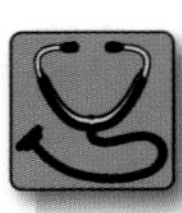

Clinical Insights

- This term encompasses a spectrum of cystic and solid lesions, histologically identifiable as CCAMs, i.e. an overgrowth of terminal bronchiolar-type tubular structures and absence of mature alveoli.
- Classified (by Stocker) on the basis of clinical and pathological presentation into cystic (older infant, child or adult), intermediate (at birth) and solid lesions (usually in the stillborn) or on prenatal ultrasound into macrocystic (>5 mm) or microcystic (<5 mm solid or cystic).
- Present with respiratory distress in the newborn or with recurrent respiratory infection later on.

Warnings

- Emergency thoracotomy and lobectomy may be life saving in the newborn that presents with respiratory distress.
- Malignancy has been reported (>200 cases).

Controversies

- Lobectomy may be indicated in all of these lesions because of the risk of malignancy.

Urgency

❑ Emergency
☑ Urgent
❑ Elective

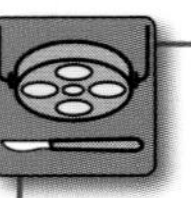

What the Surgeon Needs to Know

- Is there any co-existing pulmonary hypoplasia?
- Are there associated renal or cardiac anomalies?
- Are there any life-threatening complications such as pneumothorax or compression of the great vessels?
- Is hydrops present on ante-natal scan?

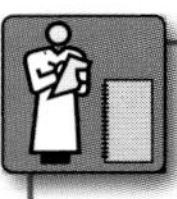

Clinical Differential Diagnosis

- Bronchogenic cyst
- Pulmonary Sequestration

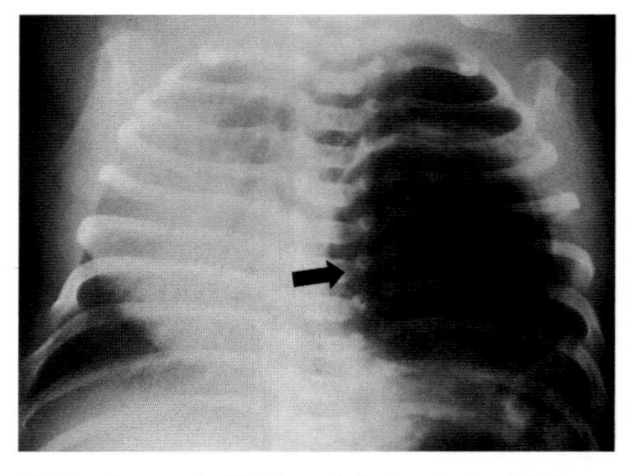

CXR – Large, air-filled cystic lesion in the left lower zone (*arrow*) with obscuration of the left hemidiaphragm. Mediastinal shift to the right with appearance of compressed lung at the superior border. Stomach bubble not clearly separated from the cystic mass

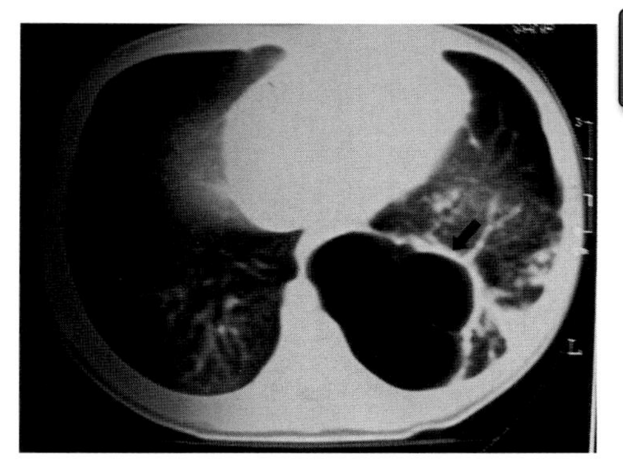

CT (lung window) – Large air-filled cystic mass containing septations within the left lower lobe (*arrow*) with mild surrounding air space disease

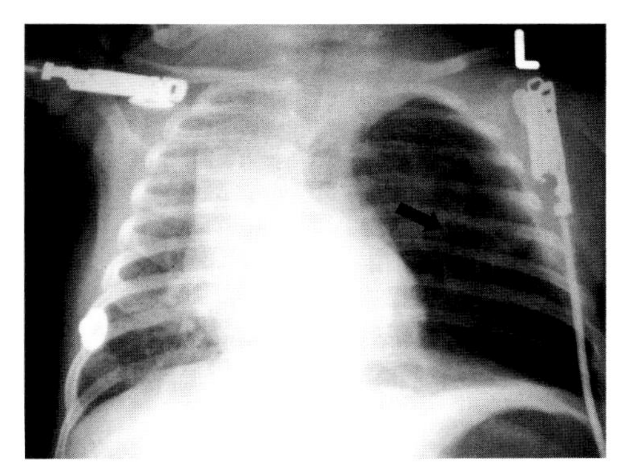

CXR – Air-filled cysts occupying most of the left lung representing a CCAM (*arrow*) with mediastinal shift to the right

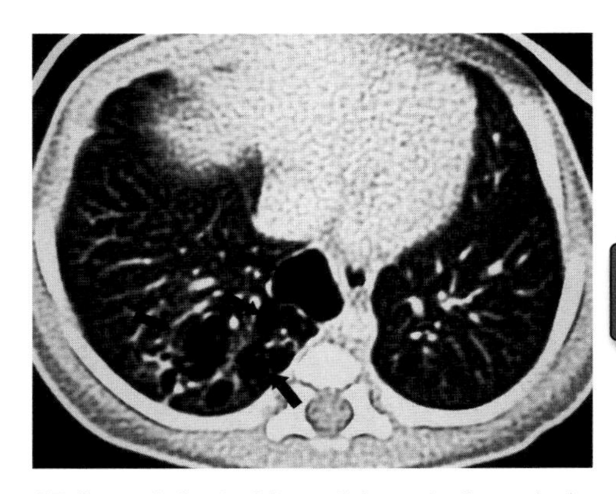

CT (lung window) – More subtle cystic change in the infero-posterior portion of the right lung (*arrows*) also within the spectrum of CCAM

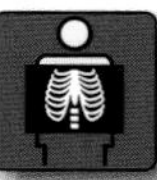

Imaging Options

- Primary: CXR/pre-natal US
- Follow-on: CT

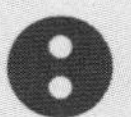

Imaging Findings

CXR

- May be normal if pre-natal diagnosis.
- Multicystic mass – Appearance depends on the size and content of cysts.
- Cysts communicate with bronchial tree at birth and fill with air early in life.
- Cysts can be radiodense immediately after birth.
- No lobar predilection but usually confined to one lobe.

CT

- Cysts of varying size containing air or fluid.

Tips

- CT is useful for characterization and pre-surgical planning.
- CT must exclude arterial supply from aorta in a hybrid lesion (IVI contrast needed).
- CT indicated if prenatal US suggestive even when CXR negative.
- AXR shows a normal gas pattern in contrast to Bochdalek hernia.

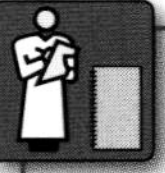

Radiological Differential Diagnosis

- Pulmonary Sequestration – Only air filled when infected
- Congenital diaphragmatic hernia – Changes appearance with time
- Cavitatory pneumonia

Congenital Lobar Emphysema (CLE)

Surgeon: A. Brooks
Radiologist: C. Ackermann

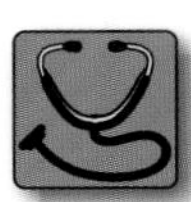

Clinical Insights

- Defined as isolated hyperinflation of a lobe in the absence of extrinsic compression, due to partial bronchial obstruction.
- Left upper lobe and right middle lobe are most often involved.
- Usually produces symptoms in infancy; mostly present before 6 months.
- Examination: Signs of mediastinal shift to contralateral side, decreased breath sounds, hyperresonance.

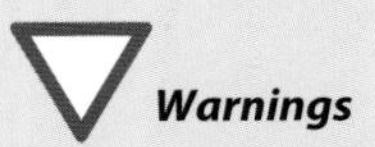

Warnings

- Careful inspection of vascular markings reduces the risk of misdiagnosis as a tension pneumothorax.
- In a newborn with respiratory distress a chest radiograph is the only investigation indicated.
- Respiratory distress may be escalated by positive pressure ventilation.

Controversy

- Lobectomy is definitely indicated in the presence of significant respiratory symptoms; most surgeons would say it is required in almost all cases, but some would prefer to follow those with minimal symptoms.

Urgency

- ❑ Emergency
- ❑ Urgent
- ☑ Elective

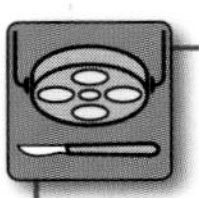

What the Surgeon Needs to Know:

- Is there an extrinsic cause for the lobar emphysema such as vascular anomaly or a mediastinal mass?

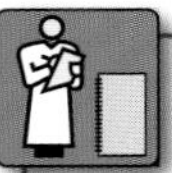

Clinical Differential Diagnosis

- Pneumothorax.
- Acquired lobar emphysema due to extrinsic compression from enlarged lymph nodes, bronchogenic cyst, anomalous blood vessels or intrinsic obstruction from catheter trauma in an infant subjected to prolonged ventilation.
- In the older child: Foreign body.

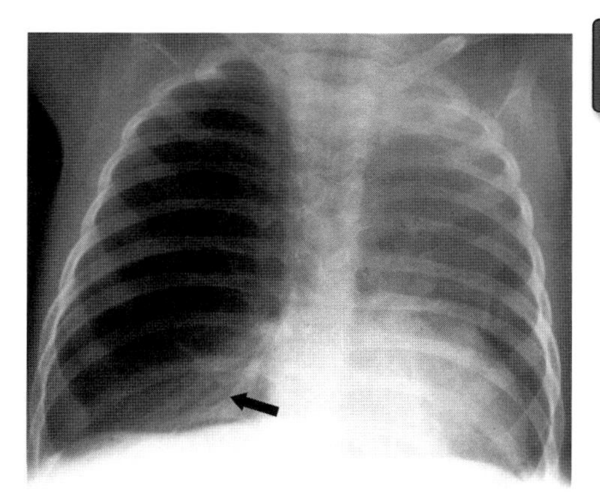

CXR – Hyperexpanded, hyperlucent right upper lobe, with compression of the right middle and lower lobe (*arrow*) and mediastinal shift to the left

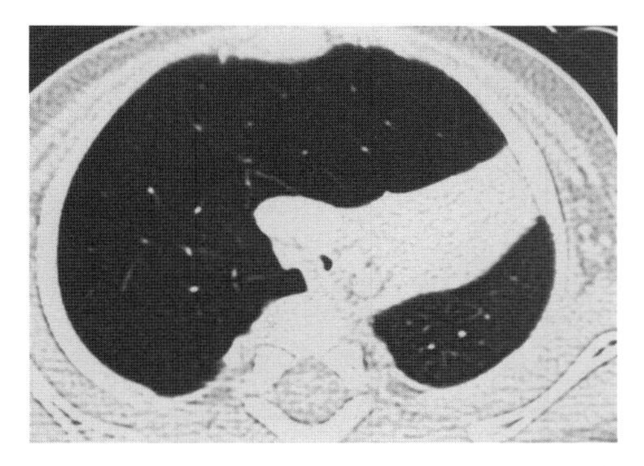

CT – CT demonstrates attenuated pulmonary vessels in the expanded right middle lobe with mediastinal shift to the left

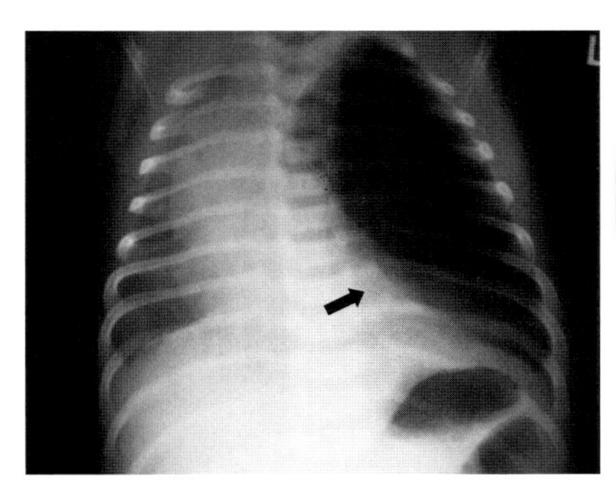

CXR – Demonstrating hyperexpansion of the left upper lobe with compression of the left lower lobe (*arrow*) and mediastinal shift to the right in keeping with CLE

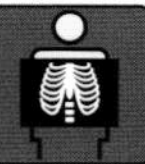

Imaging Options

- Primary: CXR
- Follow-on imaging: CT

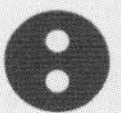

Imaging Findings

CXR

- After birth, may be filled with fluid and appear as radiodensity that shows progressive hyperlucency.
- Hyperlucent, hyperexpanded lobe.
- Mediastinal and tracheal deviation and compression of remaining ipsilateral lung.

CT

- Pulmonary vessels are attenuated or displaced.
- Left upper lobe is most commonly affected (43%).

Tips

- CT – Confirms diagnosis, defines extent and excludes other lesions.
- In contrast to pulmonary interstitial emphysema (PIE), vascular structures are at periphery of expanded air spaces rather than central.

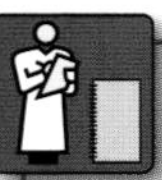

Radiological Differential Diagnosis

- Congenital adenoid malformation (CCAM)
- PIE can rarely persist and present as an expanding mass
- Congenital diaphragmatic hernia (left diaphragm not seen)
- Pneumothorax
- Foreign body in older child

Crohn's Disease

Surgeons: A. Alexander, C. Davies
Radiologist: J. du Plessis

Clinical Insights

- A chronic, transmural inflammatory process of unknown aetiology, affecting any part of the intestine, from the mouth to the anus.
- Typically patchy and usually involves the terminal ileum.
- Usually manifests in young adults but may rarely affect children.
- Clinical features include:
  - Chronic diarrhoea and intermittent pain.
  - Obstruction due to fibrosis or inflammatory mass effect.
  - Perforation causing abscess formation and fistulisation.
  - Malabsorption.
  - Perianal disease.
- Extra-intestinal manifestations worth looking for include:
  - Biliary and renal stones.
  - Hepatic cirrhosis and abscess formation.

Warning

- These patients are often on immune suppressants, and as a result, their immune function can be depressed in the presence of severe complications.
- Always ensure that they are adequately resuscitated prior to imaging.

Urgency

- ☐ Emergency
- ☐ Urgent
- ☑ Elective (unless complicated)

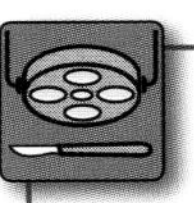

What the Surgeon Needs to Know

- Confirm the diagnosis.
- Identify complications.
- Exclude extra-intestinal manifestations.

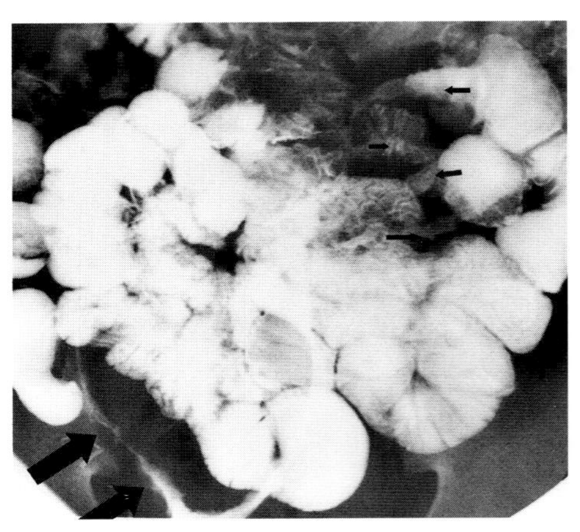

Small bowel study – Demonstrates significant stricture of the terminal ileum (*large arrows*) and separation from other bowel loops due to wall thickening. Skip lesions more proximally (*small arrows*) also show separation of loops and thickening of valvulae conniventes

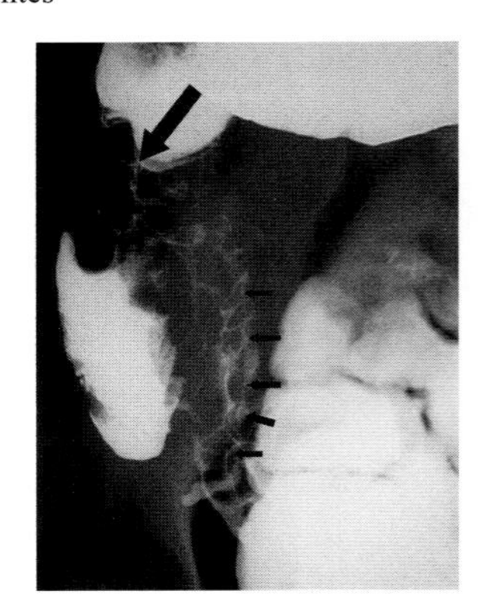

Small bowel study – Strictures involving the caecum/ascending colon (*large arrow*) and terminal ileum with large irregular nodular impressions on the lumen – "cobblestone appearance" (*small arrows*)

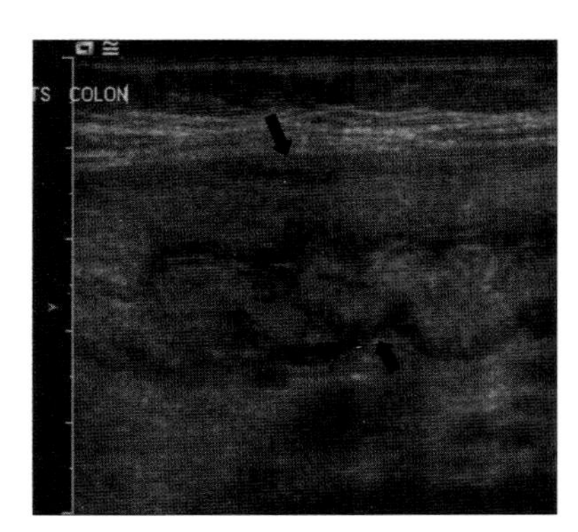

US: Linear high-resolution probe – Longitudinal representation of the transverse colon (produced by scanning transversely in the epigastrium) demonstrates the bowel wall thickening (opposing ends between arrows) and "thumb-printing" in a patient with Crohn's colitis [Image courtesy Dr. Kieran McHugh]

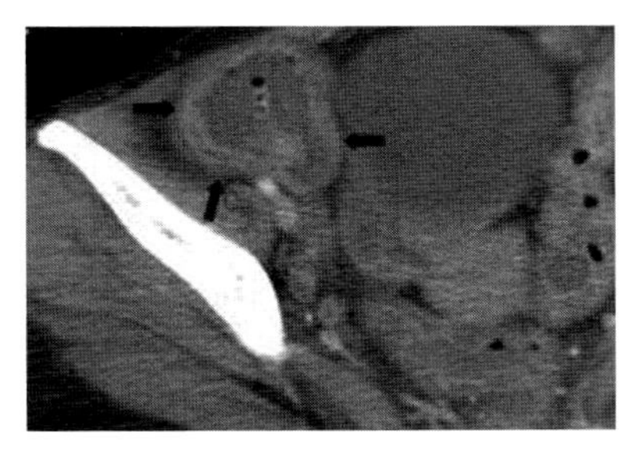

CT – Demonstrates thickening of the small bowel and caecum with a "target" sign (*arrows*)

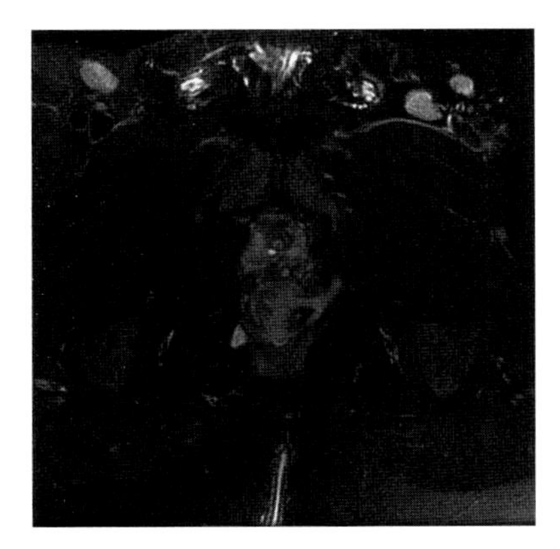

MRI STIR of the perineum demonstrates multiple sinus/fistula openings (*arrows*)

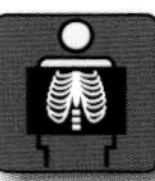

Imaging Options

- Primary: Small bowel contrast study
- Follow-on: US, CT, MRI, Nuc Med

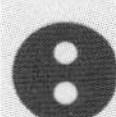

Imaging Findings

Small Bowel Contrast

- Early– Irregular, nodular thickening of bowel wall, aphthous ulcers.
- Advanced – "Skip lesions" and "cobblestone" appearance, separation and displacement of bowel loops, pseudopolyps, pseudodiverticula, and polyps.
- Complicated – Sinuses, fistulas, abscesses, strictures, malignant changes.

US

- Thick bowel wall
- Aperistaltic rigid bowel
- Echogenic surrounding mesentry

CT

- Discontinuous/asymmetric bowel wall thickening
- Target sign (enhancing mucosa, hypodense submucosa)
- Fistulae, sinuses, abscesses

MRI

- Best for peri-anal fistulas and sinuses

Tips

- Terminal ileum involved in >90%.
- Do not mistake the normal nodular terminal ileum in children for disease. The normal lymphoid tissue is seen as smaller nodules.

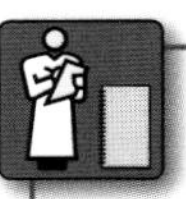

Radiological Differential Diagnosis

- Ulcerative colitis
- Infectious colitis (TB, ascaris)
- Appendicitis
- Lymphoma

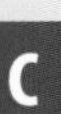

Cystic Hygroma (Lymphatic Malformation)

Surgeon: A. Darani
Radiologist: J. Naidu

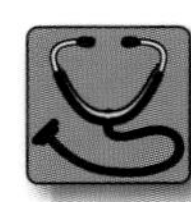

Clinical Insights

- Benign hamartomatous malformation of the lymphatic system.
- ±50% present at birth.
- Spectrum of anomalies:
  - Multiple large lymphatic cysts (cystic hygroma).
  - Multiple small cysts infiltrating tissue, with other mesodermal elements (vessels and fibrous tissue).
- Can occur anywhere: neck (75%), axillary (20%).

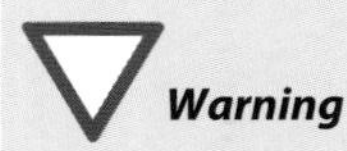

Warning

Exclude

- Airway obstruction and feeding difficulties
- Haemorrhage, infection and deformity of surrounding bone
- Recurrent pleural/pericardial effusions (sometimes chylous)

Urgency

- ☐ Emergency
- ☐ Urgent
- ☑ Elective

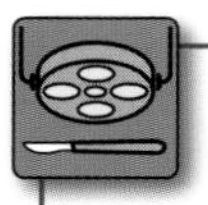

What the Surgeon Needs to Know

- Is the mass a localized macrocystic structure (cystic hygroma) or microcystic?
- Relation to surrounding structures (vascular, neural, visceral etc).

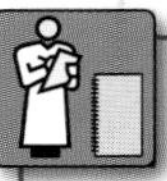

Clinical Differential Diagnosis

- Infantile fibrosarcoma
- Vascular malformation
- Branchial cleft cysts
- Neck abscess
- Other soft-tissue tumour
- Plunging ranula in the floor of the mouth or neck

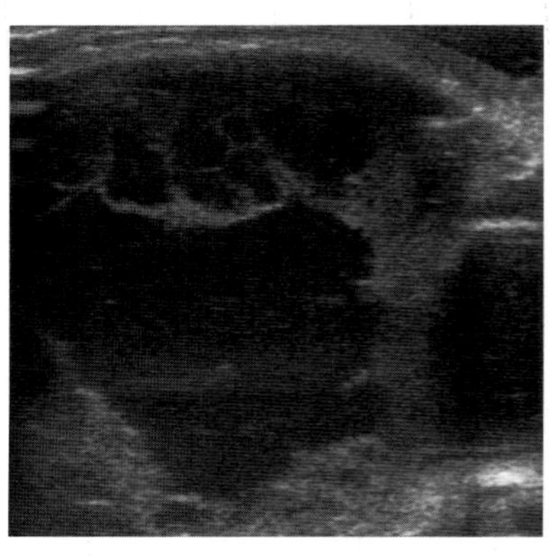

US – A lateral neck mass shows a multi-cystic appearance consistent with a cystic hygroma

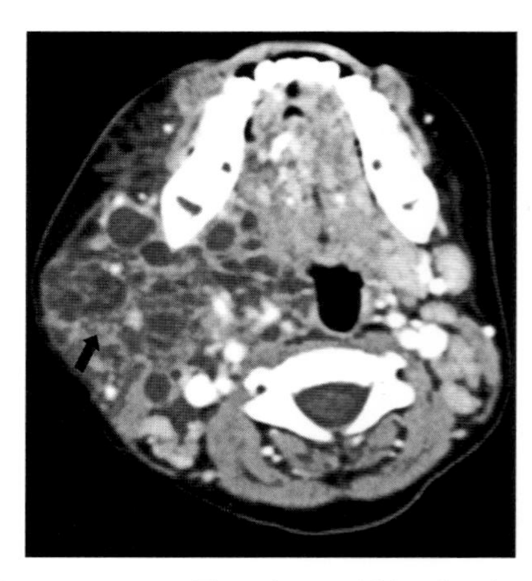

CT post-contrast – There is a multi-loculated cystic mass (*arrow*) involving the parotid space and the parapharyngeal space

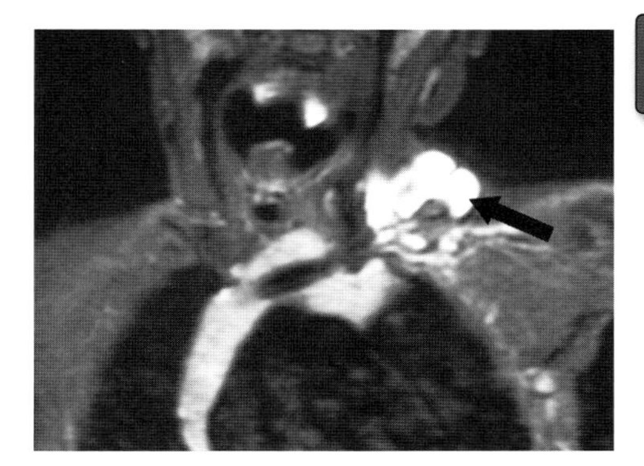

MRI Coronal T2 – Demonstrates a high signal fluid-filled mass in the left lateral neck posterior triangle (*arrow*), infiltrating between vascular structures

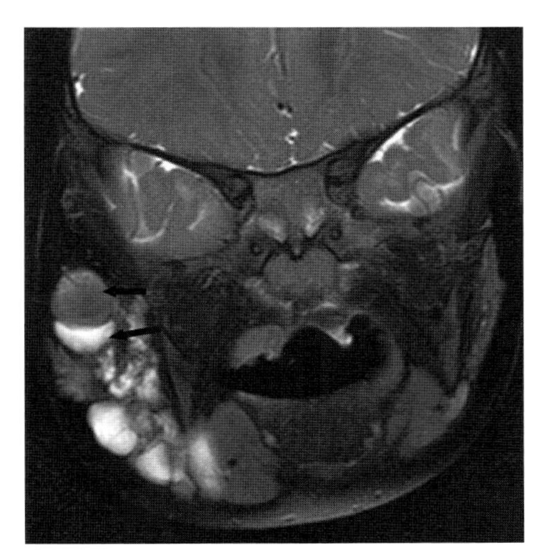

Coronal T2 MRI of the face – Demonstrates a right multi-loculated mass with varying signal intensities (*arrows*) indicating that the cystic hygroma was complicated by haemorrhage or infection

Tips

- MRI best for showing deep extension and intrathoracic extension.
- T2-weighted images – Demonstrates best tissue contrast between lymphangiomas and surrounding tissues.
- Gadolinium provides no additional information with regard to diagnosis and extent of involvement.
- Imaging guides therapeutic injections.

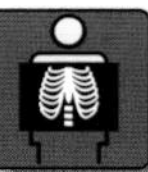

Imaging Options

- Primary: US
- Follow-on: MRI
- Back up: CT

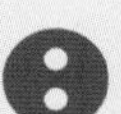

Imaging

US

- Unilocular or multilocular predominantly cystic mass with septae of variable thickness.
- Fluid–fluid levels with layering haemorrhage.
- Prenatal US may demonstrate a cystic hygroma in the posterior neck soft tissue.

MRI

- Low/intermediate signal intensity on T1-weighted images and hyperintensity on T2-weighed images.
- If hyperintense on T1, it is due to clotted blood or high lipid (chyle) content.
- Fluid–fluid levels if intralesional haemorrhage or infection.

CT

- Hypo-attenuated poorly circumscribed unilocular or multiloculated mass.
- Homogenous fluid attenuation.
- If infected may show increased attenuation.
- Usually located in the posterior triangle or submandibular space of the neck.
- These lesions are infiltrative in nature and do not respect fascial planes.

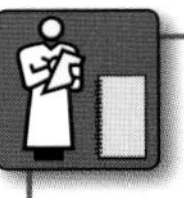

Radiological Differential Diagnosis

- Branchial cleft anomalies

Duodenal Atresia (Duodenal Stenosis, Web)

Surgeon: A. Alexander
Radiologist: G. Dekker

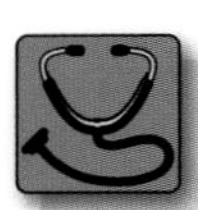

Clinical Insights

- A congenital abnormality of unknown aetiology that is characterised by complete obliteration of the duodenal lumen.
- Usually diagnosed on antenatal ultrasound, which shows the fluid-filled double bubble in the setting of polyhydramnios.
- Present with bile-stained vomiting from birth.
- Associated with:
  - Trisomy 21 in 40%.
  - Other intestinal atresias.
  - VACTERL abnormalities.
- Almost always occur in the region of ampulla of Vater and are frequently accompanied by abnormalities of the bile duct and pancreas (annular pancreas present in 20%).
- Surgical management is duodenoduodenostomy regardless of the nature of the congenital obstruction.

Warnings

- Bile-stained vomiting in a neonate is a radiological emergency.
- Delayed presentation often leads to marked fluid and electrolyte abnormalities. Resuscitation must be complete prior to imaging.

Urgency

- ☐ Emergency
- ☐ Urgent
- ☑ Elective

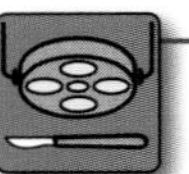

What the Surgeon Needs to Know

- Is there evidence of complete duodenal obstruction?
- Could this be malrotation with intestinal volvulus?

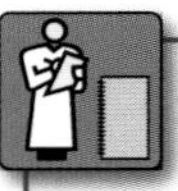

Clinical Differential Diagnosis

- Duodenal web
- Duodenal stenosis
- Malrotation and volvulus
- Annular pancreas
- Preduodenal portal vein
- Duplication of duodenum
- Haematoma of duodenum

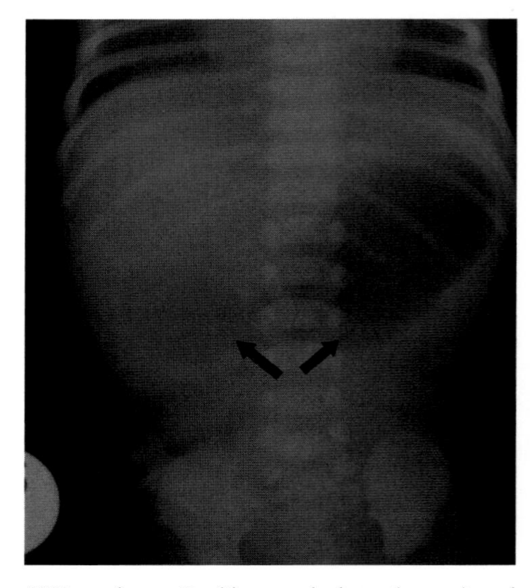

AXR supine – Double gas shadows (*arrows*) and absence of distal gas is diagnostic of duodenal atresia in a newborn and less likely to represent a malrotation

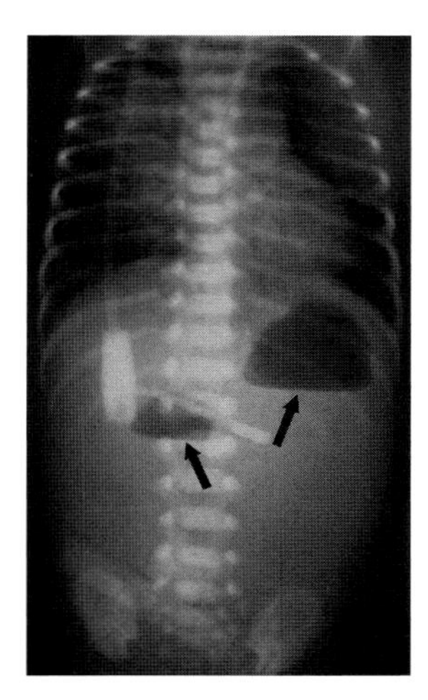

AXR erect – The traditional "double bubble" with air–fluid levels (*arrows*), representing gas in stomach and proximal duodenum and absence of gas in the distal bowel

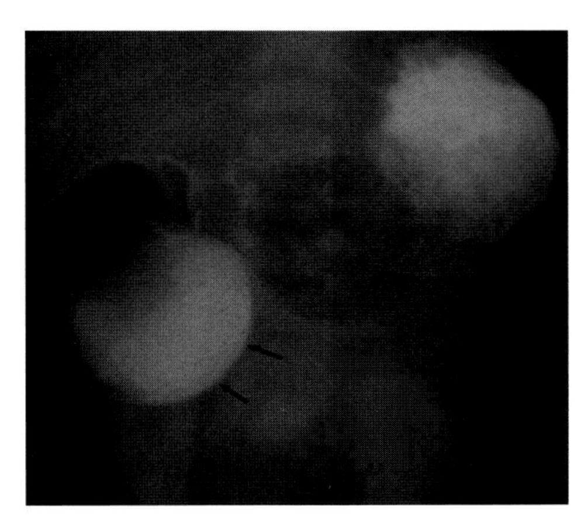

Supine UGIS is not indicated in a typical "double bubble" sign. In this study the blind ending distended proximal duodenum with rounded appearance (*arrows*) is termed a "windsock" deformity indicative of a duodenal web that is long standing

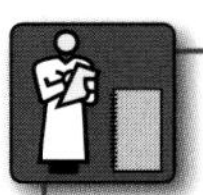

Imaging Differential Diagnosis

- Malrotation and volvulus; Ladd band
- Annular pancreas
- Duodenal duplication
- Extrinsic compression of duodenum (rare)

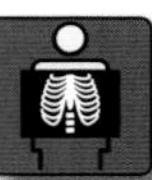

Imaging Options

- Primary: AXR, US (antenatal)
- Back-up: UGI

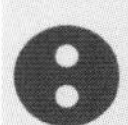

Imaging Findings

US antenatal

- May show fluid-filled double bubble

AXR

- Double bubble appearance sufficient to make diagnosis
- Represents air-filled stomach and first part of duodenum
- Gas absent in distal small and large bowel suggests atresia
- Small amounts of gas in distal bowel suggests stenosis or web

UGI

- Contrast meal unnecessary unless surgery is delayed, partial obstruction is defined or if malrotation and volvulus is suspected by the paediatric surgeon.

Tips

- Perform prenatal ultrasound in mothers with polyhydramnios
- Erect or decubitus AXR may define duodenum
- Injecting air via NGT may assist in demonstrating the "double bubble"
- Long-standing obstruction (as in duodenal atresia) results in a large D1 while malrotation with volvulus results in a less-distended relatively small D1
- Look for cardiac anomaly on CXR related to trisomy 21

Duplex Kidney

Surgeon: J. Lazarus
Radiologist: H. Viljoen

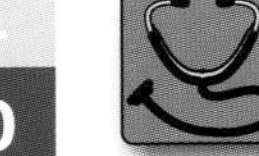

Clinical Insights

- Duplex kidneys contain two pyelocalyceal systems associated with a single ureter or double ureters.
- Two ureters may empty separately into the bladder or fuse to form a single ureteral orifice.
- Duplex kidneys can be unilateral or bilateral.
- Most patients are asymptomatic.
- Symptoms may be due to:
  - Urinary tract infection (UTI).
  - Obstructed upper moiety.
  - Vesico-ureteric reflux (VUR).
  - Ectopic upper moiety ureterocele.
  - Ectopic upper moiety ureter.
- Exclusion of VUR is necessary.
- A nuclear study often confirms a non-functional upper moiety.
- Imaging to demonstrate the ureters, and their implantation is necessary.
- Symptomatic children may benefit from partial nephrectomy, incision of an ureterocele, common sheath ureteric reimplant or ureteropyelostomy.

Warnings

- Duplex anomalies can be easily missed.
- A cystic structure at the bladder base may be interpreted as an ureterocele, while it may represent a dilated extravesical ectopic ureter. ("pseudo-ureterocele.")

Urgency

- ❑ Emergency
- ❑ Urgent
- ☑ Elective

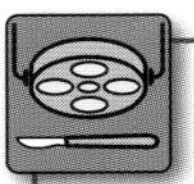

What the Surgeon Needs to Know

- Is the upper pole hydronephrotic or dysplastic?
- Is a ureterocele present?
- Is VUR present?
- What is the differential nuclear function of the two moieties?

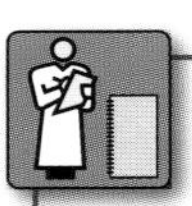

Clinical Differential Diagnosis

- Crossed fused renal ectopia

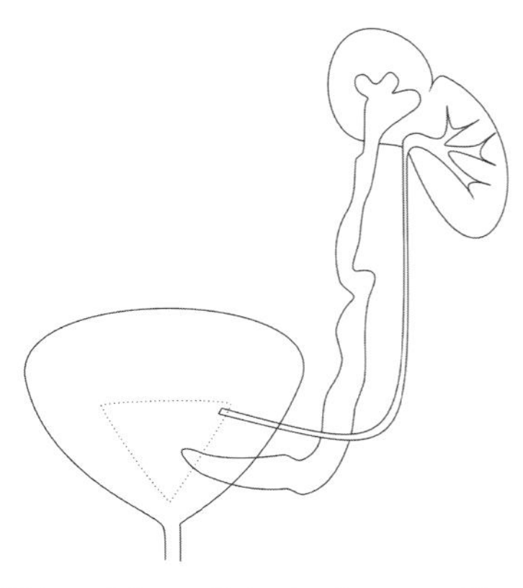

The Weigert-Meyer Rule is shown – The upper moeity ureter implants into the bladder more medially and distally

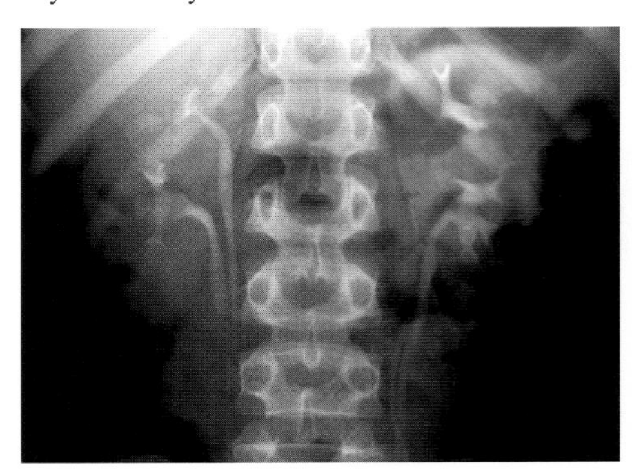

IVP – Bilateral duplex systems

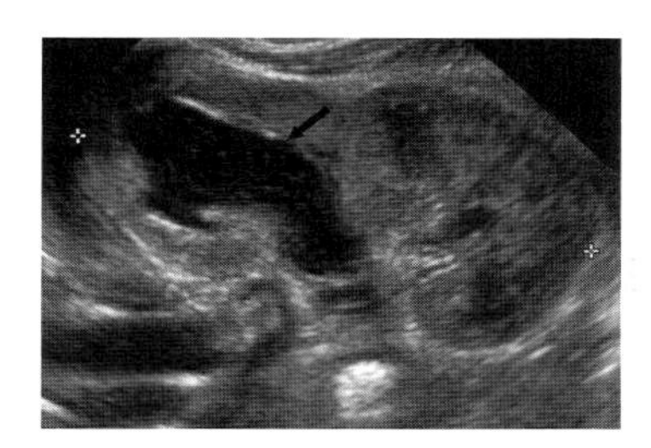

US of a duplex kidney with an obstructed upper moiety (*arrow*)

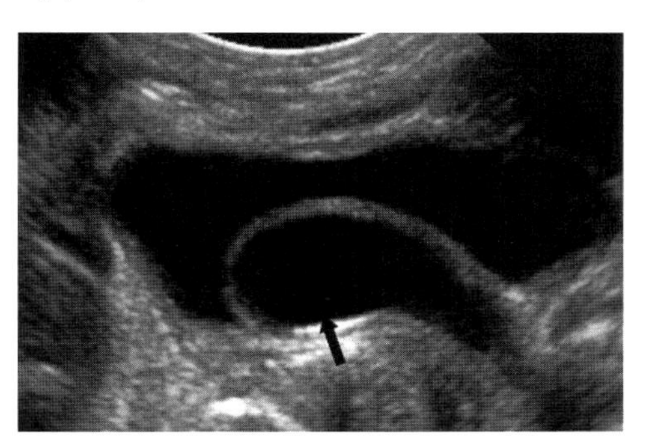

US of the bladder (transverse) showing the ureterocoele (*arrow*) associated with the upper moiety ureter

Tips

- On MCUG visualize ureterocoele during early filling after which it is obscured by contrast or collapses because of pressure (and can also evert).
- Investigate girls with enuresis (diurnal and nocturnal) for ectopic insertion of ureter associated with a duplex kidney.

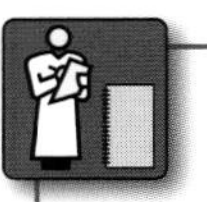

Radiological Differential Diagnosis

Ureterocoele

- Bladder mass – Rhabdomyosarcoma, hematoma, fungus ball
- Mass effect from sigmoid colon
- Bladder "Hutch" diverticulum

Calyectasis

- Hydronephrosis due to PUJ
- Renal scarring

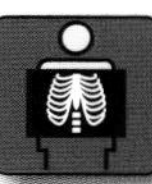

Imaging Options

- Primary: US
- Follow on: MCUG
- Backup: IVP, Nuc Med, MRU

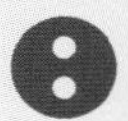

Imaging Findings

US

- An uncomplicated duplex kidney may be suspected on ultrasound when there is a large kidney unilateral, an appearance of two kidneys adjacent to each other, or when there is a prominent ridge between the upper and lower portions. Not all duplex kidneys have ureterocoeles, show obstruction or reflux.
- Upper moiety associated with ureterocoele in 75% and may be obstructed (hydronephrosis and distal ureter seen).
- Ureterocoele is anechoic, thin-walled cyst in bladder (possible connection with uereter and ureteric jet) – Should prompt investigation for duplex kidney.

MCUG

- Ureterocoele seen as filling defect in contrast-filled bladder on MCUG.
- May show reflux into ureter of lower moiety.

Nuc Med

- Mag 3 renogram may show two ureters.
- Mag 3 renogram may show an obstructed upper moiety and a scarred non-functioning lower moiety.
- Delayed voiding imaging may show VUR

IVP

- Ureterocoele is seen as a contrast-filled structure with thin radiolucent wall in contrast-filled bladder.
- "Drooping lily" represents an obstructed upper moiety drooping over the lower moiety.

Duplication Cyst (Enteric Cyst)

Surgeon: A. Numanoglu
Radiologist: L. Naidu

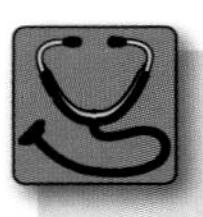

Clinical Insights

- Most present in the first 2 years of life.
- May occur anywhere from mouth to anus.
- Abdominal pain, vomiting and mass are common signs and symptoms.
- Wide variety of mass lesions, tubular or cystic in shape.
- Associated abnormalities include vertebral, pulmonary, intestinal atresias and genito-urinary malformations.
- 80% abdominal (50% jejuno-ileal, 20% colorectal, 10% other); 20% thoracic origin.

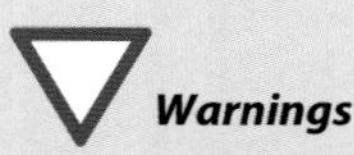

Warnings

- Cervical and thoracic duplications may have abdominal communication and are associated with vertebral anomalies (split notochord).
- Can present with volvulus of involved gut.

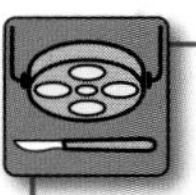

What the Surgeon Needs to Know

- Is it simple, complex or are there multiple cysts?
- Origin of the cyst.
- Relationship to neighbouring organs.
- Associated abnormalities (spinal, vertebral)

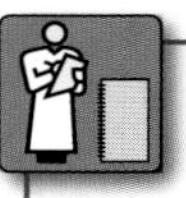

Differential Diagnosis

- Intussusception
- Other cystic lesions, i.e. urinary, lymphatic, mesenteric, hepatic, ovarian and neoplastic

Urgency

- ☐ Emergency
- ☐ Urgent
- ☑ Elective

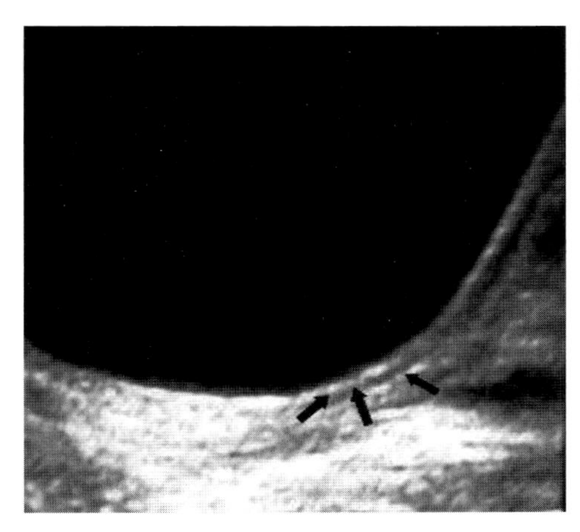

US – Demonstrating duplication cyst with "gut signature sign." Note the hyper-echoic inner and outer rims and hypo-echoic central muscular layer (*arrows*)

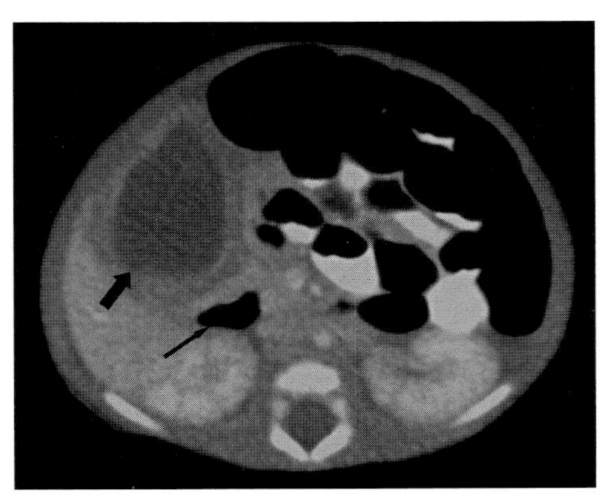

CT – Displaying a well-defined cyst with a thick wall (*thick arrow*) abutting the duodenum (*thin arrow*)

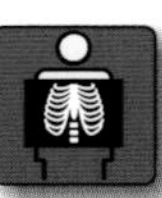

Imaging Options

- Primary: US
- Back-up: CT, MRI

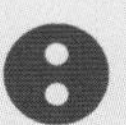

Imaging Findings

US

- Cystic lesion in abdomen
- May be mobile between examinations
- Debris common
- May see peristalsis
- Gut wall "signature" very suggestive – echogenic mucosa, hypoechoic muscular layer, echogenic serosa

CT

- Well-defined cystic mass related to bowel/pancreas
- Non-specific as gut signature not visualized
- Relatively thick enhancing wall
- ±Fluid/debris layers

MRI

- Cyst content (High T2 signal reflects simple fluid nature)

Tips

- US for abdominal imaging
- CT/MRI for thoracic imaging
- Gut signature may be lost in inflammation, ulceration, or perforation
- Enteric non-duplication cysts are rare – no double layer as they lack hypoechoic muscle layer
- Can intussuscept or cause obstruction

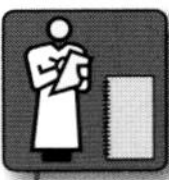

Radiological Differential Diagnosis

- Mesenteric cysts – Uni/multilocular with high protein content on MRI (no gut signature)
- Meckels diverticulum (gut signature)
- Lymphatic malformation (cystic multiseptated)
- Ovarian cyst (location similar to ileal duplication)
- Urachal cyst (connection to bladder)

Empyema

Surgeon: J. Loveland
Radiologist: D. J. van der Merwe

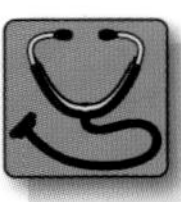

Clinical Insights

- Accumulation of infected fluid within thoracic cavity.
- Complicates underlying pneumonia.
- Cause needs to be elucidated and treated in its own right.
- Therapy may vary depending on stage of "maturation."
- Spectrum includes simple tube drainage, streptokinase fibrinolysis, thoracoscopic debridement and open thoracotomy.

Controversies

- Thoracoscopic drainage and local fibrinolysis
- Indicators for drainage: CT density > 25 HU

Urgency

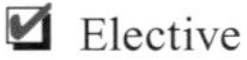

- ☐ Emergency
- ☐ Urgent
- ☑ Elective

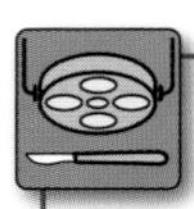

What the Surgeon Needs to Know

- Is the collection simple or does it have a more complex appearance with pleural thickening, multiple septations and numerous separate abscesses?
- If complex, is the collection amenable to percutaneous drainage?
- Can the site be marked anatomically?

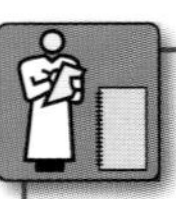

Differential Diagnosis

- Haemothorax
- Vertebral and mediastinal pathology
- Rarely, chylous, pancreatic or biliary effusion

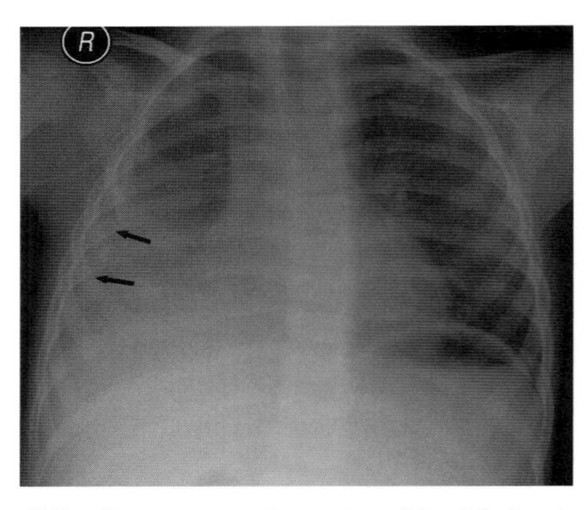

CXR – Demonstrates obscuration of the right hemidiaphragm in a patient with spiking temperatures in keeping with an empyema. Note fluid tracking along the inner thoracic margin (*arrows*)

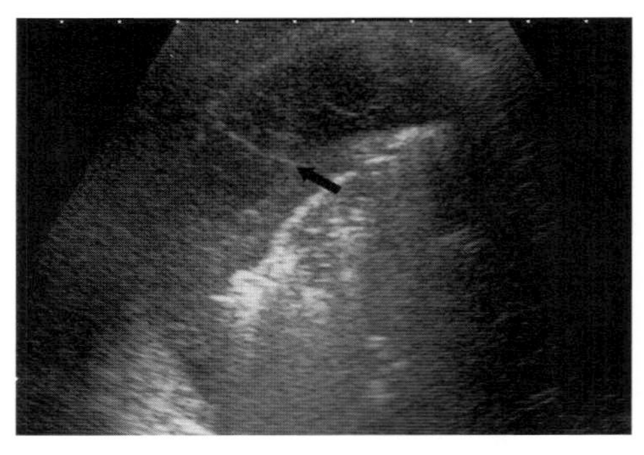

US – Demonstrates a pleural collection with numerous compartments and strands (*arrow*) diagnostic of an empyema

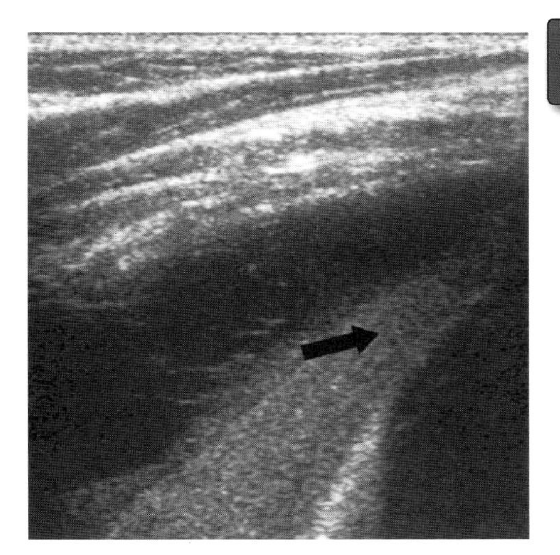

US – The consolidated lung edge (*arrow*) does not move on dynamic imaging. In conjunction with the visible debris an empyema was diagnosed

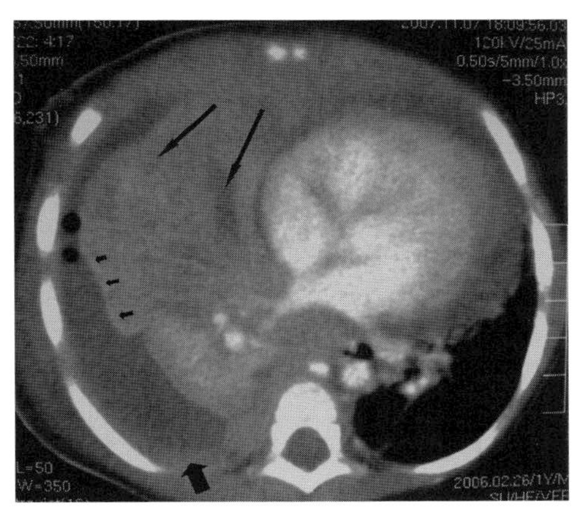

CT – Demonstrates a complex pleural collection with air pockets and an enhancing lung edge (*small arrows*). There is also a pleural "rind" (*thick arrow*) and underlying lung parenchymal consolidation and breakdown (*long arrows*)

Tips

- US – No loculation, mobile lung and minimal/no debris allows for urokinase therapy via chest tube

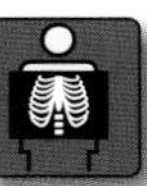

Imaging Options

- Primary: CXR
- Follow-on: US
- Back-up: CT

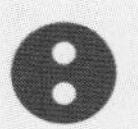

Imaging Findings

CXR

- Effusion conforms to the shape of chest; may track up the lateral margin and retain the costo-phrenic angle.
- Underlying lung compression/collapse/consolidation.

US

- US demonstrates septations and debris, which characterize empyema better than CT.
- Differentiates transudates (hypoechoic) from exudates (strands, debris).
- Mobile lung edge is in keeping with an exudate.
- Underlying non-aerated lung, or abscess can also be identified through the empyema.

CT

- Pleural thickening and enhancement (Rind)
- Split pleura sign
- Underlying parenchyma – necrosis, abscess, consolidation

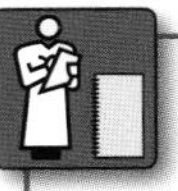

Radiological Differential Diagnosis

- Transudate: Low HU; hypoechoic
- Chylothorax: Neonates; post-thoracic surgery
- Malignancy: Lymphoma; pulmonary blastoma
- Lung abcess/cavitatory necrosis: Best defined by CT

Epididymo-Orchitis

Surgeon: A. Alexander
Radiologist: A. Bagadia

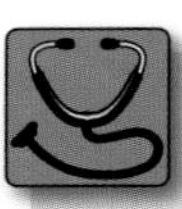

Clinical Insights

- 10–15% of acute scrotums are due to epididymo-orchitis.
- Bimodal age distribution: infants and adolescents.
- Urine analysis should be performed.
- If culture grows uropathogens then ultrasound of the kidneys, ureter and bladder should be performed.
- Consider a MCUG in complicated or recurrent cases.

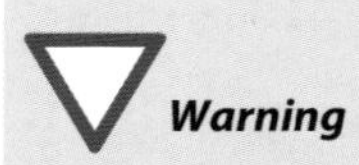

Warning

- Scrotum must be surgically explored urgently if torsion cannot rapidly and reliably be ruled out by clinical evidence or Doppler ultrasound scanning.

Controversy

- A MCUG is indicated to rule out ectopic ureter and ejaculatory duct reflux

Urgency

- [x] Emergency (if torsion suspected)
- [ ] Urgent
- [ ] Elective

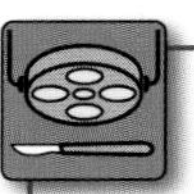

What the Surgeon Needs to Know

- Exclude other causes of acute scrotum
- Exclude associated urogenital abnormalities predisposing to infection

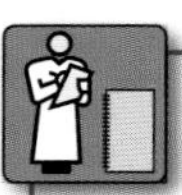

Clinical Differential Diagnosis

- Torsion testis
- Torsion of appendix epididymus/testis
- Scrotal cellulitis
- Idiopathic scrotal oedema

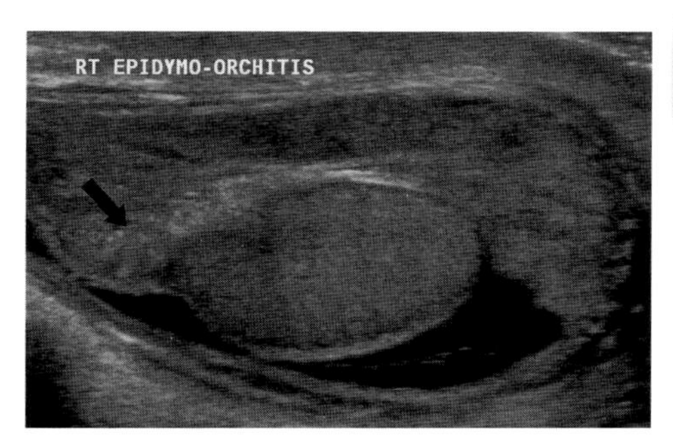

US longitudinal – Demonstrates a thickened epididymus (*arrow*) and reactive hydrocoele as well as a thick scrotal wall

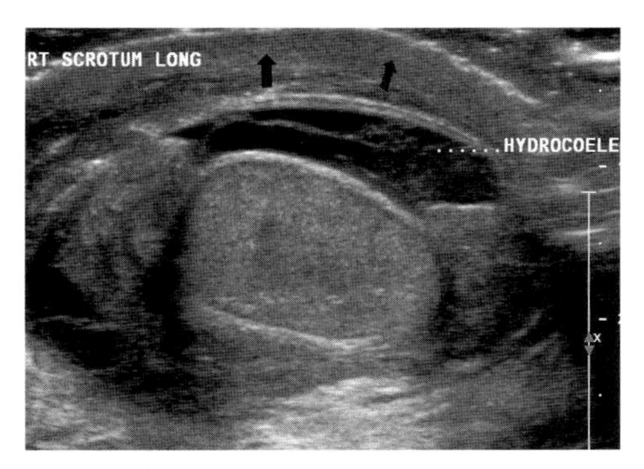

US transverse – Demonstrates the thick epididymus and hydrocoele with scrotal wall thickening (*arrows*)

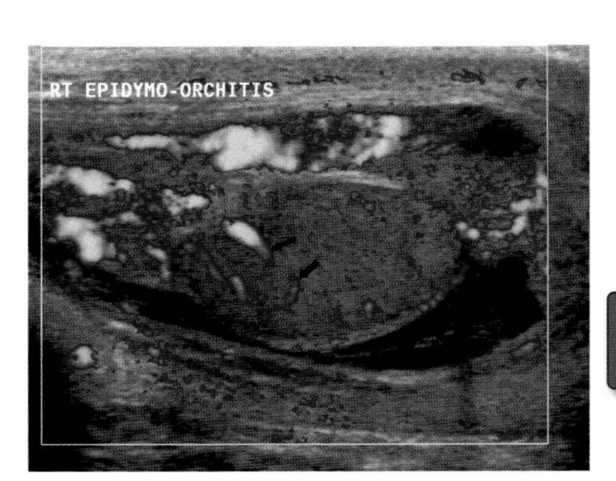

US Doppler – Demonstrates the excessive colour flow involving the epididymus and relatively normal parenchymal testicular flow (*arrows*) differentiating this from a testicular torsion

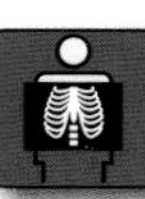

Imaging Options

- Primary: US/Doppler
- Back-up: Nuc Med
- Follow-on: MCUG

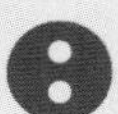

Imaging Findings

US/Doppler

- Enlarged, hypo-/hyper-echoic epididymus and/or testis
- Diffuse or focal increased Doppler flow of epididymus and testis (resistive index < 0.5)
- Thickened inflamed scrotal wall
- Reactive hydrocoele
- Complications – hypo-echoic areas may represent venous infarction

MCUG

- To check for associated abnormalities

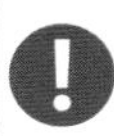

Tips

- Compare contralateral testis especially when changes are subtle.

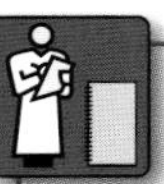

Radiological Differential Diagnosis

- Testicular torsion
- Testicular trauma
- Testicular mass
- Scrotal cellulitis

Foreign Body Aspiration

Surgeon: A. B. van As
Radiologist: H. Viljoen

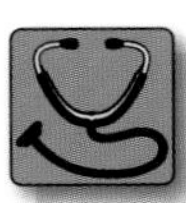

Clinical Insights

- Foreign body ingestion is the fifth commonest cause of admission in paediatric emergency.
- Peak age of presentation: 2 years.
- Most morbidity is in children less than 1 year.
- It is estimated that of all ingested foreign bodies, 80% will enter the gastrointestinal tract and 20% the tracheo-bronchial tree.
- All children presenting with a history of a sudden attack of coughing and the possibility of having aspirated a foreign body *must* be investigated by bronchoscopy.

Warning

- The clinical signs can be deceiving and a foreign body can still be present without any symptoms.
- Tracheal aspiration can be lethal.
- Most food aspirations (e.g. peanuts) are not radiodense on chest radiographs.

Controversy

- All children with suspected FB ingestion require a bronchoscopy.

Urgency

- ☑ Emergency
- ☐ Urgent
- ☐ Elective

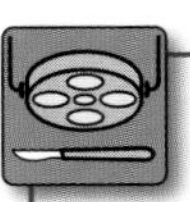

What the Surgeon Needs to Know

- Is there a foreign body present?
- What is the location?
  - Cervical or thoracic.

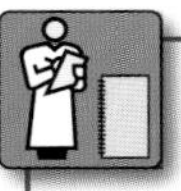

Clinical Differential Diagnosis

- Acute respiratory infection
- Ingestion of FB into GI tract
- "Scraping" of the oropharynx: It feels the FB is still there

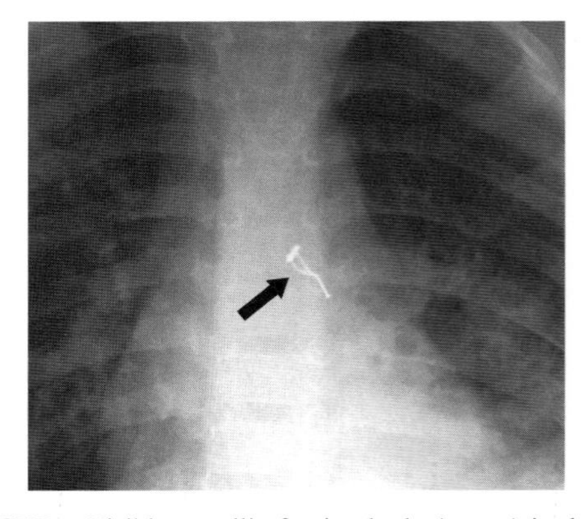

CXR – Visible metallic foreign body (*arrow*) in the left main bronchus with associated changes in the left lower lobe

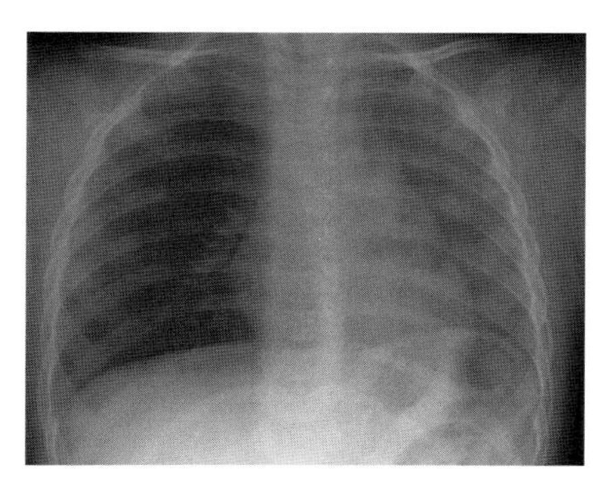

CXR expiratory – Same patient as in the previous figure during expiration confirms and exaggerates the air-trapping on the right (thereby excluding volume loss of the left). This is due to a ball valve phenomenon where the more proximal bronchi collapse on expiration and a foreign body cannot travel more proximally towards the larger calibre air-way [courtesy Ian Cowan]

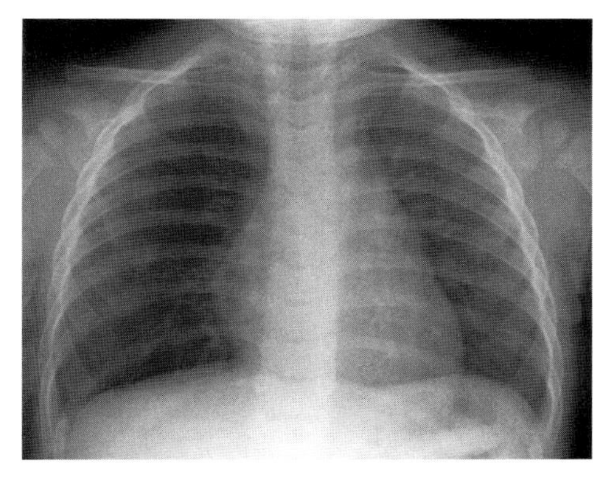

CXR inspiratory – There is differential density of the two lungs on the inspiratory view. The right lung is moderately hyperlucent suggesting air-trapping [courtesy Dr. Ian Cowan]

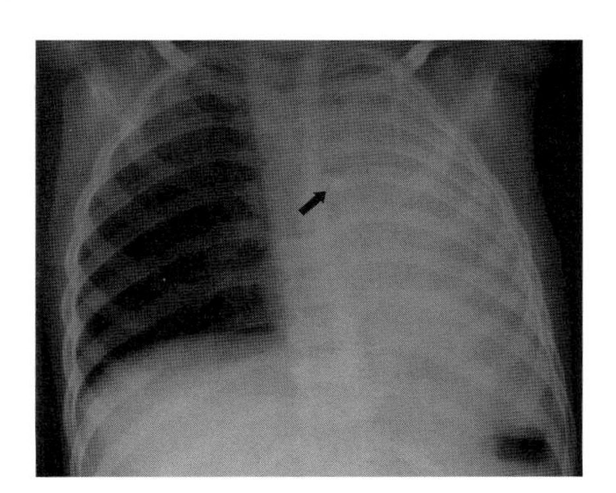

CXR – Complete collapse of the left lung due to a foreign body in the left main bronchus (*arrow*)

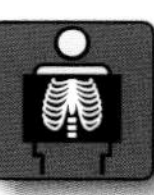

Imaging Options

- Primary: CXR (inspiratory/expiratory)
- Backup: Fluoroscopy/CT

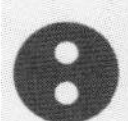

Imaging Findings

CXR

- Normal X-ray in 25% (suspicion demands bronchoscopy)
- Foreign body visible in 20%
- Hyper-expansion/lucency of lung distal to obstruction exagerated on expiratory view due to ball-valve obstruction
- Collapse/consolidation distal to bronchus when complete occlusion

CT

- To assess the extent of destruction prior to surgery in long-standing obstruction.

Tips

- Expiratory film or dynamic fluoroscopy demonstrates air-trapping on affected side if there is a ball-valve obstruction.
- Expiratory views in young non-cooperative children can be obtained using two lateral decubitus views – The side down is expiratory.

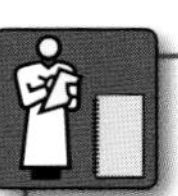

Radiological Differential Diagnosis

- Refractory asthma
- Extrinsic airway compression, e.g. TB glands, bronchogenic cyst
- Endobronchial tumour – carcinoid/mucoepidermoid
- CLE
- Hypoplastic lung with contralateral hyperexpansion

Foreign Body Ingestion (Oesophageal FB)

Surgeon: A. Darani
Radiologist: A. Maydell

Clinical Insights

- Peak at 24 months; 50% < 4 years.
- More common in boys.
- History must raise suspicion (parents, children, teacher).
- Coins, toys and batteries are common.
- Asymptomatic in nearly 35%.
- Usual symptoms: Dysphagia, poor feeding, choking, pain, irritability and drooling.
- Fever, sepsis in case of perforation and mediastinitis.
- Anatomical narrowing: Cricopharyngeus, carina and lower oesophageal sphincter.
- Oesophagoscopy is the safest option for removal and permits post-removal assessment of oesophageal integrity.

Warnings

- History of choking episode or coughing implies tracheobronchial foreign body until proven otherwise (bronchoscopy!)
- Button batteries can cause necrosis and perforation. Emergency removal from the oesophagus is indicated.

Controversy

- Foley catheter can be used for removal with the aid of fluoroscopy: Risk of airway obstruction in non-prepared environment!

Urgency

- ❑ Emergency
- ☑ Urgent
- ❑ Elective

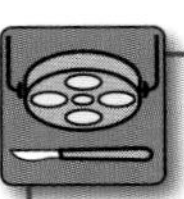

What the Surgeon Needs to Know:

- Is the foreign body in the oesophagus or in the tracheobronchial tree?
- Are there any signs of complication?

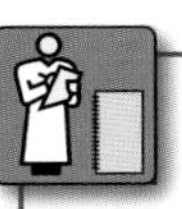

Clinical Differential Diagnosis

- Tracheobronchial foreign body
- Consider foreign bodies lying outside the patient in clothing or bedding

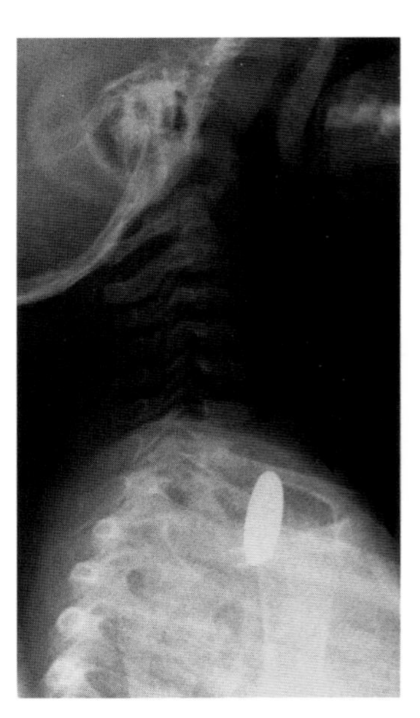

Lateral X-ray – Demonstrates the coin to be situated in the oesophagus, posterior to the airway (*arrow*) that is clearly visualized anterior to this

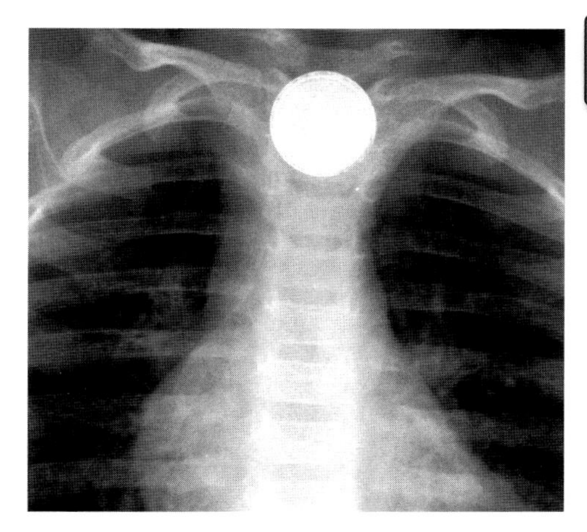

CXR – A radiodense FB in the form of a coin has lodged in the oesophagus at the thoracic inlet. There are no visible complications

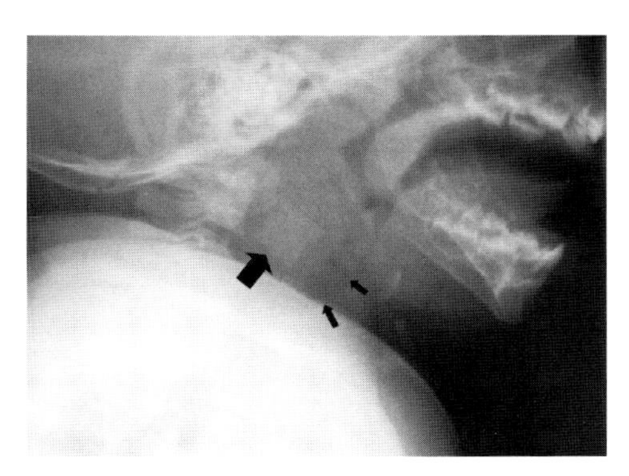

Lateral X-ray – The square structure swallowed (*large arrow*) represents a dice. The airway is seen anteriorly to this (*small arrows*)

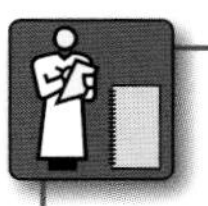

Radiological Differential Diagnosis

- FB in the airway
- Airway obstruction (abscess, croup, asthma, vascular ring)
- Oesophageal stricture
- Achalasia

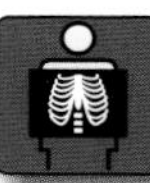

Imaging Options

- Primary: X-ray
- Follow-on: Contrast swallow (UGI)/CT

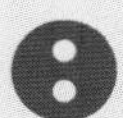

Imaging Findings

X-ray

- Radio-opaque FB in the region of oesophagus [common at thoracic inlet, aortic arch, GOJ]
- Tracheal narrowing/bowing due to inflammation of oesophagus and trachea
- Dilated oesophagus
- Complications include pneumomediastinum and abscess (air–fluid level)

Contrast Swallow (UGI)

- For non-radio-opaque FB
- To diagnose underlying stricture/cause
- Irregular mucosa implies oesophagitis, fistula, perforation

CT

- Demonstrates complications [mediastinitis, abscess, oesophageal leak]

Tips

- Initial survey should include lateral neck, CXR and if not visualized, then AXR.
- Use water-soluble contrast for swallow.
- Once FB in stomach it will invariably pass through the GIT unless sharp.
- Magnets are particularly dangerous as they attract each other across bowel walls and cause a chemical reaction that affects the Bowel wall.
- Batteries are also dangerous inciting an inflammatory reaction predisposing to perforation.

Gallstones

Surgeon: S. Cox
Radiologist: S. Theron

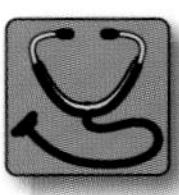

Clinical Insights

- Gall bladder calculi are uncommon in children, but the incidence is increasing.
- The incidence of cholelithiasis in children is 0.15–0.22% and it is more common in girls.
- Predisposing factors include hemolytic diseases, hepatobiliary disease, sepsis, prolonged total parenteral nutrition, trauma and abdominal surgery.
- Children may have cholesterol, pigment or mixed-type gallstones.
- Clinical presentation is of biliary colic, acute cholecystitis, choledocholithiasis, biliary obstruction with or without cholangitis, and biliary pancreatitis.
- The frequency of cholelithiasis in children with sickle-cell disease is almost double that of the general population.

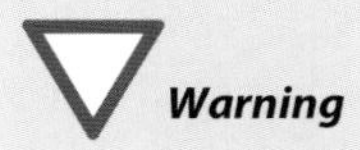

Warning

- Patients with acute cholecystitis or biliary pancreatitis need resuscitation prior to imaging.

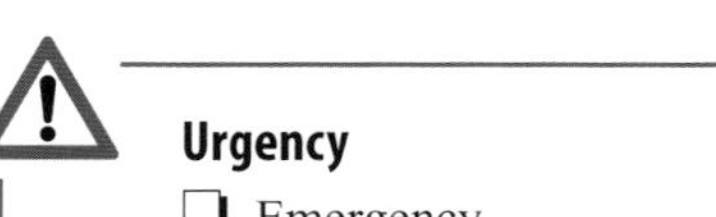

Urgency

❑ Emergency
❑ Urgent
☑ Elective

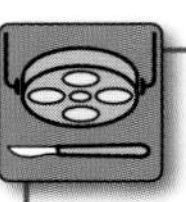

What the Surgeon Needs to Know

- Are there gallstones in the gallbladder or bile ducts?
- Is there any associated biliary dilatation?
- Exclude associated cholecystitis or pancreatitis
- Note hepatomegaly and splenomegaly. They may be a clue to hepatic disease or hemolytic processes.

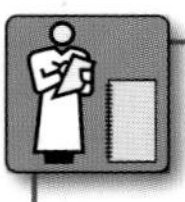

Clinical Differential Diagnosis

- Biliary ascariasis
- Acalculous cholecystitis
- Biliary dyskinesia
- Idiopathic fibrosing pancreatitis

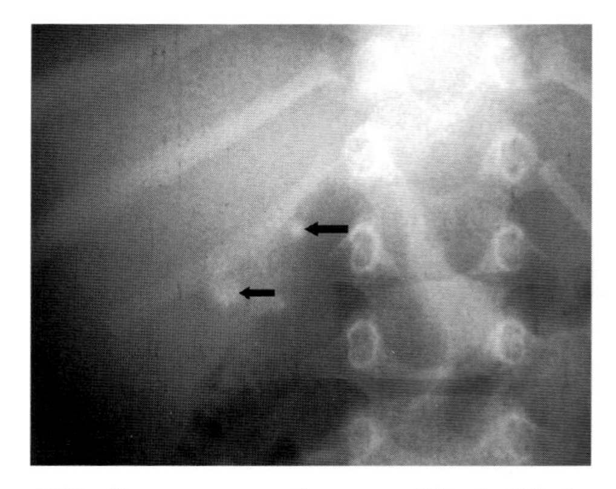

AXR – Demonstrates radio-opaque GB calculi in the right hypochondrium (*arrows*)

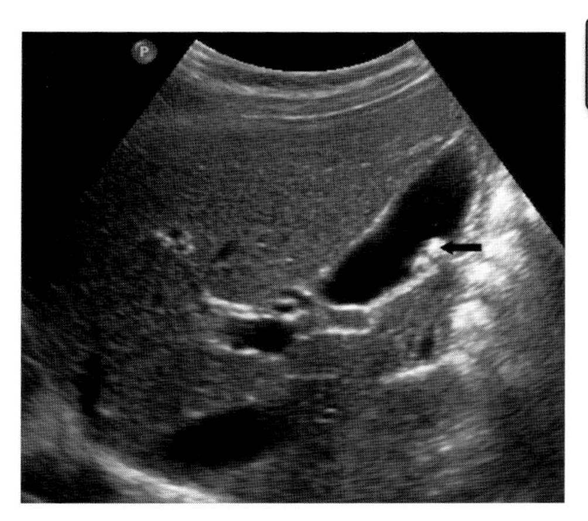

US – Shows a hyperechoic gallstone within the gallbladder (*arrow*) without an acoustic shadow

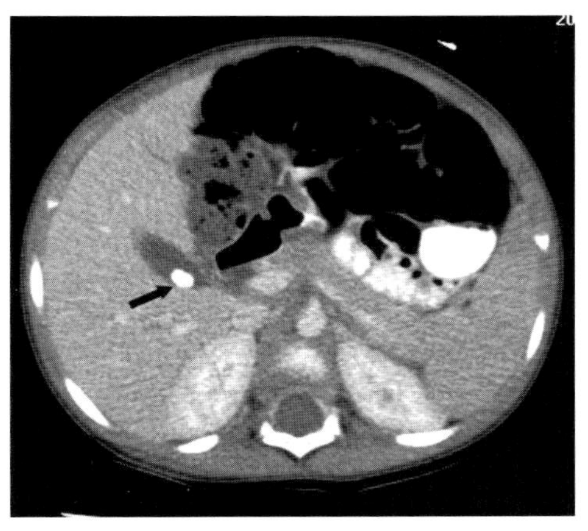

CT Abdomen – Demonstrates an incidental finding of a hyperdense stone within the gallbladder (*arrow*)

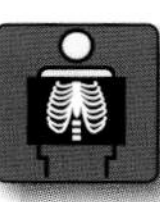

Imaging Modalities

- Primary: US
- Back-up: CT/MRCP

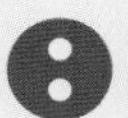

Imaging Findings

US

- Echogenic intra-luminal structure with acoustic shadowing.
- Usually clean shadows, but gas can cause comet-tail or reverberation artifact.
- Dependent unless gas or cholesterol containing.
- Mobile unless adherent/impacted.
- If GB is packed with calculi then echogenic replacement of the gall bladder with acoustic shadowing.
- Wall thickening, tenderness, pericholecystic fluid indicate cholecystitis.

CT

- Reserved for complications, e.g gallstone pancreatitis, biliary obstruction

MRCP

- Heavily T2 weighted – Hyperintense bile with hypointense filling defect

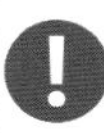

Tips

- Gallstones are mobile on ultrasound
- Gallstones often isodense to bile on CT
- Look for complications: obstruction, pancreatitis

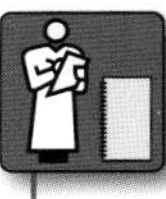

Radiological Differential Diagnosis

- Gallbladder polyp – non-mobile
- Sludge
- Hemobilia
- Inflammatory debris
- Gas

Gastro-Oesophageal Reflux

Surgeon: J. Loveland
Radiologist: P. J. Greyling

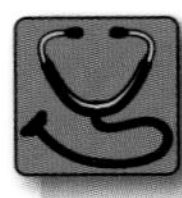

Clinical Insights

- Consider gastro-oesophageal reflux as a normal finding in the infant; when it causes pathology it is defined as a disease.
- Effortless, non-projectile vomiting not necessarily related to feeds.
- Associated poor feeding history.
- Occurs from neonatal period into infancy and later childhood.
- Untreated, 95% settle by 24 months of age.
- May require an urgent investigation and surgical intervention for life-threatening complications – aspiration, apnoea, recurrent pneumonia, oesophagitis with bleeding and stenosis.

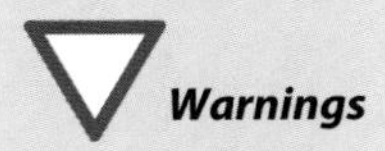

Warnings

- Life-threatening episodes, namely "Near-Sudden Infant Death Syndrome" and pulmonary aspiration, warrant urgent surgical intervention.
- Always visualize stomach and duodenum to exclude distal obstruction.

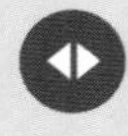

Controversy

- Majority of GORD settles on conservative management.

Urgency

- ❑ Emergency
- ❑ Urgent
- ☑ Elective

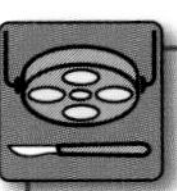

What the Surgeon Needs to Know

- Are there any anatomical abnormalities?
- Is there evidence of gastro-oesophageal reflux disease (GORD)?
  - Aspiration with pneumonia
  - Chronic oesophagitis with dysmotility and/or strictures
  - Chronic ENT infections or inflammation
  - Is there distal obstructing disease or delayed gastric emptying?

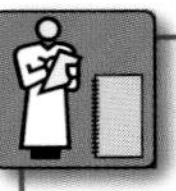

Clinical Differential Diagnosis

- Infantile hypertrophic pyloric stenosis
- Malrotation
- Pyloric web or atresia
- Duodenal stenosis or atresia
- Vomiting from intracranial pathology

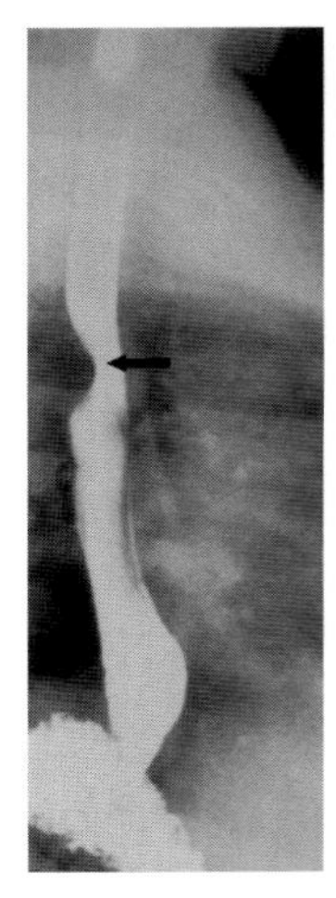

UGI lateral– Demonstrates an aberrant right subclavian artery (a posterior impression on the oesophagus – (*arrow*)) discovered while investigating a patient suspected of GOR

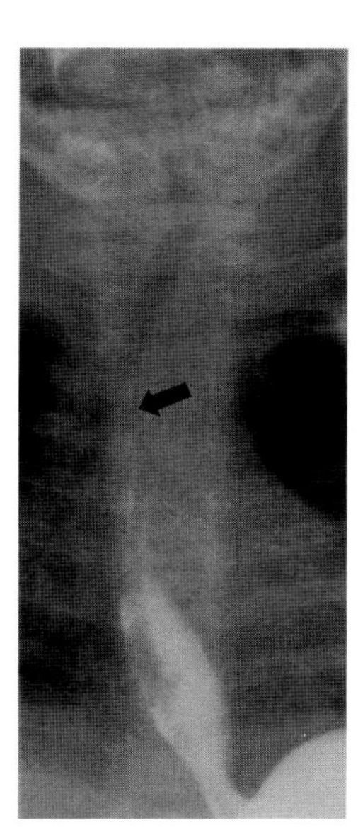

UGI – Demonstrates relatively mild GOR well below the level of the carina (*arrow*)

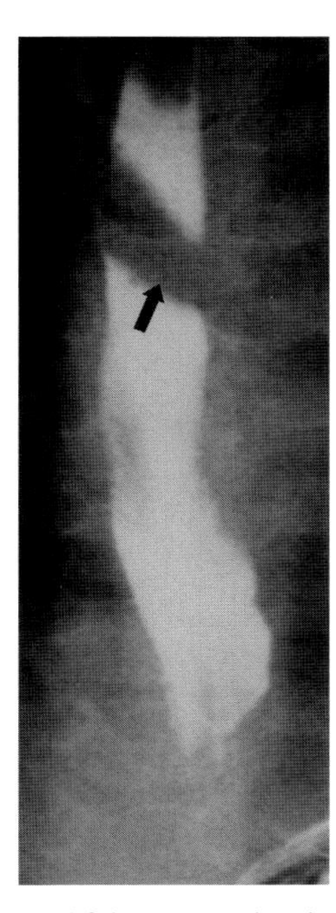

UGI AP view – Of the same patient in the previous figure confirms the vascular impression (*arrow*) and by its oblique orientation is consistent with an aberrant right subclavian artery

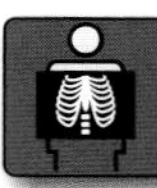

Imaging Options

- Primary: 24-h pH monitoring (use CXR for positioning)
- Secondary: Milk scan
- Back-up: UGI

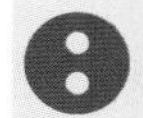

Imaging Findings

UGI:

- Detection of anomalies and pathology [e.g. vascular impressions]
- Reflux of barium seen from stomach during UGI
- Grade 1: Into distal oesophagus
- Grade 2: Up to level of carina
- Grade 3: Reflux into mouth

CXR:

- Position of pH monitor tip – T8 to T10

Tips

- All children reflux (developmental phenomena).
- 80% of children <1 year have reflux (decreases with advancing age).
- Investigate only children with pathogenic reflux/complications of reflux.
  - Oesophageal: Oesophagitis or swallowing difficulties.
  - Pulmonary: Aspiration or recurrent chest infections.
  - Constitutional: Failure to thrive/poor weight gain.
- Trial of therapy is an alternative to imaging.
- UGI is the best modality to demonstrate anatomy/rule out anomalies.
- UGI useful in evaluating swallowing mechanism.
- Grading reflux is not very helpful.
- Radiology reports should clearly state that demonstration of reflux during fluoroscopy does not equate to GORD.
- Fluoroscopy time should not be prolonged to attempt to demonstrate GOR during barium contrast radiography.

A B C D E F G **H** I J K L M N O P Q R S T U V W X Y Z

Hemangioma – Infantile Soft Tissue/Cutaneous (Strawberry Nevus)

Surgeon: A. Potgieter
Radiologist: A. Maydell

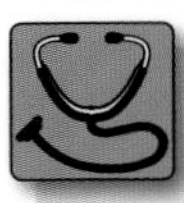

Clinical Insights

- Characterized by proliferation of endothelial cells.
- Most common tumour of childhood – 4–10% of white infants.
- Increased frequency in premature infants, 23% in neonates <1,200 g.
- 3–5 times more common in females.
- Characteristic behaviour of hemangiomas:
  - Grow rapidly (proliferative phase – 0–1 year).
  - Slowly regress (involuting phase – 1–7 years).
  - Never recur (involuted phase – after 7 years).
- Commonest sites – Craniofacial region (60%), trunk (25%), extremities (15%).
- Their appearance is "heralded" (30–50%) by a telangiectatic, macular, red spot.

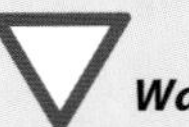

Warnings

- Beware of possible visceral lesions, e.g. hepatic hemangiomas (30–80% mortality).
- Be vigilant and cautious with visceral lesions and those affecting the airway or orbit.

Controversy

- When to intervene, if at all, and what treatment is most appropriate.

Urgency

- ❑ Emergency
- ❑ Urgent
- ☑ Elective unless vital structures involved

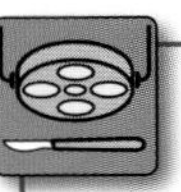

What the Surgeon Needs to Know

- What is the extent of the lesion?
- Is it solid or cystic?
- Is there high or low flow within it?

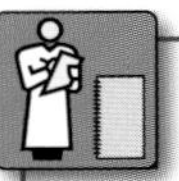

Clinical Differential Diagnosis

- Vascular malformations (capillary, venous or lymphatic)
- Other infantile vascular tumours (hemangioendothelioma, tufted angioma, hemangiopericytoma, fibrosarcoma)
- Pyogenic granuloma
- Kassabach-Merritt (Kaposiform Hemangioendothelioma) – Consumptive coagulopathy

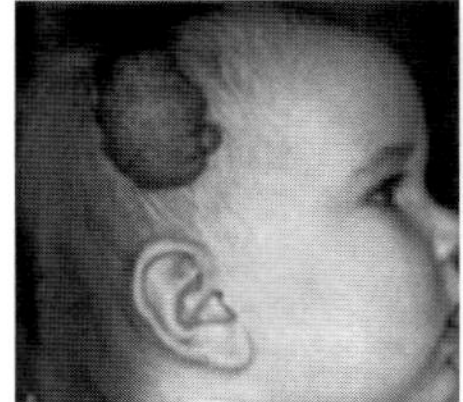
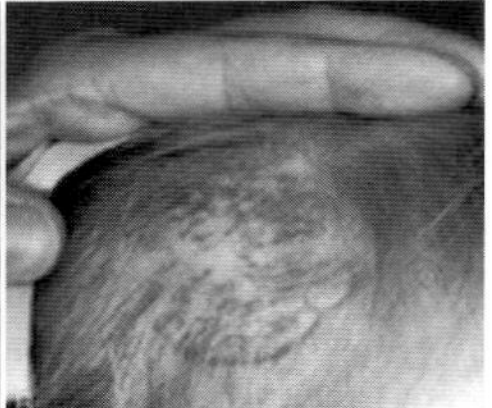

A child at 6 months of age with a scalp hemangioma and the same lesion at 2 years with advanced involution

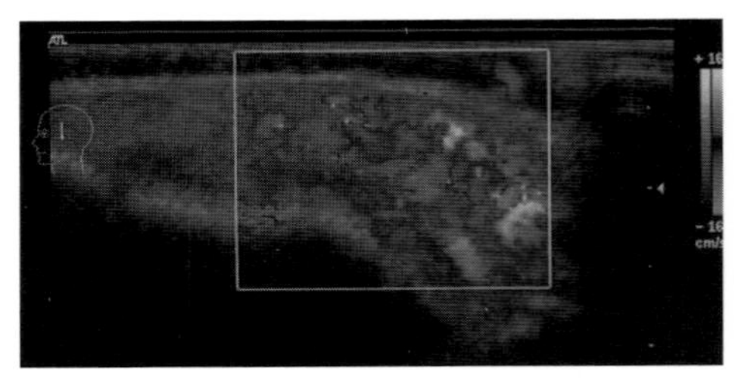

US colour Doppler – Demonstrates a high concentration of vessels in this solid subcutaneous lesion of the scalp [courtesy Irene Borzani]

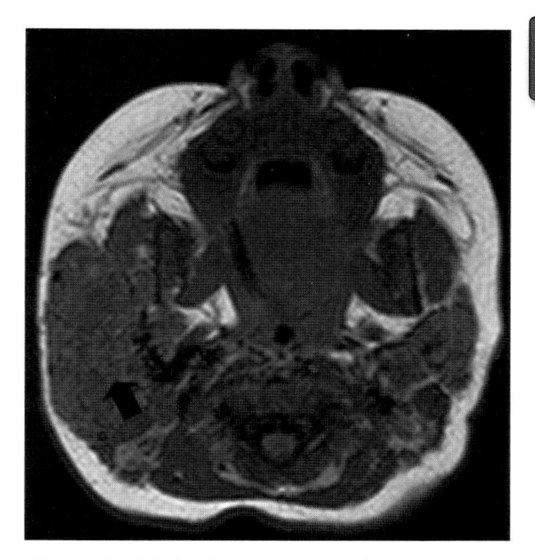

T1-weighted MRI demonstrates an isointense right parotid mass (*arrow*) with feeding vessels

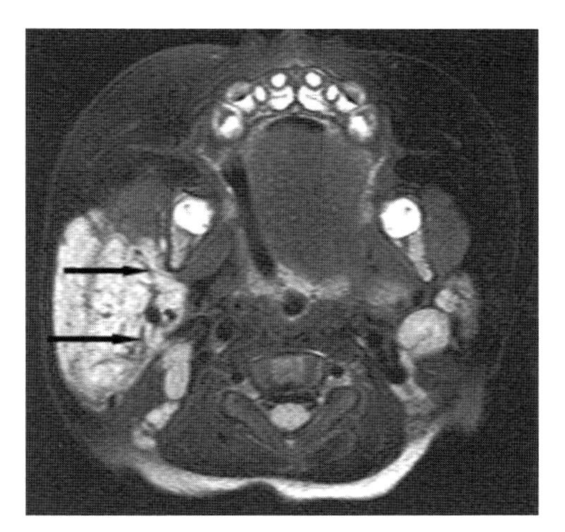

STIR MRI demonstrates the right parotid hemangioma to be of high signal intensity and contain what appear to be multiple low signal septations, which in fact represent multiple vessels (*arrows*) seen as flow voids

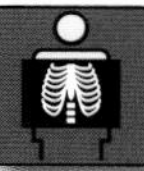

Imaging Options

- Primary: MRI/US Doppler

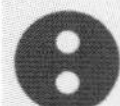

Imaging Findings

MRI

- Lobulated mass.
- High signal on T2 with multiple flow voids.
- Iso-intense to muscle on T1.
- Intense enhancement with Gadolinium.
- Involuting mass may contain fat and calcium.

Doppler US

- High vessel density (>5 vessels/cm^2)
- High peak arterial Doppler shift (exceeding 2 kHz)
- Lobulated mass

Tips

- Complications requiring management: airway obstruction, high output cardiac failure, Kassaback Merrit (platelet consumption), vision impairment
- Most are benign and involute spontaneously and completely
- During involution lesions may show calcification, fat and cystic changes
- Large segmental lesions rarely associated with multi-system congenital malformation syndromes

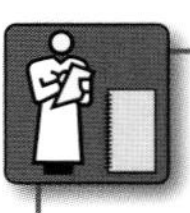

Radiological Differential Diagnosis

- Venous malformation
- Soft-tissue sarcoma (rhabdomyosarcoma)
- Kaposiform hemangioendothelioma

Hemangioma – Liver (Hemangioendothelioma)

Surgeon: A. Numanoglu
Radiologist: S. Theron

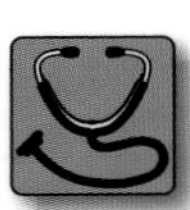

Clinical Insights

- Commonly found incidentally.
- Cardiac failure may be seen in severe forms.
- Can be isolated or multiple.
- Cutaneous involvement occurs in up to 60% of cases.
- Usually follow proliferation/involution sequence.

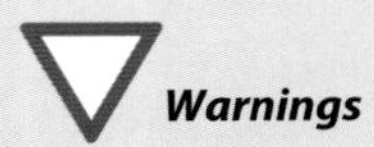

Warnings

- May be associated with Beckwith-Wiedemann, hemihypertrophy and multiple cavernous angioma syndromes.
- May increase rapidly in size leading to abdominal compartment syndrome.
- Occasionally associated with profound hypothyroidism.

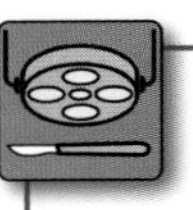

What the Surgeon Needs to Know

- Location in liver.
- Size; localized/diffuse; single/multiple?
- Size of distal aorta – Decreased if significant "steal" phenomenon from hepatic artery
- Is there a significant portal vein contribution?
- Degree of reduction in size during follow-up

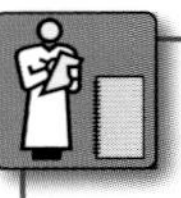

Clinical Differential Diagnosis

- Congenital hepatic arterio-venous fistulas

Urgency

- ❑ Emergency
- ❑ Urgent
- ☑ Elective

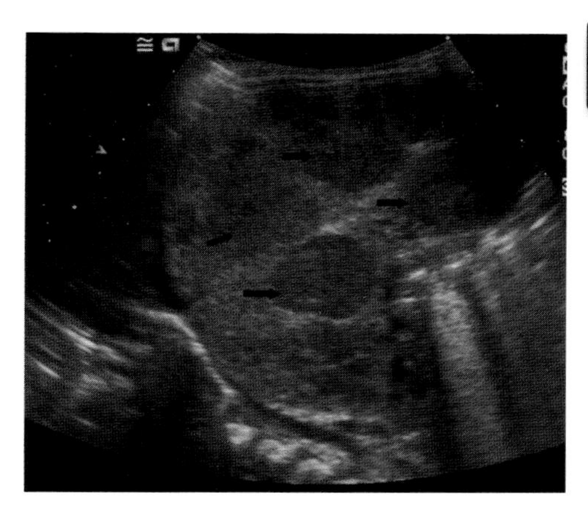

US longitudinal – Of the liver demonstrates multifocal low echogenicity lesions representing haemangiomata (*arrows*) [courtesy Dr. Kieran McHugh]

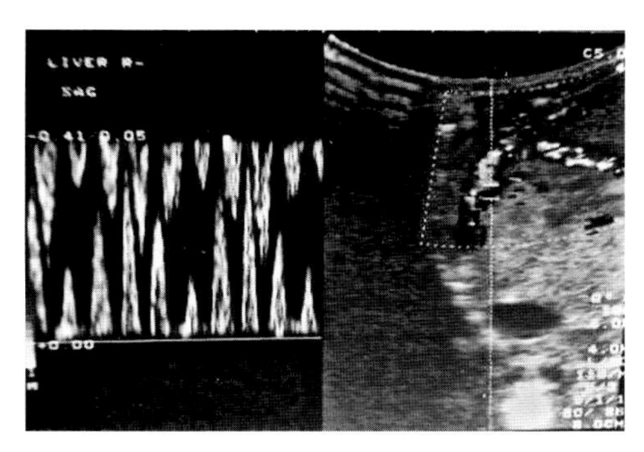

US Doppler – There are large vascular channels demonstrating high flow in these haemangiomata

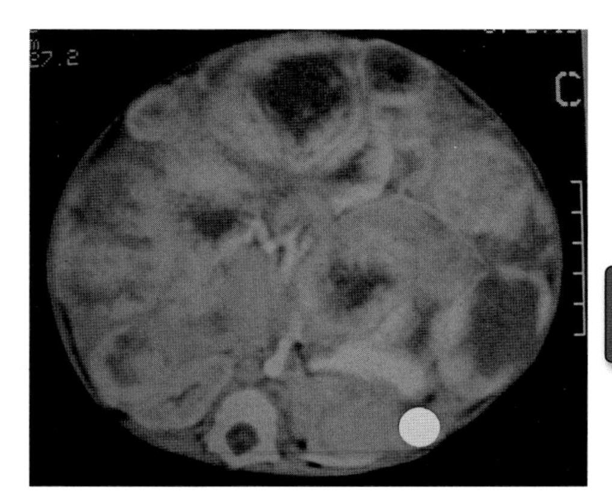

Contrasted CT abdomen – The liver parenchyma is replaced by diffuse, heterogeneously enhancing masses, causing hepatomegaly. Multifocal early peripheral enhancement is present consistent with multiple liver haemangiomata

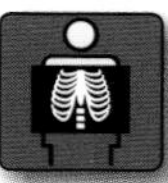

Imaging Options

- Primary: US
- Follow on imaging: CT
- Back-up: MRI

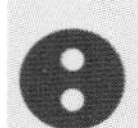

Imaging Findings

US

- Heterogenous hypoechoic masses
- High flow vascular structures

CT

- Low-density masses precontrast
- Early peripheral, late central or diffuse enhancement (characteristic)

MRI

- Heterogenous masses, T1 low, T2 high
- Prominent vascular flow voids
- Post-gadolinium enhancement like CT

Tips

- Solitary or multiple, heterogenous liver masses.
- Mass well-defined or diffusely infiltrative.
- Lesion contains large vascular structures.

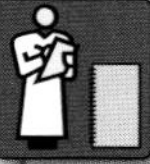

Radiological Differential Diagnosis

- Hepatoblastoma: Usually well-defined, solitary, can be hypervascular
- Neuroblastoma metastases: Multiple liver masses, or diffuse heterogeneity
- Mesenchymal hamartoma: Multilobulated, well-defined, cystic mass

Hematometrocolpos (Hydrometrocolpos)

Surgeon: A. Alexander
Radiologist: S. Przybojewski

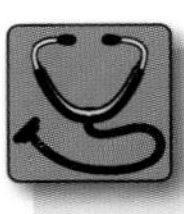

Clinical Insights

- Haematometrocolpos is defined as the retention of blood within the uterus and vagina.
- Because of menstruation, it is dependent on menarche and caused by:
  - Imperforate hymen.
  - Vaginal atresia.
  - Vaginal tumours.
- Hydrometrocolpos is fluid in the obstructed genital tract usually due to imperforate hymen associated with:
  - Complex urogenital sinus abnormalities and with perineal level obstruction.
  - Cloacal abnormalities giving rise to genital dilatation of varying degrees.
- Clinically they can present as an abdominal or perineal mass.

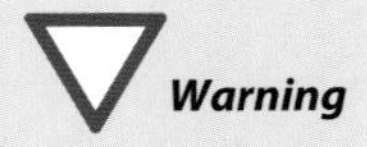

Warning

- Hydrocolpos associated with congenital abnormalities (VACTERL).

Urgency

- ☐ Emergency
- ☑ Urgent
- ☐ Elective

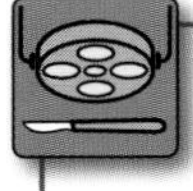

What the Surgeon Needs to Know

- Are the vagina and uterus involved (hydrometrocolpos vs. hydrocolpos)?
- At what level is the obstruction?
- Are there associated abnormalities: Renal dysgenesis; dysplasia; obstruction?

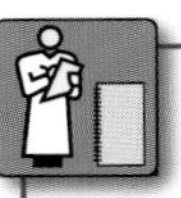

Clinical Differential Diagnosis

- Prolapsing ureterocoele
- Bartholin's cyst/abscess
- Pelvic duplication cyst
- Ovarian cyst
- Meconium cyst
- Full bladder

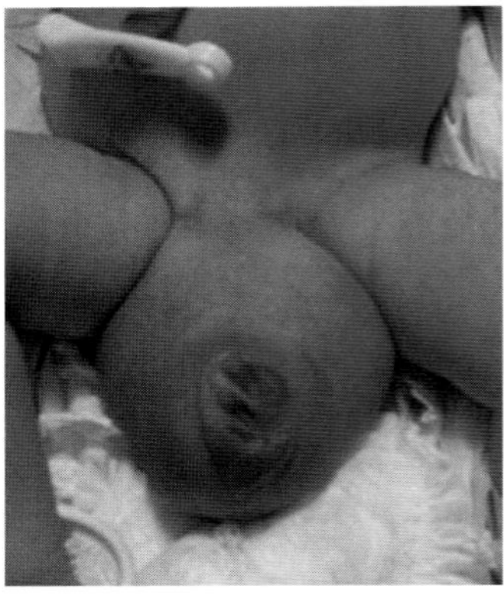

Hydrocolpos – Prolapsing perineal mass in a female neonate

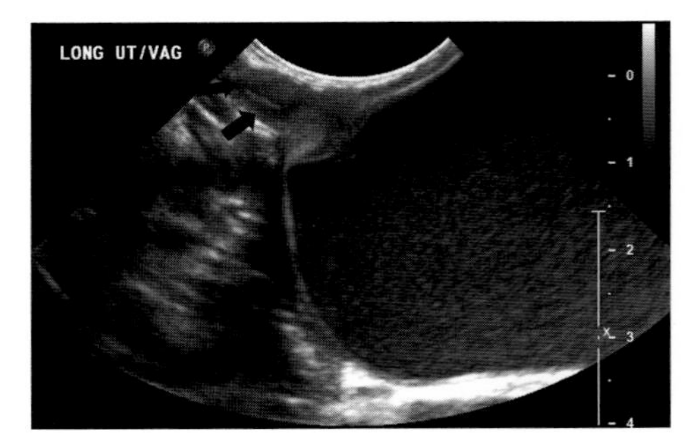

US longitudinal – The uterus is cephalad to the distended vagina and not (or less) distended (arrows)

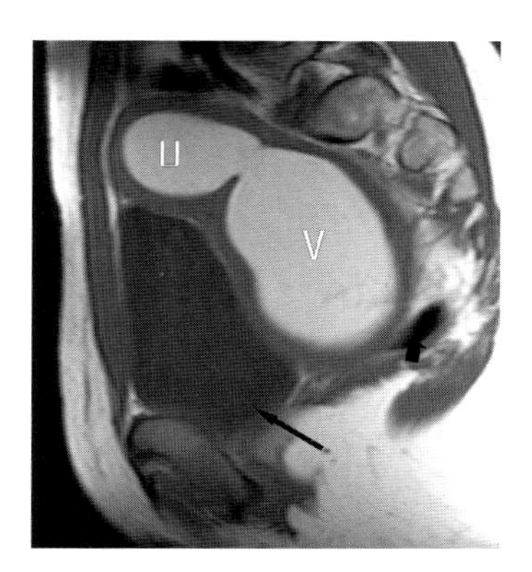

MRI – Sagittal T1 – Hyperintense blood within a distended uterus (U) and vagina (V). The blood filled cavity is located between the bladder (*long arrow*) and air-filled rectum (*short arrow*)

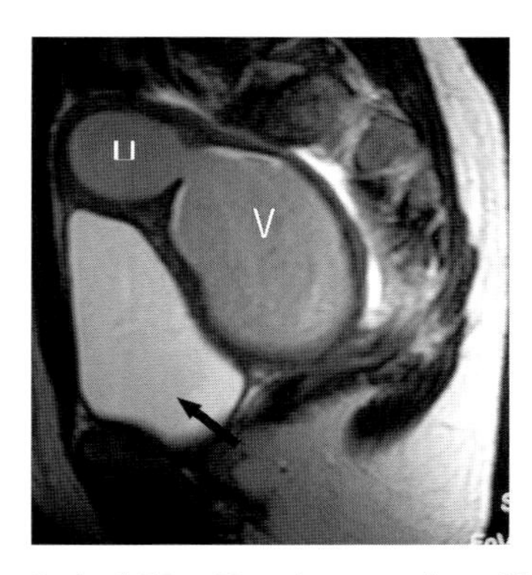

MRI – Sagittal T2 – Hyperintense urine within the bladder (*arrow*) is located anterior to the distended uterus (U) and vagina (V)

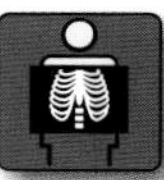

Imaging Options

- Primary: US
- Follow on: MRI
- Alternative: CT

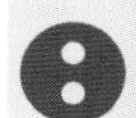

Imaging Findings

Ultrasound

- Echogenic debris in discrete cavity between rectum and bladder.
- Variably distended uterus arises from dome of collection.
- Secondary hydronephrosis.

MRI

- Aging blood products have typical signal intensity – High on T1.
- Content often high signal on T2 but blood degradation may cause a variable decrease in signal.

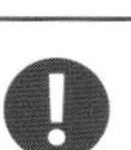

Tips

- Elastic vagina dilates more than uterus.
- Multiplanar MRI useful.
- MRI to assess for associated genitourinary anomalies not detected by ultrasound.
- High T1 products suggest haemorrhage and should prompt questioning/examination re telarche to assist diagnosis.
- Renal US should look for urinary anomalies (solitary kidney).

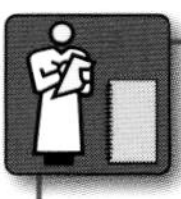

Radiological Differential Diagnosis

- Pelvic abscess – Seen in sexually active adolescents
- Ovarian neoplasm, torsion – Separate from uterus
- Fallopian tube obstruction, torsion, cyst – Separate from uterus
- Pelvic rhabdomyosarcoma

Hepatoblastoma

Surgeon: A. Numanoglu
Radiologist: S. Theron

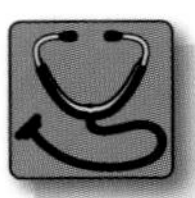

Clinical Insights

- Enlarging abdominal mass or distension.
- Mean age 3 years.
- Serum alphafetoprotein levels elevated in almost all.
- Single or multi-centric.
- If tumour is not resectable at initial presentation surgery is postponed to allow shrinkage with preoperative chemotherapy.

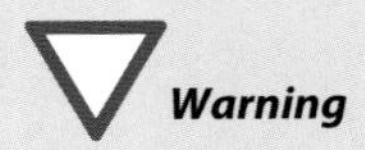

- A common site of metastatic disease is the lung.

Controversies

- Extensive hepatic resection for localized but extensive tumour.
- Intraoperative ultrasound may help improve tumour clearance.
- Irresectable tumour localized to the liver (post-chemotherapy) can do well with liver transplantation.

Urgency

- ❑ Emergency
- ❑ Urgent
- ☑ Elective

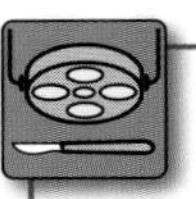

What the Surgeon Needs to Know

- Pre-TEXT staging
- Status of vascular involvement
- Post-chemotherapy resectability (centricity; portal vein involvement; hepatic venous drainage)

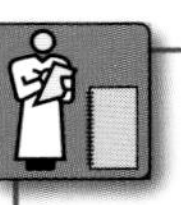

Clinical Differential Diagnosis

- Hepatocellular carcinoma
- Mesenchymal hamartoma

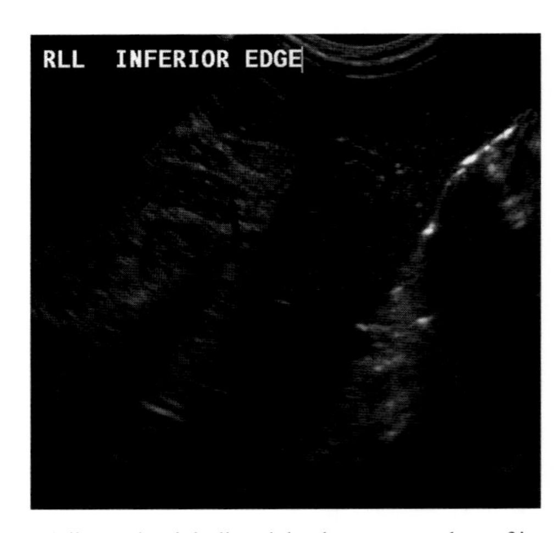

US liver. The right liver lobe demonstrates loss of its normal morphology and echogenicity due to a hepatoblastoma (*arrows*)

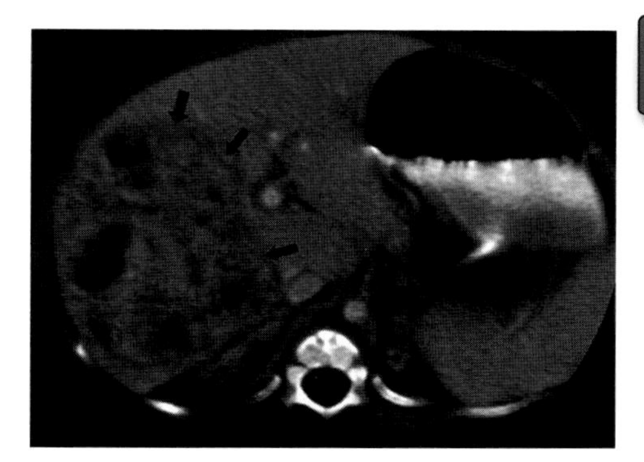

CT axial post-contrast – There is a fairly well-defined, heterogeneously hypodense (compared with normal liver) mass in the right lobe of the liver (*arrows*) with heterogenous enhancement

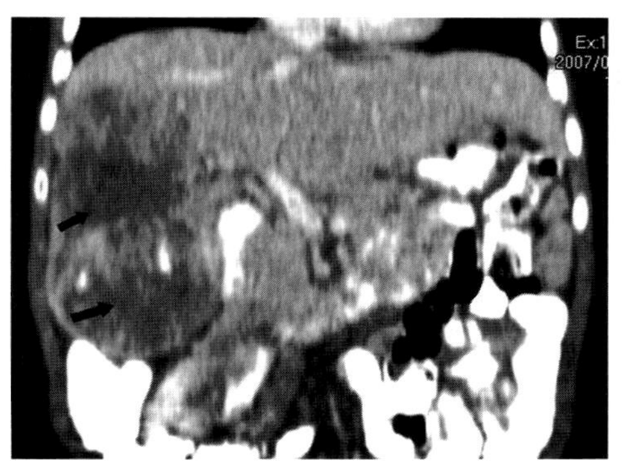

CT coronal reconstruction – The mass involves liver segments 5–8 (*arrows*), causing architectural distortion and hepatomegaly

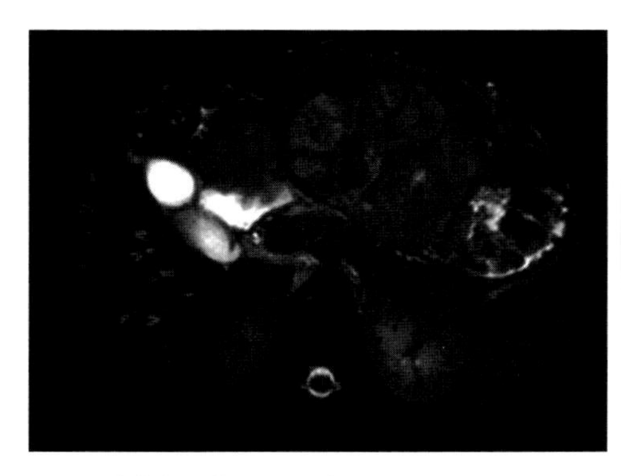

MRI axial heavily T2 weighted – Demonstrates a hepatoblastoma in segments 3 and 4b (*arrows*) of heterogenous signal intensity

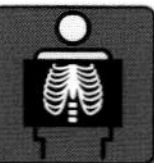

Imaging Options

- Primary: US
- Follow-on: CT
- Follow-on: MRI

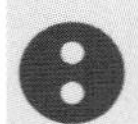

Imaging Findings

US

- Heterogenous mass due to haemorrhage/necrosis
- Typically hypervascular

CT

- Well-defined, heterogenous, hypodense mass
- Enhances less than normal liver

MRI

- T2 high, but can be low due to haemorrhage.

Tips

- CT chest to identify any metastases.
- Usually single mass, can be diffusely infiltrating or multifocal.
- Doppler good for assessment of venous invasion but usually require CT with MPR for surgical planning.
- Calcification in up to 50% of cases.

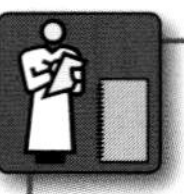

Radiological Differential Diagnosis

- Hemangioendothelioma (<1 year, heart failure)
- Neuroblastoma metastases (<2 years)
- Hepatocellular carcinoma (>5 years)
- Mesenchymal hamartoma (predominantly cystic)

Hiatus Hernia

Surgeon: S. Cox
Radiologist: S. Cader

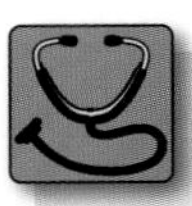

Clinical Insights

- A hiatal hernia occurs when a portion of the stomach prolapses through the diaphragmatic oesophageal hiatus.
- Symptoms are those associated with gastro-oesophageal reflux and dysphagia:
  - Regurgitation.
  - Vomiting.
  - Recurrent chest infections.
  - Failure to thrive.
  - Chronic ENT infections.
  - Dyspepsia.
  - Anaemia.
- Overall, a sliding hernia is most common:
  - Oesophago-gastric junction rises into thorax.
- Para-oesophageal hernia occurs in 3–5%:
  - Oesophago-gastric junction remains in position below the diaphragm: minimal reflux usually.
  - Fundus of stomach migrates into extra-pleural thorax: anterior and to the right.
- Partial thoracic stomach:
  - Oesophago-gastric junction and much of fundus lie in the posterior mediastinum.
  - Commonest variety in infants.

Warnings

- Aspiration of contrast is possible if there is associated severe reflux.
- Beware of labelling a fundal wrap as a hiatus hernia in patients with anti-reflux surgery.

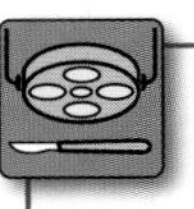

What the Surgeon Needs to Know

- Is there a hiatus hernia?
- Is there associated reflux and aspiration?
- Position of the oesophago-gastric junction
- Distal anatomy including duodenal C-loop

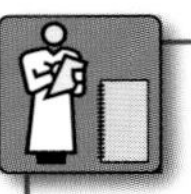

Clinical Differential Diagnosis

- Slipped anti-reflux procedure wrap

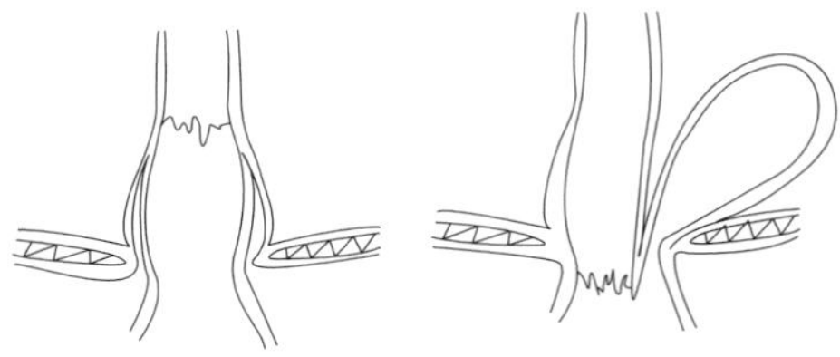

Differentiation between sliding and rolling hiatus hernia

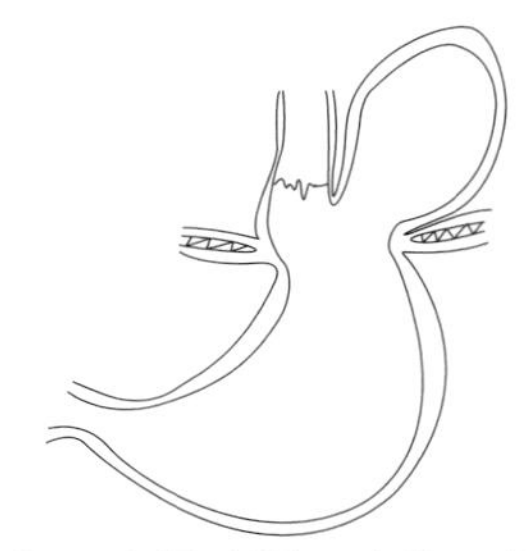

Neonatal hiatal hernia – Partial thoracic stomach type

Urgency

- ☐ Emergency
- ☐ Urgent
- ☑ Elective

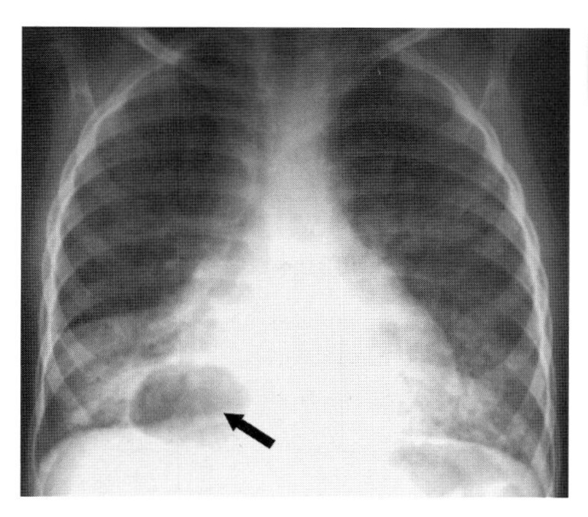

Frontal chest radiograph demonstrates the hiatus hernia as an oval lucency behind the heart on the right (*arrow*)

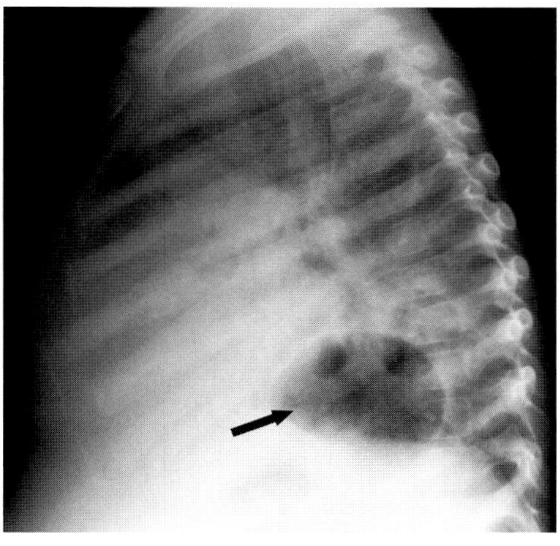

The lateral radiograph confirms the position of the hernia in the middle mediatinum (*arrow*)

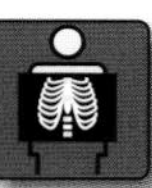

Imaging Options

- Primary: CXR, AXR, UGI
- Secondary: CT

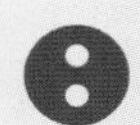

Imaging Findings

AXR/CXR

- Visible if large but may be normal.
- Large posterior retrocardiac mass that may contain an air–fluid level.
- Sometimes extends to the lateral chest wall.
- Very large hiatus hernia usually extend into the right hemithorax with gastric volvulus.

UGI

- Gastric folds more than 2 cm above the diaphragm.
- Sliding type (Type 1):
  - The oesophogus may be short and kinked.
  - The gastro-oesophageal junction is in the mediastinum above the diaphragm.
- Rolling type (Type 2/para-oesophageal):
  - The gastro-oesophageal junction is in its normal location but the fundus is located within the mediastinum.

CT

- Extension of portion of the proximal stomach into the lower mediastinum and abnormally wide oesophageal hiatus.
- Saggital and coronal reformatted images often help demonstrate the hernia and hiatal defect.

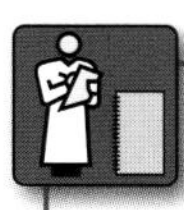

Radiological Differential Diagnosis

- Moragagni hernia
- Oesophageal diverticulum
- Mediastinal/pericardial cyst
- Bronchogenic cyst
- Aortic aneurysm
- Loculated pleural effusion

Hirschsprung's Disease (Colonic Aganglionosis)

Surgeon: S. Moore
Radiologist: P. J. Greyling

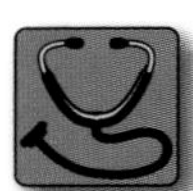

Clinical Insights

- The most common cause of lower intestinal obstruction in a neonate.
- Male babies (M:F ratio 4:1).
- Regarded as a genetic disease (mostly RET gene).
- Two forms of clinical presentation:
  - Neonatal – Delay in passage of meconium (>24 h); low intestinal obstruction; abdominal distension
  - Late– Abdominal distension; constipation (no overflow); Hirschsprung's associated enterocolitis (HAEC)

Warnings

- Check if enema/rectal washout has taken place (may distort imaging).
- Total colonic aganglionosis may not show typical clinical or radiological features.
- In the presence of HAEC patient may be extremely ill (septicaemic with friable bowel wall).

Controversies

- The role of imaging is to suspect diagnosis and suggest the level of obstruction.
- Ultimate diagnosis is based on histological aganglionosis and abnormal acetyl cholinesterase positive nerves in submusoca (Meier-Ruge).
- Anal achalasia/ultra-short segment Hirschprung – diagnosed by ano-rectal manometry and histology.
- Relationship to intestinal neuronal dysplasia.

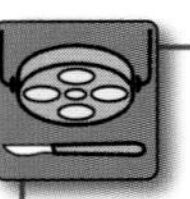

What the Surgeon Needs to Know

- Is there discrepancy of size in bowel loops?
- What is the level of obstruction?

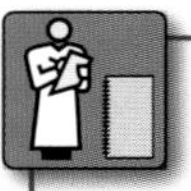

Clinical Differential Diagnosis

- Obstruction due to other causes
- Colonic motility disturbances other than Hirschsprung's
- Chronic constipation

Urgency

- ☐ Emergency
- ☐ Urgent
- ☑ Elective

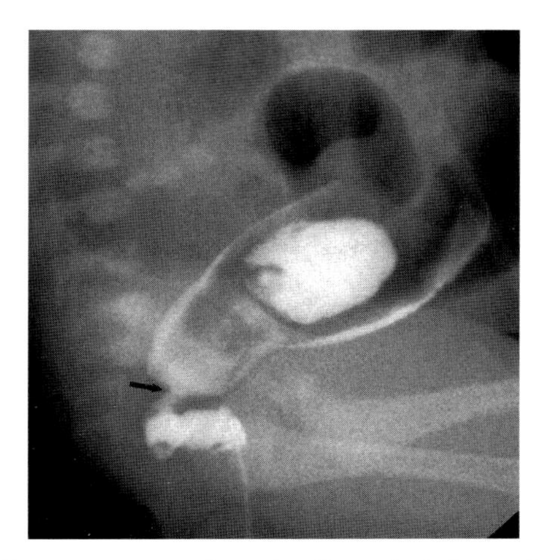

Contrast enema – Lateral radiograph during early (slow) filling shows that the caliber of the rectum is smaller than that of the sigmoid colon. There is a clear transition zone (*arrow*) from small rectum to dilated (normal) sigmoid

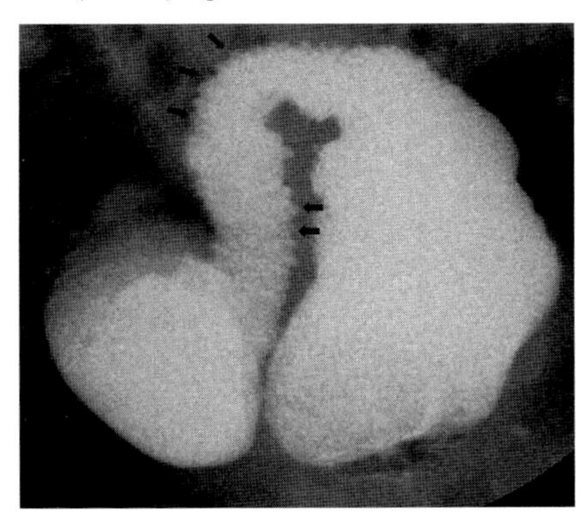

Contrast enema – Demonstrates secondary signs of a "saw-tooth" appearance (*arrows*) to mucosa from spasm. The rectal diameter has been affected in this patient by rectal examination and excessive pressure infusion of the contrast during the enema

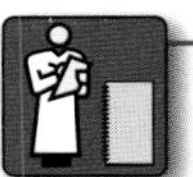

Radiological Differential Diagnosis

(As for any distal bowel obstruction)

- Anorectal malformation – Evident clinically
- Meconium plug/small left colon syndrome
- Meconium ileus
- Ileal atresia

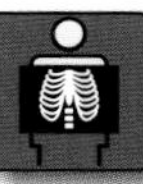

Imaging Options

- Primary: Contrast enema
- Back up: AXR

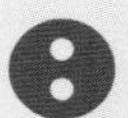

Imaging Findings

Contrast Enema

- Findings not always typical, particularly in the neonatal period.
- Normal – rectum has the largest diameter of the left hemi-colon.
- Hirschprung's disease – Lateral projection shows smaller caliber rectum compared with sigmoid.
- Transition zone between distal and proximal dilated colon
- Secondary signs are fasciculations or "saw-tooth" appearance to mucosa from spasm.
- In total colonic aganglionosis. The colon may have a "microcolon" appearance.

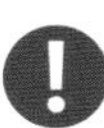

Tips

- Purpose of contrast enema – Determine other aetiology causing distal obstruction, and if Hirschprung's disease, to demonstrate the disease extent [site of transition zone].
- Use water-soluble contrast for all studies.
- Start contrast enema in lateral position.
- Fill rectum slowly.
- Use small caliber catheter and no balloon.
- Delay study to next day if rectal examination has been performed.
- Treat as a relative emergency – a dilated colon may result in a colitis with perforation.

Horseshoe Kidney

Surgeon: J. Loveland
Radiologist: H. von Bezing

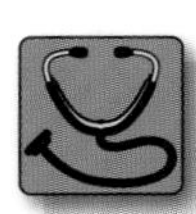

Clinical Insights

- The most common renal fusion anomaly.
- Ninety percent involve fusion of the lower pole.
- Male:female ratio of 2:1.
- Mid and upper pole variants may occur.
- Kidney located inferior to normal position, with isthmus caught between aorta and inferior mesenteric artery.
- Connected by fibrous or parenchymal bridge that may contain dominant vessel.
- Arterial anatomy may be aberrant.
- Risk of nephrolithiasis secondary to stasis.

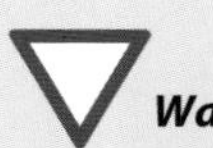

Warning

- Look for associated sacral and cloacal anomalies as well as gonadal dysgenesis

Urgency

- ❑ Emergency
- ❑ Urgent
- ☑ Elective

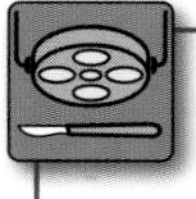

What the Surgeon Needs to Know

- Exclude associated renal anomalies
  - Vesico-ureteric reflux
  - Pelvi-ureteric junction obstruction
  - Ureteral duplication

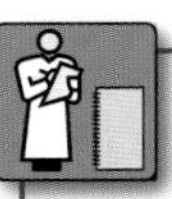

Clinical Differential Diagnosis

- Tumour

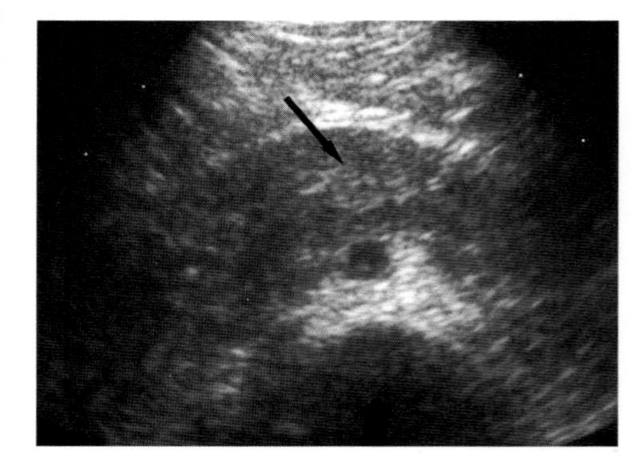

Transverse US to the lower poles of the “kidneys” demonstrates the isthmus of the horseshoe kidney (*thin arrow*) overlying the spine (*thick arrow*)

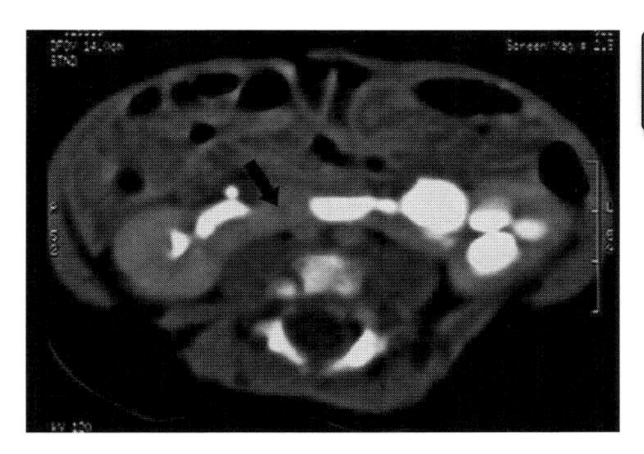

Delayed post-contrast CT demonstrates the isthmus of the horseshoe kidney (*arrow*) extending over the vertebral column with associated hydronephrosis

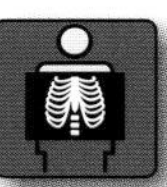

Imaging Options

- Primary: US
- Back-up: nuclear medicine, IVP, MRI, CT

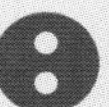

Imaging Findings

- One kidney/moiety appears small because of asymmetrical position.
- One or both moieties lie in an unusual location, anterior to the spine.
- Usually one moiety is more normally positioned in the flank; normal size.
- Bridging renal tissue anterior to spine (isthmus).
- Hydronephrosis present in 30%.
- Urolithiasis present in 20%.

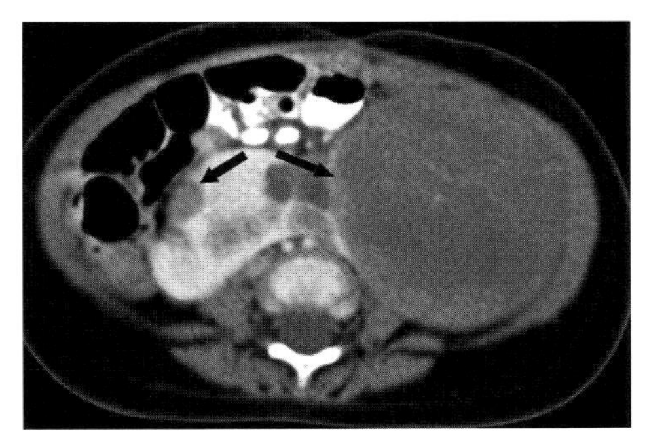

Early post-contrast CT demonstrates a horseshoe kidney complicated by Wilm's tumour on both sides (*arrows*)

Tips

- US – Always scan all children's kidneys in the transverse plane and identify end of each kidney to exclude a horseshoe.
- Higher incidence in trisomy 18 and Turner syndrome.
- Exclude VUR in all patients.
- Increased incidence of Wilm's tumour requires monitoring and vigilance.

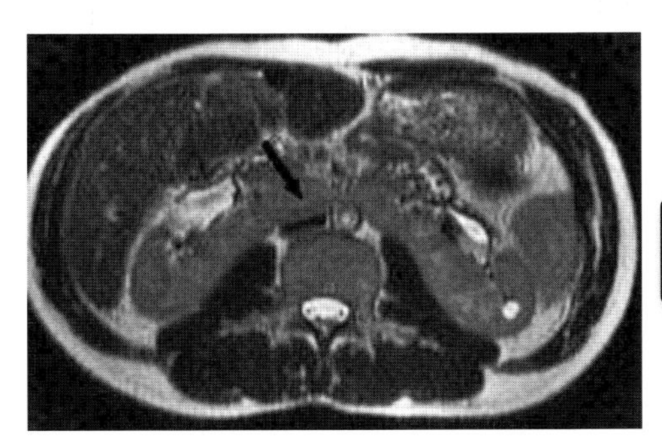

Transverse MRI demonstrates the orientation of the lower poles (note the renal pelves) of the two moieties and the isthmus (*arrow*)

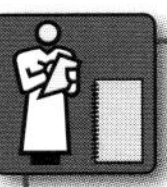

Radiological Differential Diagnosis

- Crossed fused ectopia – Part of the same spectrum of anomaly
- Intussusception or pseudokidney of GIT pathology

Hydatid Cysts (*Echinococcus* Cyst)

Surgeon: M. Arnold
Radiologist: J. W. Lotz

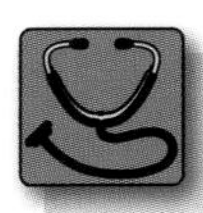

Clinical Insights

- Caused by *Echinococcus granulosis* (tapeworm) – majority.
- Endemic in Southern and East Africa, Mediterranean, Middle East, Australasia and South America.
- Slow growing thus fewer present in childhood.
- Liver and lungs are the most commonly involved – Exclude brain involvement.
- Symptoms can be due to primary mass effect in any organ or secondary to rupture or infection.

Warnings

- Acute rupture can cause anaphylaxis, which can be fatal if massive.
- Chemotherapy with albendazole or mebendazole must be started 4 days before drainage and continued for a month after.

Controversies

- 2–25% risk spillage with surgical excision, but complete excision is curative.
- Some respond to albendazole alone and do not require surgery.

Urgency

- ☐ Emergency
- ☐ Urgent
- ☑ Elective

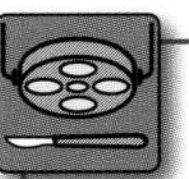

What the Surgeon Needs to Know

- Exact anatomical location.
- Size of cyst.
- Presence and location of cysts in other organs.
- Is it super-infected?
- Local pressure effects e.g. portal hypertension, biliary or urinary tract obstruction.
- Follow-up imaging: Is the cyst getting smaller, is there separation of germinal layer, is there calcification within the cyst?

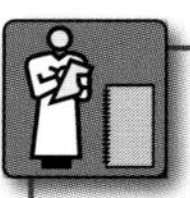

Clinical Differential Diagnosis

Abdominal

- Abscesses
- Mesenteric cysts
- Cystic Wilm's tumour
- Cystic teratoma
- Cystic liver tumour (mesenchymal hamartoma)
- Tuberculosis
- Choledochal cysts
- Hepatic cysts
- Congenital cysts (enteric, lymphangioma)

Chest

- Tumour (metastasis)
- Congenital cyst (bronchogenic)
- Abscess

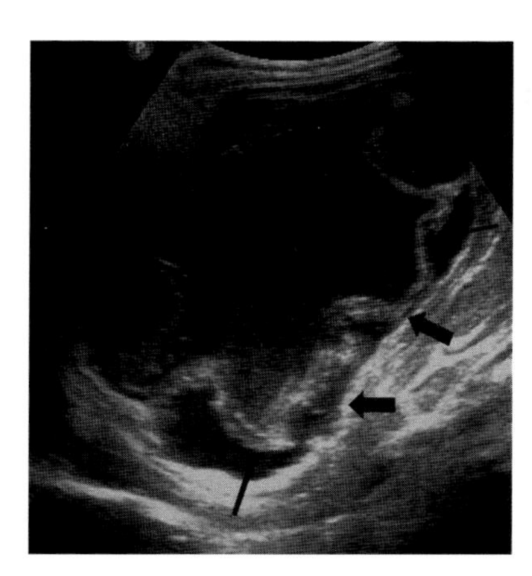

US of a dying hydatid cyst demonstrates separation of the ecto and endo cysts (*long arrows*) from the pericyst (*short arrows*), which allows for a confident diagnosis

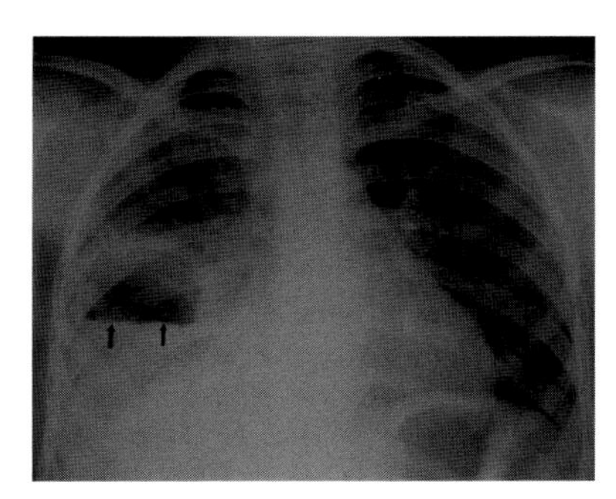

An intrathoracic hydatid cyst that has complicated by eroding a bronchus results in an air–fluid level with a floating membrane often called a "floating lily" (*arrows*)

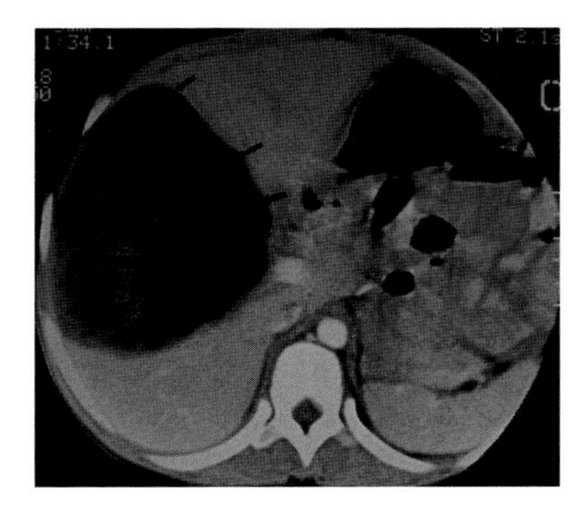

CT scan demonstrates a hepatic hydatid cyst with typical daughter cysts (*arrows*) allowing for a confident diagnosis

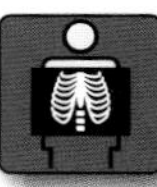

Imaging Options

- Primary: US
- Back-up: CT/MRI
- Alternative: AXR

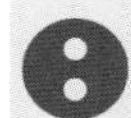

Imaging Findings

US/CT

- Hepatic cyst containing "hydatid sand" representing membranes and other debris.
- "Water lily" sign due to detachment of laminated membrane.
- Multi-septated cyst containing daughter cysts ("cogwheel" appearance).
- Single or multiple unilocular or septated cysts containing fluid (3–30HU on CT).
- Separation of these layers on imaging is specific.

MRI

- Single or multiple cysts with hyperintense signal centre and hypo-intense rim on T2 (often in liver but can be anywhere)

AXR

- Curvilinear calcification (20–30%) (usually hepatic)

Tips

- Super infection may produce peripheral rim echogenicity indistinguishable from abscess.
- Look elsewhere: CXR, CT/MRI brain – hydatid cysts can occur anywhere.

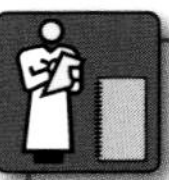

Radiological Differential Diagnosis

- Benign hepatic cyst, e.g. with tuberous sclerosis, von Hippel Lindau
- Hepatic abscess
- Primary or metastatic cystic hepatic neoplasm (e.g. mesenchymal hamartoma)

Hydronephrosis

Surgeon: A. Alexander
Radiologist: H. von Bezing

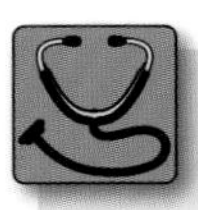

Clinical Insights

- Dilated pelvi-calyceal system.
- Often detected ante-natally.
- Of itself the entity is not necessarily pathological.
- The concern is that it can be a surrogate marker of distal obstruction.
- This is the premise for further investigation of the *entire* urogenital tract (from the UPJ to the tip of the penis/labia).

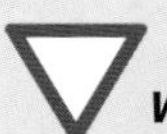

Warnings

- Always consider extrinsic compression from masses in the pelvis.
- Always investigate the anatomy and function of the contra-lateral kidney.

Urgency

- ❑ Emergency
- ❑ Urgent
- ☑ Elective

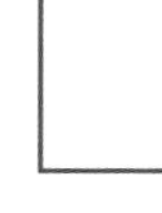

Clinical Differential Diagnosis

- Extrarenal pelvis
- Peripelvic cyst
- Congenital megacalyces
- Calyceal diverticula

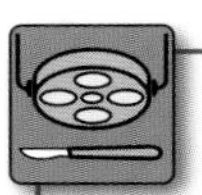

What the Surgeon Needs to Know

Pelvis

- Is there dilation of the pelvi-calyceal region?
- Is it pathological?

Ureter

- Is there associated hydroureter?

Kidney

- What is the state of the kidney parenchyma: scars, cortico-medullary differentiation, cystic or dysplastic?
- Is there evidence of a duplex system and which pole is affected?

Bladder

- Is it hypertrophied, small capacity?
- Is there evidence of an ureterocoele?
- Is there evidence of PUV?
- Is there a significant post-void residual volume?

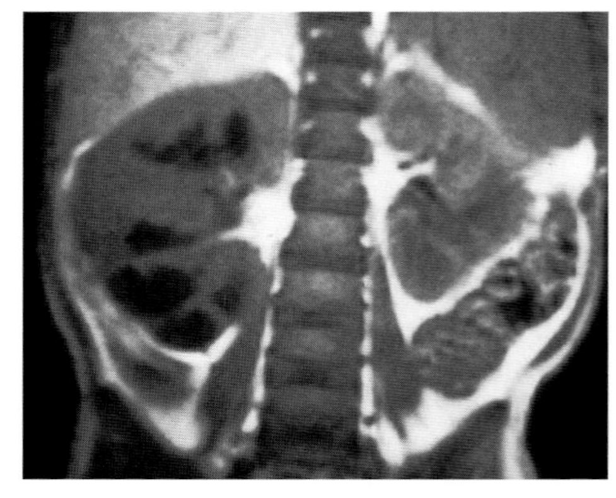

MRI Coronal T1 – Incidental demonstration of right hydronephrosis and cavitation in a child with renal TB

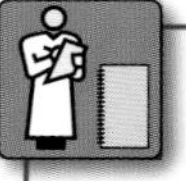

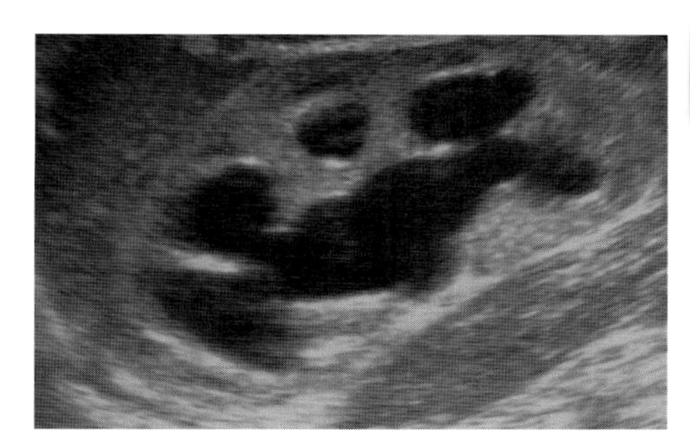

Longitudinal US of a hydronephrotic kidney demonstrates multiple fluid-filled distended calyces that show clear communication with each other

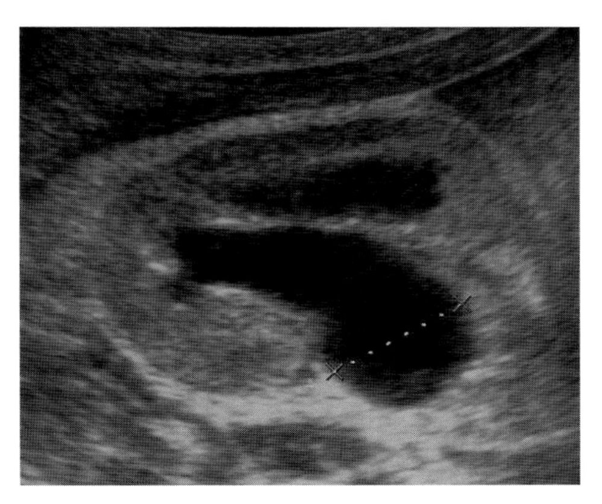

Transverse US allows measurement of the AP renal pelvis diameter (calipers), which is a reproducible measure for follow-up of hydronephrosis

Tips

- "Calyceal separation" means visible calyces but not pathologically enlarged. Within normal limits; AP pelvis < 10 mm.
- Real-time US confirms the communicating nature of fluid-filled spaces in hydronephrosis compared with MCDK (non-communicating).
- MAG 3 renogram determines if hydronephrosis is due to obstruction.

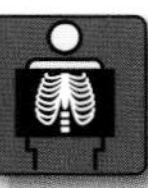

Imaging Options

- Primary: US
- Follow-on: MAG 3 renogram (to prove obstruction and site)/MCUG (to show VUR or exclude PUV as a cause)
- Alternative: MRI/MRU/CT (non-contrast for calculi)

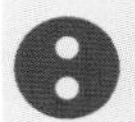

Imaging findings

US

- Calyectasis/pyelectasia.
- AP renal pelvis diameter > 10 mm.
- Visible dilated renal pelvis and distal ureter suggests that obstruction is at VUJ, bladder or urethra.
- Dilated renal pelvis without visible ureter suggests obstruction at the renal pelvis (PUJ obstruction).
- US cannot differentiate any of the above from VUR; therefore, MAG 3 indicated to prove obstruction and level.

MAG 3

- Delayed excretion demonstrated over time and plotted on a graph after a frusemide challenge.

MRI/MRU

- Replaces IVU for demonstrating anatomy of ureter in cases of ureteric obstruction.

CT

- Usually demonstrates hydronephrosis as a complication when imaging for calculus or a mass.

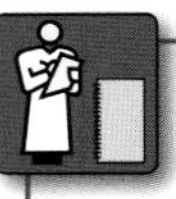

Radiological Differential diagnosis

- PUJ
- VUR
- Megaureter
- MCDK (contralateral PUJ)
- Complicated duplex kidney
- Neurogenic bladder

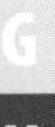

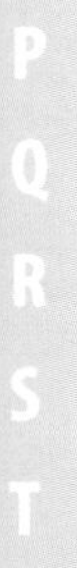

Hypertrophic Pyloric Obstruction (HPO)

Surgeon: A. Alexander
Radiologist: A. Brandt

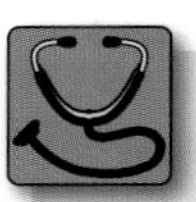

Clinical Insights

- The most common surgical cause of non-bilious vomiting in infancy.
- White, male babies.
- 2–8 weeks of age.
- Forceful vomiting (Projectile).
- Hungry after a vomit.
- May have a palpable pylorus ("olive" tumour).

Warnings

- Usually dehydrated with hypochloraemic, hypokalaemic metabolic alkalosis – Image only after resuscitation
- Strangely, up to 10% may vomit bile

Controversy

- A palpable tumour ("olive") in the right clinical setting does not need US; just operate

Urgency

- ☐ Emergency
- ☐ Urgent
- ☑ Elective

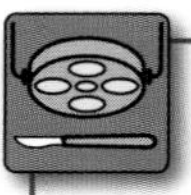

What the Surgeon Needs to Know

- Is the pylorus hypertrophied?
- Is there evidence of a more distal duodenal obstruction?
- Exclude major respiratory and urinary infection (both increased incidence).

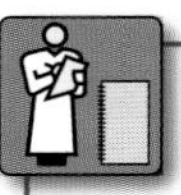

Clinical Differential Diagnosis

- Gastro-oesophageal reflux
- Duodenal or antral webs/stenosis – Symptoms usually present from birth
- Duodenal duplications

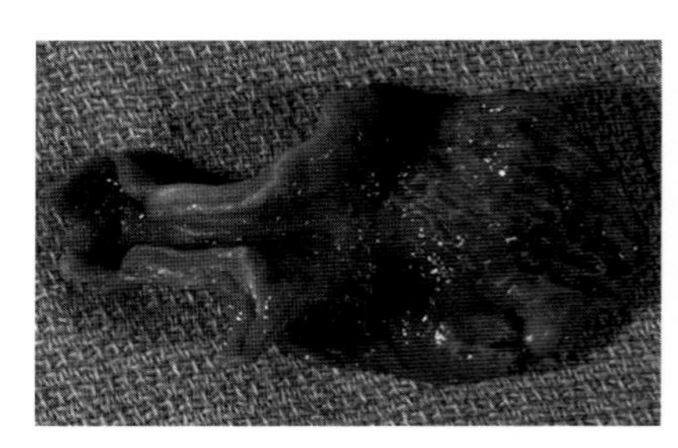

Post-mortem specimen demonstrating hypertrophy of the pylorus

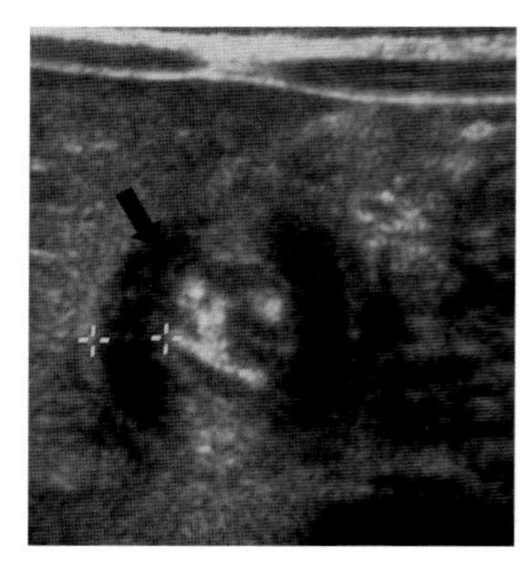

US (Longitudinal view of the abdomen) – Transverse view of the pylorus (*arrow*) – "doughnut" used to measure the thickness of the wall (hypo-echoic – calipers) and the total diameter

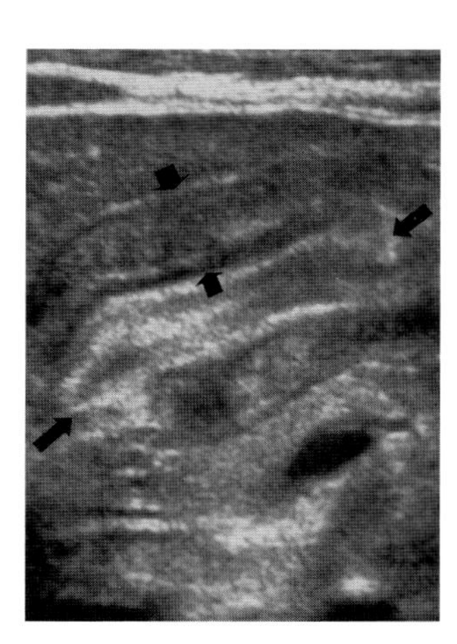

US – Pylorus shown in length –Note that use of a high-frequency linear probe results in an iso-echoic muscle wall and hyper-echoic mucosa. View used to measure length (*long arrows*) and wall thickness (*short arrows*)

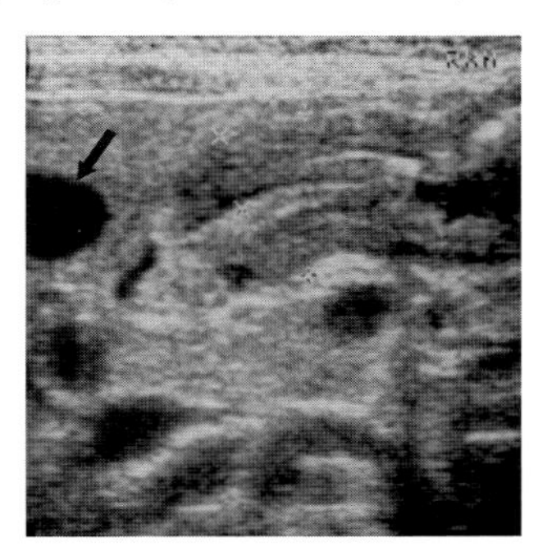

US – Pylorus shown in length to demonstrate the close relationship with the gall bladder (*arrow*), which is used as an anatomical landmark

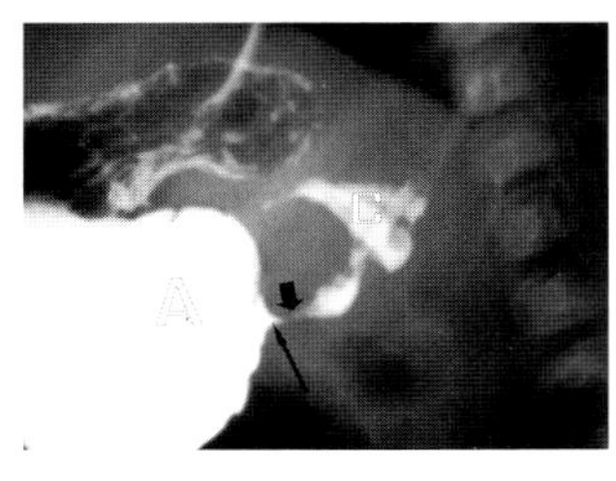

UGI (prone oblique) – Demonstrates beak (*long arrow*) and string signs (*short arrow*) as well as an impression on the antrum (A) and duodenal cap (C) (shouldering)

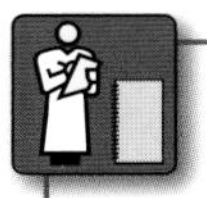

Radiological Differential Diagnosis

- Pylorospasm – Resolves over time

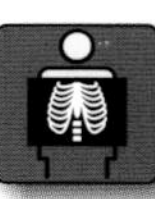

Imaging Options

- Primary: US
- Back-up: UGI

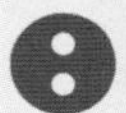

Imaging Findings

US

- Muscle wall is thickened and elongated
- Appearance of a "doughnut" in its transverse orientation (longitudinal scans of the body are used to get this view)
- Muscle – Hypo-echoic on the curved array and may be iso-echoic on linear array (depending on transducer frequency)
- Mucosa – Hyper-echoic
- Rule of thumb for abnormality
  - Muscle thickness > 5 mm
  - Total diameter > 15 mm
  - Length > 20 mm

UGI

- Beak sign – Narrowing of the pyloric lumen/channel to a point
- String sign – Persistence of a very narrow pyloric channel outlined by contrast
- Shoulder sign – Impression on the antrum and/or duodenal cap by the thick muscle
- Double tracking – When the narrow pyloric channel is lined on opposing luminal surfaces with contrast

Tips

- US – Ensure the stomach is not over-distended as this may obscure pylorus
- US – Start with curved array probe and convert to linear when pylorus identified
- US – Scan longitudinally in the midline below xiphisternum and work towards the liver (the gall bladder is the lateral marker)
- Dynamic scanning will show decreased gastric emptying
- Contrast study not indicated unless a diagnostic dilemma.
- UGI – Best view is the prone oblique

Ileal Atresia

Surgeon: A. Alexander
Radiologist: B. Khoury

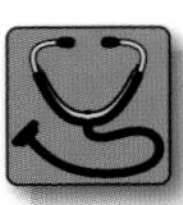

Clinical Insights

- Common cause of neonatal bowel obstruction.
- Ante-natally presents as polyhydramnios.
- Post-natally it presents with bilious vomiting, abdominal distension and failure to pass meconium.

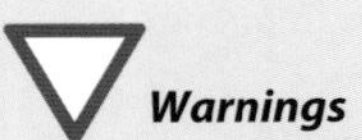

Warnings

- Any child with bilious vomiting must be investigated as an emergency to exclude possible midgut volvulus.
- Noenates should be adequately resuscitated prior to imaging.
- A tender/peritonitic abdomen should preclude further imaging – Emergency surgery is indicated.

Controversy

- Preoperative contrast enema for excluding colonic atresias

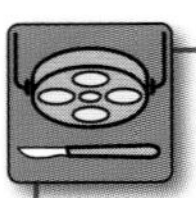

What the Surgeon Needs to Know

- Volvulus must be excluded
- Inguinal hernias and Hirschprung's disease should be excluded
- The level of the obstruction
- Is there evidence of complications: antenatal or post-natal perforation

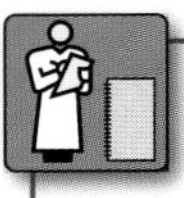

Clinical Differential Diagnosis

- Malrotation with or without midgut volvulus
- Colonic aganglionosis
- Meconium ileus
- Intestinal duplication
- Internal hernia
- Colonic atresia

Urgency

- ☐ Emergency
- ☐ Urgent
- ☑ Elective

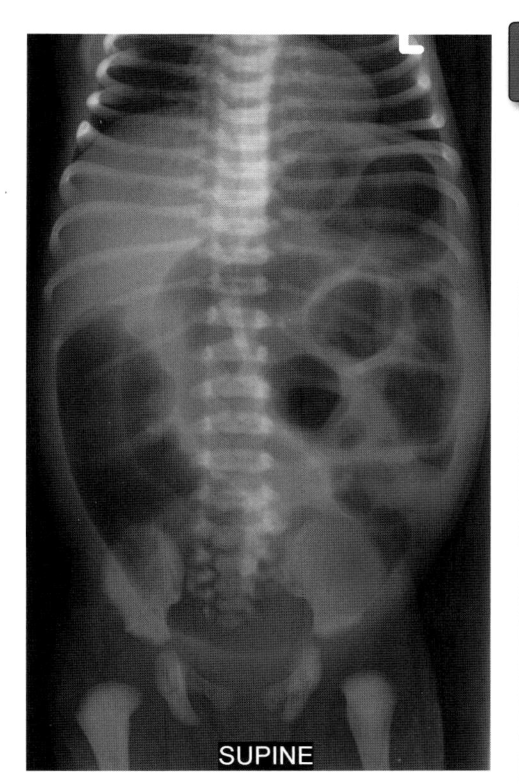

AXR – Multiple dilated loops of bowel in keeping with a distal obstruction

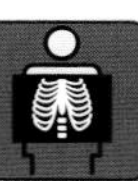

Imaging Options

- Primary: AXR
- Follow-on: Water-soluble contrast enema
- Back-up: US

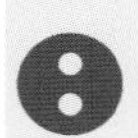

Imaging Findings

AXR

- Multiple dilated loops of bowel
- Erect/lateral decubitus/lateral shoot-through radiograph may reveal multiple air–fluid levels

Contrast Enema

- Colon has a small caliber in distal ileal atresia (functional microcolon).
- Normal to slightly small colon in proximal ileal atresia.

US

- Limited utility: Shows dilated fluid-filled loops of bowel; does not show site of obstruction.
- Useful to differentiate between small bowel and colonic obstruction.

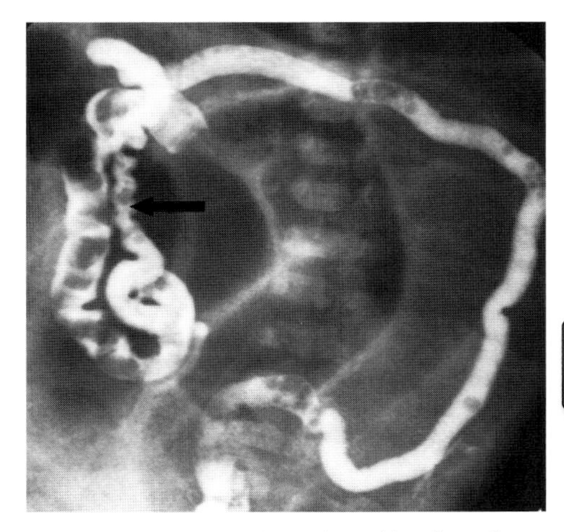

AP contrast enema – Microcolon with reflux of contrast into terminal ileum (*arrow*). There are numerous plugs of meconium noted as filling defects particularly in the ascending colon but no colonic strictures. The bowel more proximally is distended with gas

Imaging Tips

- Water-soluble non-ionic contrast to be used in contrast enema as this is nearly iso-osmotic to body fluids and avoids fluid shifts

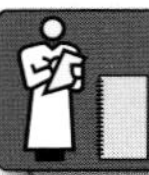

Radiological Differential Diagnosis

- Meconium ileus
- Meconium plug syndrome/functional immaturity of the colon
- Hirschprung's disease
- Ileal duplication cyst
- Incarcerated inguinal/umbilical hernia

Inguinal Hernia

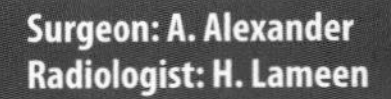

Surgeon: A. Alexander
Radiologist: H. Lameen

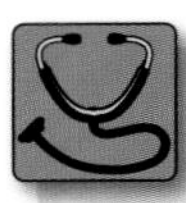

Clinical Insights

- Always an indirect hernia: Bowel or fluid contained in a patent processus vaginalis.
- One of the most common causes of neonatal bowel obstruction.
- The younger the child, the greater is the risk of complication (irreducibility and strangulation).
- Inability to get above the sac at the external ring differentiates it from a hydrocoele.

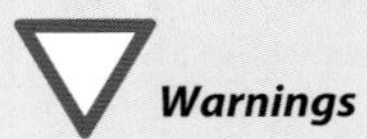

Warnings

- Oedema of the overlying skin and subcutaneous tissue is an indication of impending strangulation – Immediate exploration and repair is required.
- In the absence of diagnostic uncertainty, imaging should not delay manual reduction.

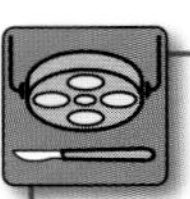

What the Surgeon Needs to Know

- Is this a hernia or a hydrocoele?
- What is in the hernial sac?
- Is there perfusion of the incarcerated bowel and/or ipsilateral testicle?

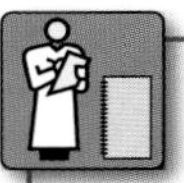

Clinical Differential Diagnosis

- Hydrocoele
- Scrotal mass
- Un-descended testis with torsion
- Inguinal lymphadenopathy
- Cord lipoma
- Hydrocoele of the cord

Urgency

- ☑ Emergency
- ☐ Urgent
- ☐ Elective

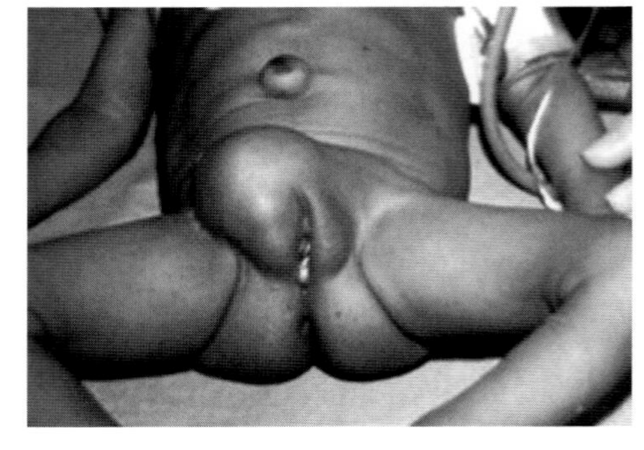

Inguinal swelling on the right representing an inguinal hernia

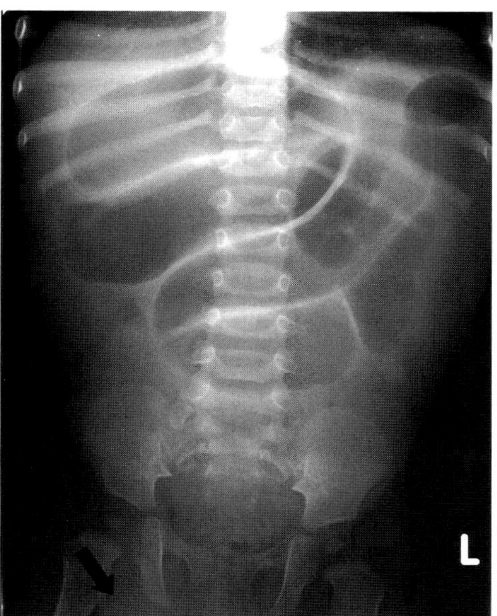

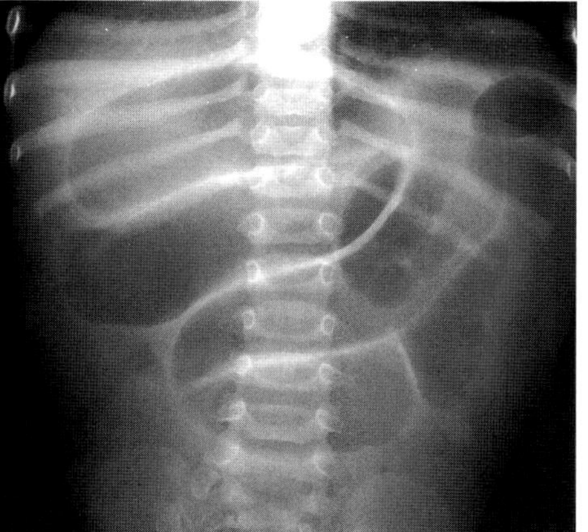

AXR – Distal obstruction with a right soft-tissue inguinal/scrotal mass (*arrow*)

Imaging Options

- Primary: AXR
- Follow on: US

Imaging Findings

AXR

- Soft-tissue swelling in inguinal region, which may show gas (with or without bowel obstruction).
- Multiple dilated bowel loops suggestive of distal bowel obstruction.
- If bowel compromise, may see wall thickening or perforation.

US

- Inguinal/scrotal swelling with fluid-filled bowel loop ± peristalsis

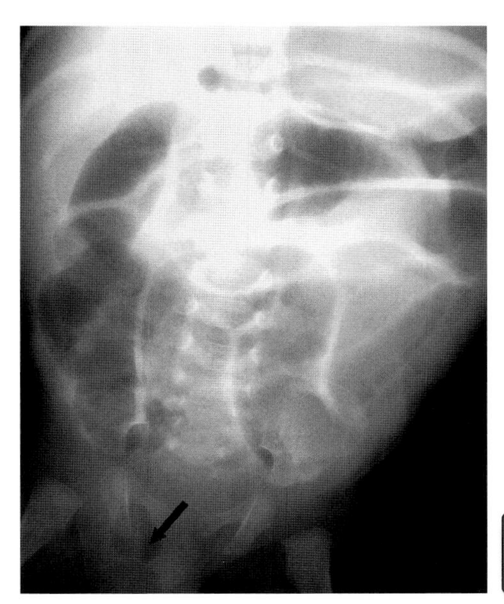

AXR – Distal obstruction with air in a right scrotal mass (*arrow*)

Tips

- Inguinal region should be included on all supine AXR's.

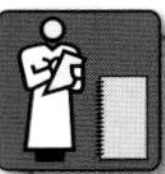

Radiological Differential Diagnosis

- Neonates: Other causes of distal intestinal obstruction
- Child: Other causes of SB obstruction appendicitis, intussusception, etc.

A B C D E F G H I J K L M N O P Q R S T U V W X Y Z

Intussusception

Surgeon: A. Alexander
Radiologist: M. Hayes

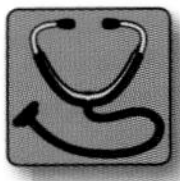

Clinical Insights

- Peak incidence at 1 year
- Male predominance 3:1
- Usually a well-nourished infant with a preceding viral illness
- Eighty percent are ileo-colic intussusceptions
- Ninety percent are primary (due to lymphoid hyperplasia acting as a lead point)
- Clinical presentation
  - Episodic, cramping abdominal pain
  - Bowel obstruction
  - Classic "red currant jelly" stools are a late feature
  - Sausage-shaped abdominal mass

Warnings

- Peritonitis is a contraindication to reduction as it suggests a complication such as necrosis or perforation.
- All babies must have fluid resuscitation and a dose of broad spectrum antibiotics before radiological reduction.
- Intussusception identified on US may be ileo-ileal, would not be evident on air enema and is not amenable to pneumatic reduction.

Controversies

- Provided there are no contraindications and progress is demonstrated, up to three separate attempts at air enema reduction can be made.
- These attempts should be 4–6 h apart.

Urgency

- ❑ Emergency
- ☑ Urgent
- ❑ Elective

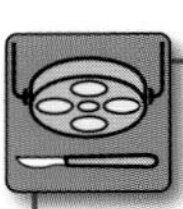

What the Surgeon Needs to Know

- Is this an intussusception?
- Are there any radiological features suggestive of a complication?
  - Free air
  - *Pneumotosis intestinalis*
  - Established small bowel obstruction with distention
- Can a cause be identified?
  - Meckel's diverticulum
  - Polyps
  - Mural masses (duplication cysts, hematomas in Henoch Schonlein purpura)

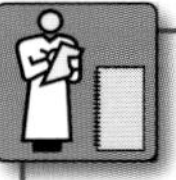

Clinical Differential Diagnosis

- Incarcerated inguinal hernia
- Volvulus about a Meckel's band
- Adhesive bowel obstruction

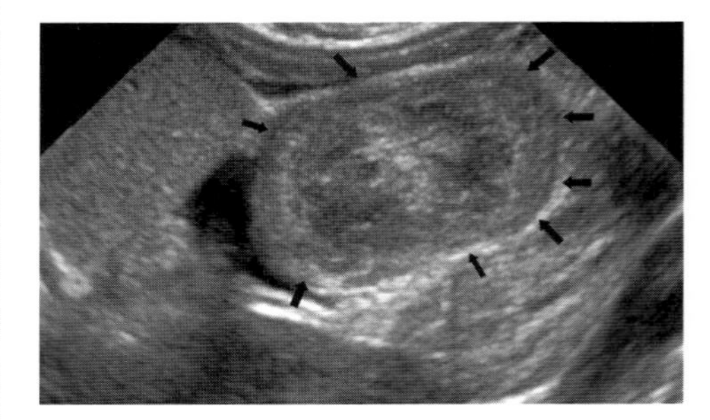

US – "Swiss-roll"/pseudokidney appearance (*arrows*) of intussusception on US

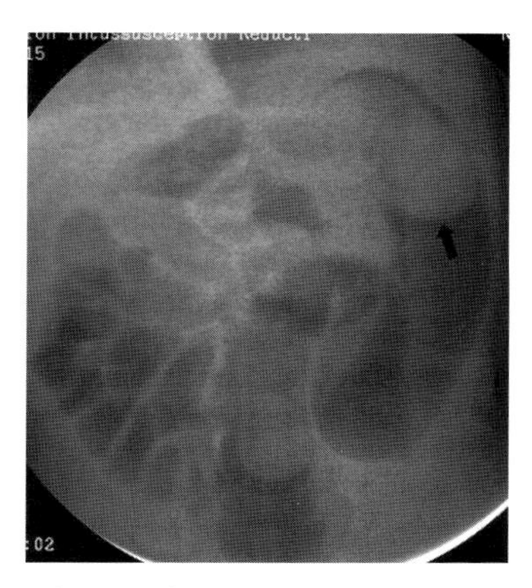

Pneumatic reduction – During early phase of air reduction, the convex end of the intussusceptum (*arrow*) is demonstrated in the descending colon as it is reduced towards the ileo-caecal valve. Note the relative paucity of Bowel gas centrally

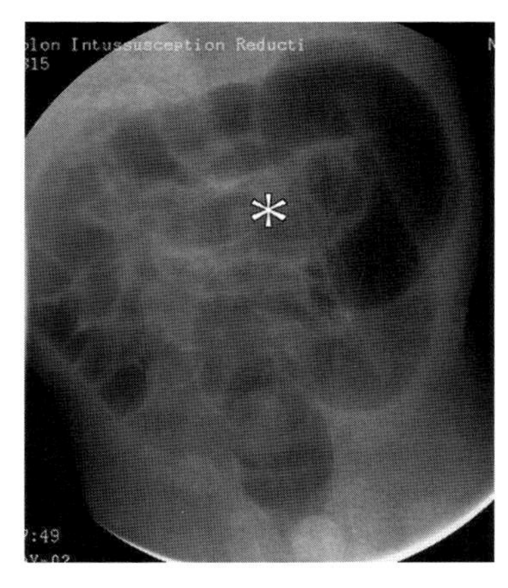

Pneumatic reduction – Successful reduction of the intussusception is indicated by visualized free flow of air into the central small bowel (*asterisk*)

Tips

- Diagnostic US scanning starts in RIF and works around full length of colon.
- Absent Doppler flow and prolonged history carries a danger of perforation.
- Perforations are emergencies as diaphragms are elevated under pressure. Do not hesitate to insert a large bore needle below the umbilicus.
- Any concern of perforation, perform proper X-ray exposure on the table.

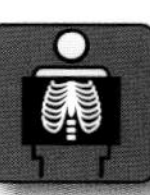

Imaging Options

- Primary: Ultrasound, AXR
- Follow-on: Fluoroscopic-guided pneumatic reduction
  Ultrasound guided fluid reduction

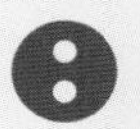

Imaging Findings

AXR

- Paucity of gas RLQ and non-visualization of caecum
- Sometimes small bowel obstruction
- Soft-tissue mass surrounded by meniscus of gas
- Free air if perforated

US

- Mass with alternating layers of hyper/hypoechogenicity (“Swiss roll”)
- “Pseudokidney” appearance on longitudinal view
- Free fluid

Air / (Fluid) enema

- Pre-procedure: Ensure hydration, IV access, surgeon present, decompression needles in hand and contraindicated if perforation.
- Foley catheter with balloon inflated and buttocks strapped.
- Clamp buttocks by squeezing them together with one hand.
- Store image prior to air insufflation for comparison with last image.
- Insufflation of air under steady pressure for multiple short periods (<1 min).
- Try not to exceed 120 mm Hg at rest.
- Lookout for perforation (remember, air is white on fluoroscopy – opposite of X-ray).
- Watch as air pushes intussusception (direct visualization of air entry from rectum).
- Intussusceptum often holds up at ileo-caecal valve.
- Reduction only complete when free flow of air into small bowel centrally.
- No limit to the number of attempts, but unsuccessful attempts can be repeated the next morning.

Jejunal Atresia

Surgeon: A. Alexander
Radiologist: B. Khoury

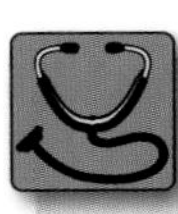

Clinical Insights

- Common cause of neonatal bowel obstruction.
- Four types are described.
- Ante-natally presents as polyhydramnios.
- Postnatally it presents with bilious vomiting, abdominal distension and failure to pass meconium.

Warnings

- Any child with bilious vomiting must be investigated as an emergency to exclude possible volvulus.
- They should be adequately resuscitated prior to imaging.
- A tender/peritonitic abdomen should preclude further imaging – Emergency surgery is indicated.

Controversy

- Preoperative contrast enema for excluding colonic atresias

Urgency

- ❑ Emergency
- ❑ Urgent
- ☑ Elective

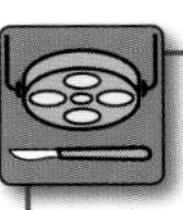

What the Surgeon Needs to Know

- Volvulus must be excluded.
- The level of the obstruction.
- Is there evidence of complications: Antenatal or post-natal perforation?

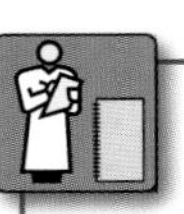

Clinical Differential Diagnosis

- Malrotation with or without midgut volvulus
- Intestinal duplication
- Internal hernia

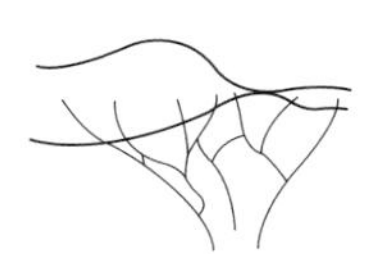

Stenosis

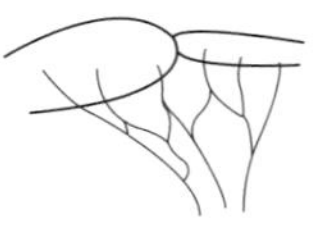

Type I - Mucous Web

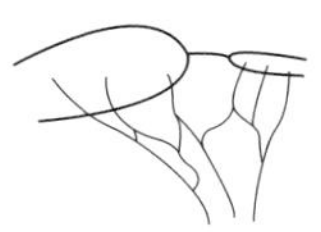

Type II - Fibrous Chord

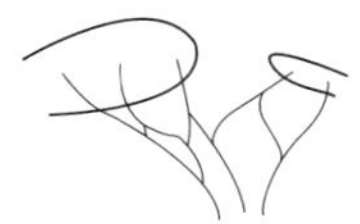

Type IIIa - Mesenteric Defect

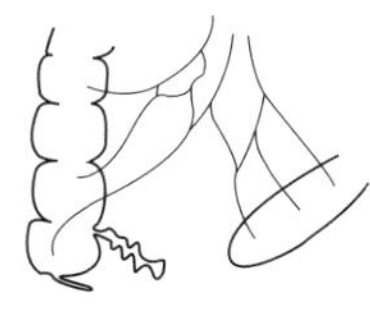

Type IIIb - Apple Peel

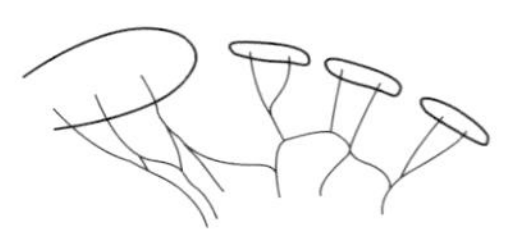

Type IV - Multiple Segments

The four broad types of atresia

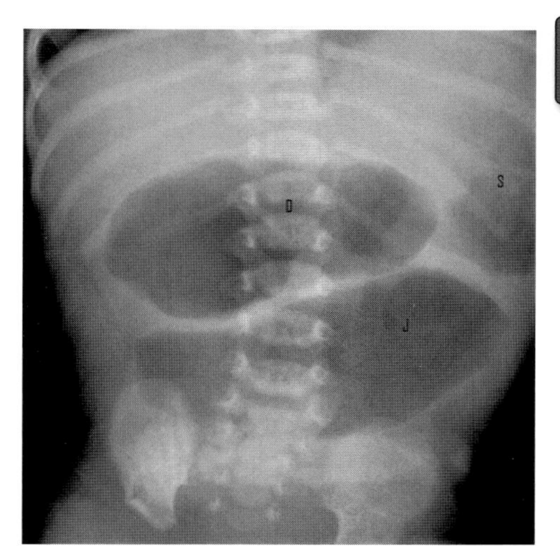

Supine AXR showing markedly distended stomach (*S*), duodenum (*D*) and jejunum (*J*). Note the absence of distal small bowel and large bowel gas shadows

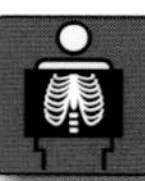

Imaging Options

- Primary: AXR
- Follow-on: Contrast enema

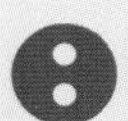

Imaging Findings

AXR

- Dilated gastric bubble, duodenum and small bowel loops.
- Triple bubble for proximal jejunal atresia.
- The loop just proximal to the atresia is disproportionately dilated and has a bulbous end.
- If fluid-filled may result in a soft-tissue density with a mass-like appearance.

Contrast Enema

- Performed to exclude co-existent colonic strictures not easily visualised during surgery (controversial).

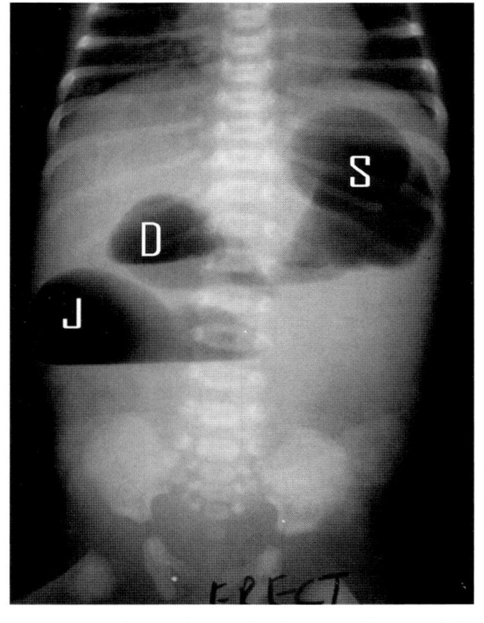

Erect AXR shows the proximal obstruction. A triple bubble appearance is present (*S* stomach, *D* duodenum, *J* jejunum) and air–fluid levels with no distal gas. Alternative views would be lateral decubitus or lateral shoot through

Imaging Tips

- Plain films are usually diagnostic.
- Triple bubble sign indicates proximal atresia (made up of stomach bubble, duodenum and proximal jejunum).
- A high index of suspicion when antenatal sonar demonstrates dilated bowel.

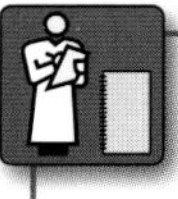

Radiological Differential Diagnosis

- Duodenal atresia/stenosis/web (including annular pancreas)
- Midgut volvulus
- Ladd bands – Often associated with malrotation

Lung Abscess

Surgeon: A. Brooks
Radiologist: A. Mapukata

Clinical Insights

- Defined as a sub-acute pulmonary infection with a chest radiograph that shows a cavity within the pulmonary parenchyma.
- Defined as acute when duration is less than 6 weeks.
- May be classified as primary or secondary.
- Treatment is medical in the first instance.
- External drainage is indicated if conservative therapy does not lead to improvement.
  - CT-guided percutanous catheter drainage
  - Chest tube thoracostomy
  - Open pneumonostomy

Warnings

- Always keep the diagnosis of foreign body aspiration in mind.
- There may be an underlying broncho-oeosophageal fistula.

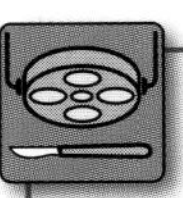

What the Surgeon Needs to Know

- Is there an underlying condition such as a bronch-oeosophageal fistula?
- Is there a radiological resolution in response to conservative therapy?
- Are there any complications such as empyema?
- Are there predisposing conditions, e.g. immune deficiency, HIV, leukaemia, endocarditis?

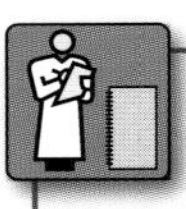

Clinical Differential Diagnosis

- Tuberculosis or fungal disease
- Empyema with bronchopleural fistula
- Diaphragmatic hernia – congenital or acquired

Urgency

- ☐ Emergency
- ☑ Urgent
- ☐ Elective

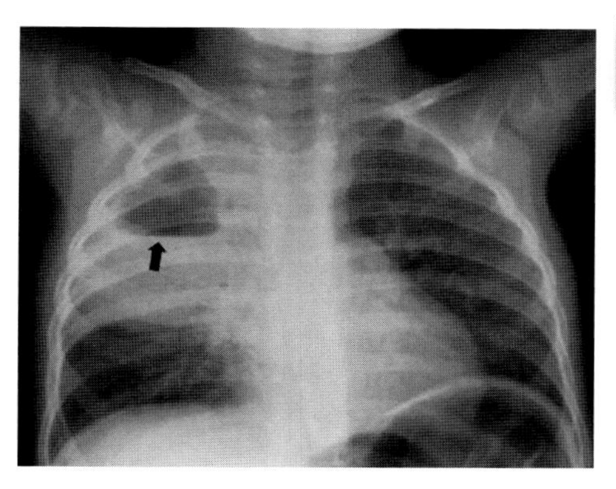

CXR demonstrating a lung abscess with an air–fluid level (*arrow*) [courtesy Ian Cowan]

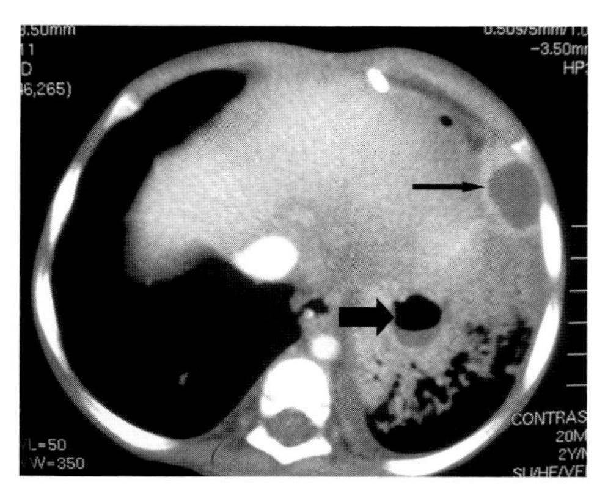

CT demonstrates a central lung abscess with an air–fluid level (*thick arrow*) and surrounding consolidation with associated pleural collections (*thin arrow*)/ empyema

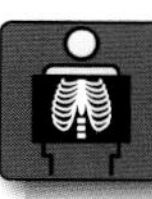

Imaging Options

- Primary: CXR
- Follow-on: CT

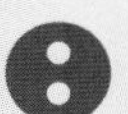

Imaging Findings

CXR

- Circumscribed oval lesion with an air–fluid level and thick wall
- Surrounding consolidation

CT

- Well-defined cavity usually with an air–fluid level, enhancing wall and surrounding consolidation
- Non-enhancing, low density, no bronchograms, no vessels
- Typically no necrosis in lung surrounding an abscess
- Often associated with empyema

Tips

- Primary abscesses are usually solitary
- CT with IV contrast can differentiate an early abscess (no central enhancement) from consolidated lung (enhances)

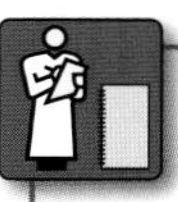

Radiological Differential Diagnosis

- Pneumatocoele – Thin walled and non-enhancing
- Complicated hydatid cyst
- Complicated foregut duplication cyst/ bronchogenic cyst

Lymphoma

Surgeon: C. Davies
Radiologist: T. Kilborn

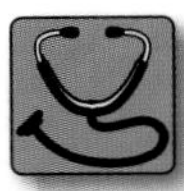

Clinical Insights

- An uncontrolled growth of cells of lymphoid origin.
- Second only to brain tumours in paediatric incidence.
- Two groups:
  - Hodgkin's (40%)
    - Painless lymphadenopathy
    - Contiguous spread – cervical and supraclavicular
    - Mediastinal disease common-airway compromise
    - Older children
  - Non Hodgkin's (60%)
    - Most common lymphoma < 11 years
    - Associated with Epstein-Barr virus (Burkitt's – involving the jaw)
    - Extranodal disease
    - Spread not contiguous
    - Abdominal disease common in young children
- Both types are chemosensitive.
- Surgery rarely indicated beyond diagnosis and IVI access.

Warnings

- Chest X-ray always required to exclude occult critical airway compromise prior to sedation or anaesthesia.
- HIV, TB and NH lymphoma frequently co-exist.

Urgency

- ❑ Emergency
- ☑ Urgent
- ❑ Elective

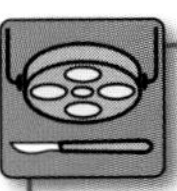

What the Surgeon Needs to Know

- Suspected epicenter of disease
- Extent of gland/organ involvement
- Presence of complications – bowel obstruction, perforation, intussusception

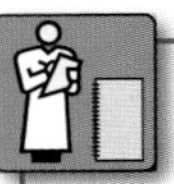

Clinical Differential Diagnosis

- Pyogenic lymphadenitis/abscess
- Reactive lymphadenitis
- TB
- HIV/AIDS
- *Mycobacterium* other than TB
- Mesenteric adenopathy
- Cat scratch disease (Bartonella Henselae infection)

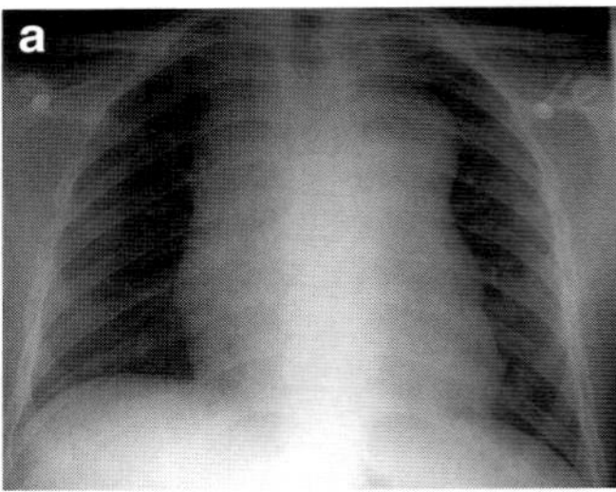

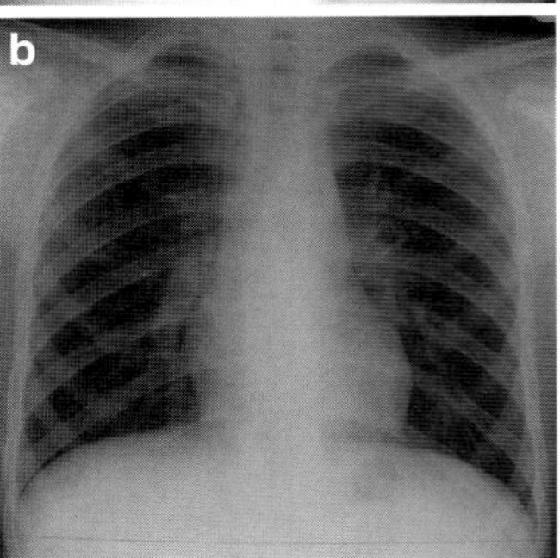

CXR pre- and post-therapy. (**a**) Widening of superior and middle mediastinum due to lymphadenopathy in child with HD. (**b**) Rapid and significant reduction of the mediastinal mass and relief the tracheal compression post-therapy

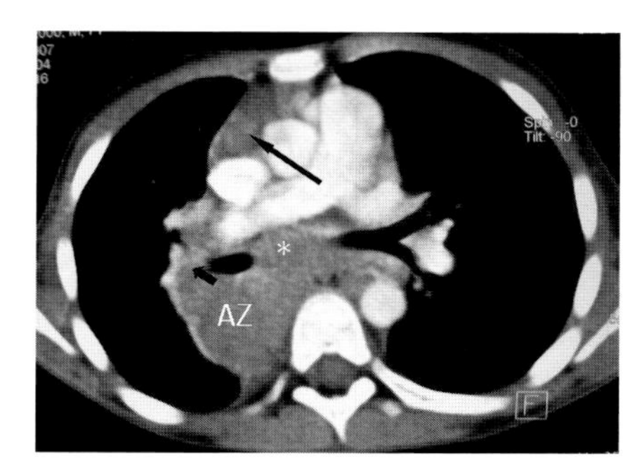

CT axial post-contrast – Non-enhancing prevascular (*short arrow*), subcarinal (*asterisk*), right hilar (*long arrow*) and azygo-oesophageal lymphadenopathy (*AZ*)

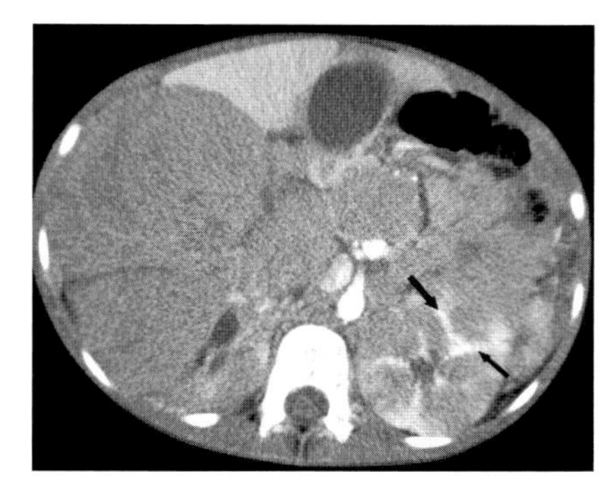

CT axial post-contrast – Low-density lesions involving right lobe of liver with large para-aortic and coeliac nodes in a child with NHL. The appearance of the kidneys that are enlarged and show streaks of normal tissue enhancement (tigroid) is typical of lymphoma/leukaemia (*arrows*)

Tips

- An enlarged thymus is not normal in a child over 7 years and may represent lymphomatous disease in the thymus or mediatinal adenopathy (mimicking thymic enlargement).
- Persistently enlarged nodes on ultrasound require biopsy.
- Staging CT should only be done post-contrast.
- STIR MRI best demonstrates lymphadenopathy as bright signal structures.
- Pelvic nodes and lack of central low density differentiate from TB.

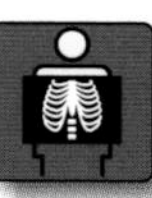

Imaging Options

- Primary: CXR/US
- Follow on: CT/MRI/PET

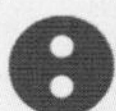

Imaging Findings

US/CT/MRI

- Show enlarged nodes and extent of disease.
- CT is the best for assessing extranodal disease – single or multiple low-density lesions in spleen, liver, kidneys and GI tract.
- MRI is the best for head and neck involvement (whole body MRI is viable).

Hodgkin's Disease, HD (40%)

- Intrathoracic nodes in 85% at presentation, usually superior prevascular and paratracheal; half have tracheobronchial compression.
- Pulmonary parenchyma involved in 10% (solid mass).
- Mesenteric nodes rarely involved, whereas paraaortic and coeliac adenopathy is common.
- PET scanning now routinely used as part of staging and to assess response (affected nodes show increased activity).

Non-Hodgkin's Lymphoma, NHL (60%)

- Lymphoblastic – Supradiaphragmatic and presents as mediastinal mass.
- Undifferentiated – Usually abdominal disease (commonly ileocaecal).
- Large cell – Occurs anywhere but is seldom mediastinal.
- >70% NHL is disseminated at the time of diagnosis, most cases extranodal.

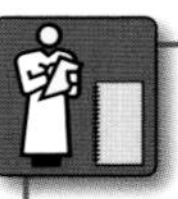

Radiological Differential Diagnosis

- Chest – TB, HIV, LCH, sarcoid
- Abdomen – HIV/TB

Malrotation and Volvulus

Surgeon: J. Loveland
Radiologist: G. Dekker

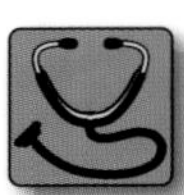

Clinical Insights

- Malrotation results in poor fixation of the intestine and a narrow mesenteric base that predisposes to torsion and volvulus of the midgut.
- It is one of the most common causes of bilious vomiting in infancy.
- Not every malrotation will undergo volvulus with strangulation, but this potentially fatal event can occur at any time.
- Fifty percent of cases present within the first month of life.
- Eighty percent will present within 6 months.
- Any infant with bile-stained vomiting is a diagnostic emergency until volvulus has been ruled out.
- The most devastating consequence of midgut volvulus is strangulation infarction of most, if not all, of the midgut.

Warnings

- Children with volvulus without strangulation can appear remarkably well with a clinically bland abdomen.
- When clinical signs are evident, strangulation is usually advanced.
- Bilious vomiting in the presence of peritonism requires emergency laparotomy.

Controversy

- Ultrasonic evaluation of the anatomical relationship of the superior mesenteric artery and vein

Urgency

- ☑ Emergency
- ☐ Urgent
- ☐ Elective

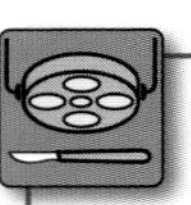

What the Surgeon Needs to Know

- Is malrotation present?
- Is there evidence of existing volvulus?

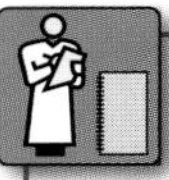

Clinical Differential Diagnosis

- Intestinal obstruction
- Duodenal stenosis/atresia
- Distal atresia
- Hernia
- Meconium disease
- Hirschsprung's disease

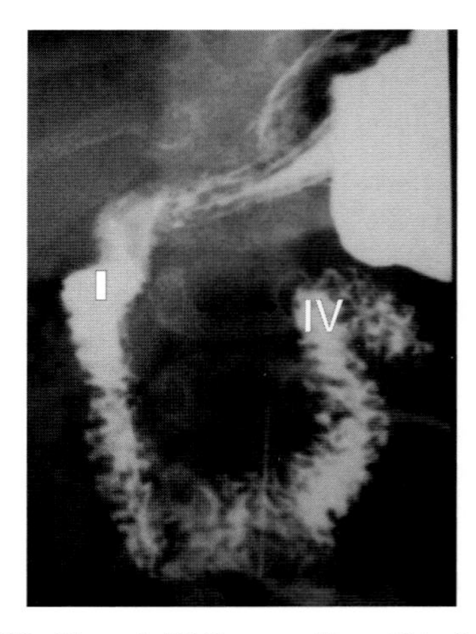

AP UGI – Normal: DJ flexure with part I to the right of the midline, part IV to the left of the left pedicle (*arrow*) and at the same cranio-caudal level as part I

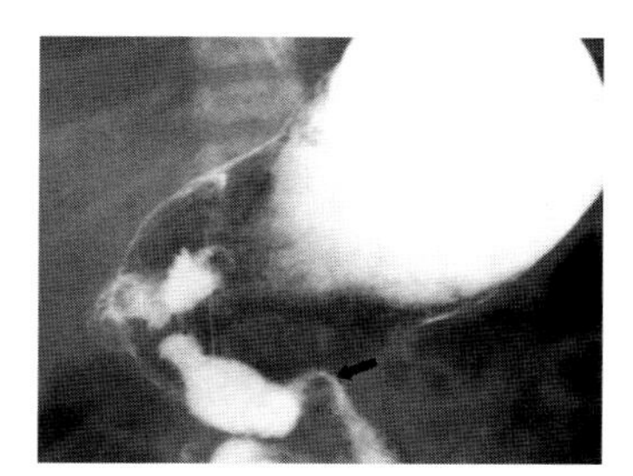

AP UGI – Malrotation: DJJ below level of pylorus and in the midline (*arrows*)

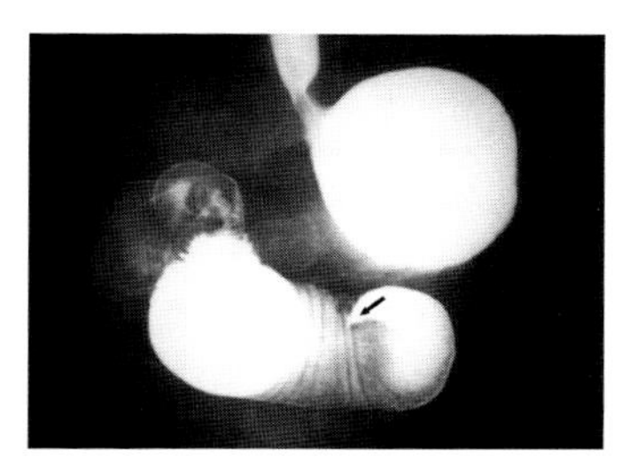

AP UGI – Small bowel volvulus: birds-beak cut-off (*arrow*) and proximal distension

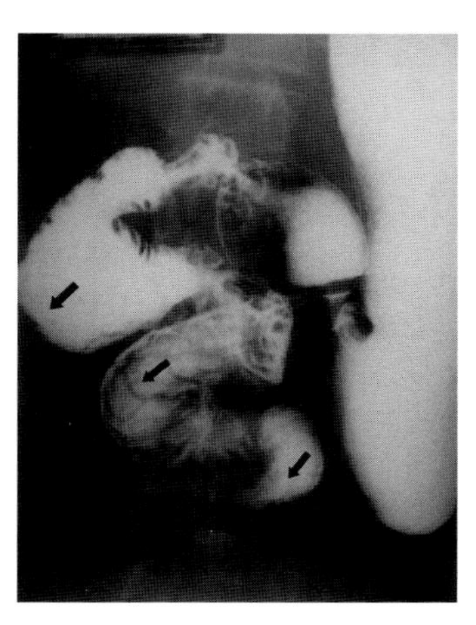

AP UGI – Left-sided pylorus with cork-screw appearance of the right-sided jejunum (*arrows*)

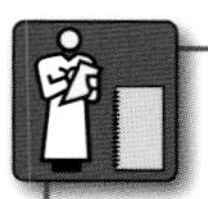

Radiological Differential Diagnosis

- Duodenal atresia/stenosis/web
- Annular pancreas
- Gastro-oesophageal reflux

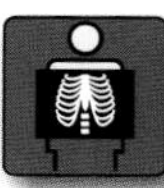

Imaging Options

- Primary: UGI/AXR
- Back-up: Contrast enema/US

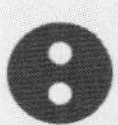

Imaging Findings

AXR

- Non-specific; may be normal; show distended stomach and proximal duodenum; small bowel obstruction or diffuse distention from ischaemia/necrosis.

UGI

- Normal DJJ should be to the left of left pedicle at the same level or superior to the first part of the duodenum.
- Malrotation is diagnosed when the DJ flexure misplaced to the right or below the normal position.
- Midgut volvulus shows complete duodenal obstruction; 'bird-beak' cut-off; or 'cork-screw' pattern of twisted bowel.

Contrast Enema

- When UGI inconclusive, may show caecal malposition [not in R lower quadrant]

US (Doppler)/CT

- Malrotation: SMV to left of SMA [neither sensitive nor specific].
- Volvulus: Bowel demonstrates a swirling pattern around SMA.

Tips

- Even when AXR normal, UGI indicated with bile stained vomit.
- Correct positioning mandatory when performing UGI [coning should allow visualisation of lower chest]

Meckel's Diverticulum

Surgeon: A. Alexander
Radiologist: H. Lameen

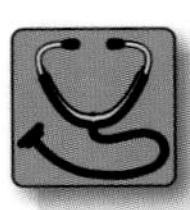

Clinical Insights

- The most common congenital malformation of the small intestine.
- The rule of two's:
  - Two percent of the population (4% will be symptomatic).
  - Two years is the peak age of presentation.
  - Two feet from the ileo-caecal valve.
  - Two centimeters in diameter.
  - Two inches in length.
- Only become symptomatic if they:
  - Ulcerate and bleed because of ectopic gastric mucosa (40–60%).
  - Cause intussusception.
  - Obstruct due to twisting about a fibrous remnant or herniation into the inguinal canal (25%).
  - Develop diverticulitis (10%).

Warnings

- May be dehydrated and should always be resuscitated prior to imaging.
- Bleeding must be active for red cell scans and angiography to be diagnostic.

Controversy

- Incidentally discovered (surgical not radiological) Meckel's diverticulum should be resected.

Urgency

- ☐ Emergency
- ☐ Urgent
- ☑ Elective

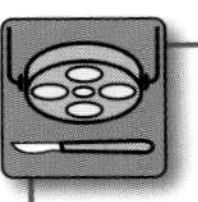

What the Surgeon Needs to Know

- Is there ectopic gastric mucosa or an intussusception?
- Are there complications of the obstruction (strangulation and perforation)?

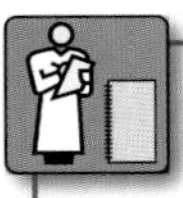

Clinical Differential Diagnosis

- Pain: Appendicitis and terminal ileal disease must be excluded.
- Bleeding: A vascular malformation or a polyp.
- Obstruction: Causes of distal obstruction.

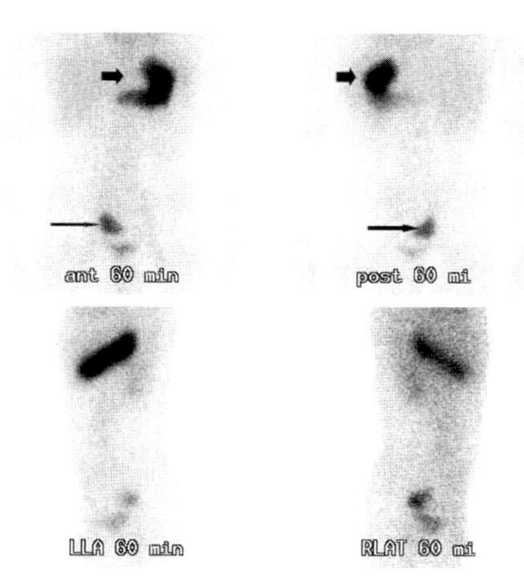

Nuc Med Tc 99 m – Simultaneous uptake of radiopharmaceutical in the right iliac fossa (*thin arrows*) and of equal amount to the stomach (*thick arrows*) is consistent with a Meckel's diverticulum [Courtesy Anita Brink]

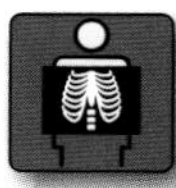

Imaging Options

- Primary: US
- Alternative: AXR/CT/contrast studies
- Backup: Nuc Med Tc99m

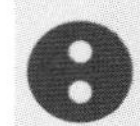

Imaging Finding

Nuclear Scentigraphy

- Focal accumulation of Tc-99 m in the ectopic gastric mucosa of the diverticulum RLQ (same time and intensity as stomach)

US

- Hetrogenous mass in RLQ (if inflamed may be cystic with hyperaemia)

AXR/CT

- RLQ mass or displacement of bowel loops, obstruction or may be normal.

Tips

- Painless rectal bleeding is diagnosed with nuclear medicine studies.
- Tc-99m scintigraphy is most accurate.
- Pain and vomiting are usually investigated with US or CT and may yield a Meckel's diverticulum.
- May complicate with bleeding, intussusception, bowel obstruction or perforation.

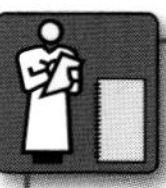

Radiological Differential Diagnosis

- Intestinal duplication containing gastric mucosa
- Hemangioma (as a cause of GIT bleeding)
- Appendicitis
- Crohn's disease

Meconium Ileus

Surgeon: D. Sidler
Radiologist: A.M. du Plessis

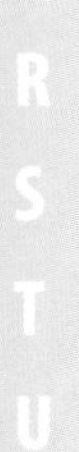

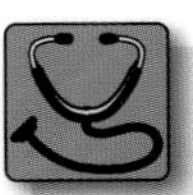

Clinical Insights

- Meconium ileus describes a neonatal intestinal obstruction caused by abnormally thick, tenacious plugs of inspissated mucus and tar-like meconium in the terminal ileum.
- It is most commonly the first manifestation of cystic fibrosis.
- Rarely it occurs with pancreatic abnormalities, total colonic aganglionosis and prematurity.
- It is classified into two groups – simple or complicated e.g.:
  - Meconium peritonitis
  - Pseudocyst
  - Volvulus
  - Small bowel atresia
- A contrast enema is diagnostic and potentially therapeutic.
- Operative therapy is reserved for failure of conservative measures and complicated cases.

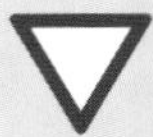

Warning

- Rehydration prior to and after a therapeutic enema is indicated to compensate for the hygroscopic effect of the contrast.

Controversy

- Choice of contrast medium (new non-ionic water soluble vs. classical descriptions with Gastrograffin)

Urgency

- ❑ Emergency
- ☑ Urgent
- ❑ Elective

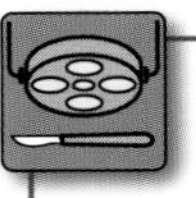

What the Surgeon Needs to Know

- Differentiate between simple and complex presentation that needs early surgery.

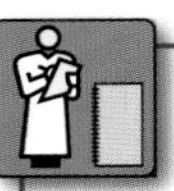

Clinical Differential Diagnosis

- Hirschsprung's disease
- Left colon syndrome
- Meconium plug syndrome
- Small bowel atresia
- Functional immaturity of the bowel.

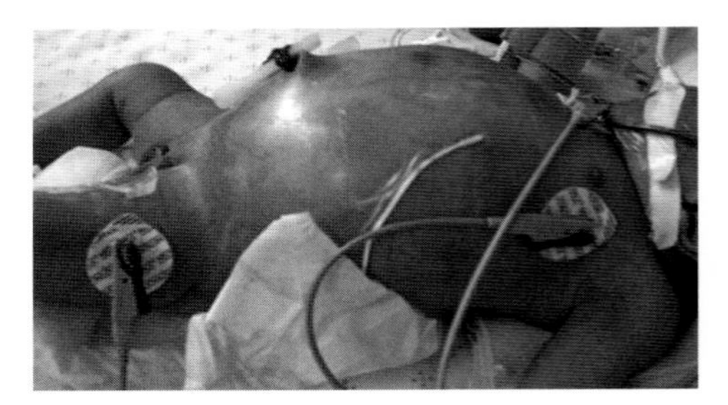

Neonate in intensive care with meconium ileus demonstrating abdominal distension

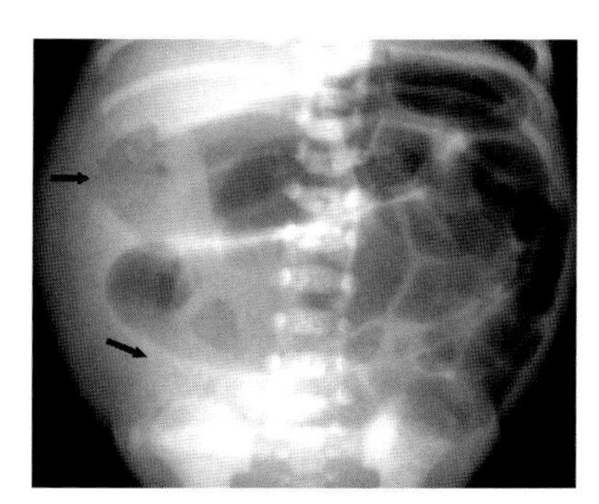

AXR – Shows distal bowel obstruction with mottled lucencies at the right iliac fossa and right upper quadrant (*arrows*) suggesting the diagnosis of meconium ileus

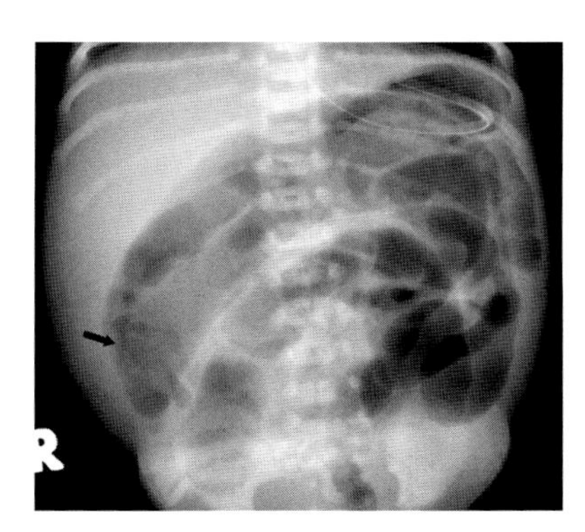

AXR – Demonstrates a neonatal distal bowel obstruction and suggestive mottled lucencies in the right iliac fossa (*arrow*)

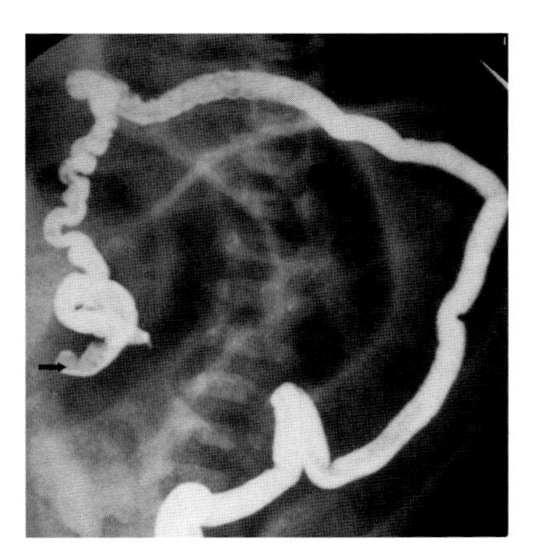

Contrast enema – Shows a microcolon with inspisated meconium as multiple filling defects in the terminal ileum (*arrow*). Contrast has not been passed into the dilated more proximal ileum

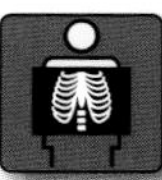

Imaging Options

- Primary: Contrast enema
- Back-up: AXR

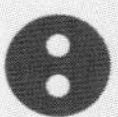

Imaging Findings

Contrast Enema

- Microcolon (entire colon <1 cm)
- Distal ileum is small with multiple filling defects. More proximally the ileum is dilated.
- Meconium seen as multiple filling defects within colon and terminal ileum

AXR

- Findings of distal bowel obstruction (multiple dilated loops of bowel)
- Bubble-like lucencies in RIF are an unreliable sign

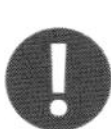

Tips

- Perform neonatal enemas with non-balloon tip catheter
- Use ionic, water-soluble contrast and attempt to reflux into terminal ileum
- Gastrograffin is not indicated
- If water soluble contrast fails to relieve obstruction, other agents such as "Mucomyst" are useful

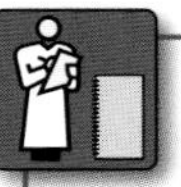

Radiological Differential Diagnosis

- Meconium plug syndrome (only left colon is small).
- Hirschsprung's disease (rectum diameter smaller than sigmoid).
- Ileal atresia (loops proximal to atresia do not opacify; also have a microcolon).

Meconium Peritonitis

Surgeon: D. Sidler
Radiologist: L. Naidu

Clinical Insights

- Describes the presence of meconium in the peritoneal cavity.
- Due to any antenatal bowel perforation.
- Usually secondary to complicated meconium ileus, but there are other causes.
- Four types – relating to timing, amount of contamination and spontaneous healing:
  - Adhesive meconium peritonitis (MP)
  - Giant cystic MP
  - Meconium ascites
  - Infected MP

Warnings

- Neonates may present in extremis and will require resuscitation prior to imaging.
- Complicated meconium ileus is a contraindication to therapeutic enema.

Urgency

- ❑ Emergency
- ☑ Urgent (may be)
- ☑ Elective

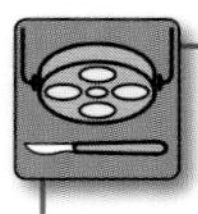

What the Surgeon Needs to Know

- Type of meconium peritonitis
- Underlying cause of perforation
- Status of the distal bowel

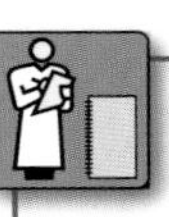

Clinical Differential Diagnosis

- Duplication cysts
- Small bowel atresias
- Hirschprung's disease

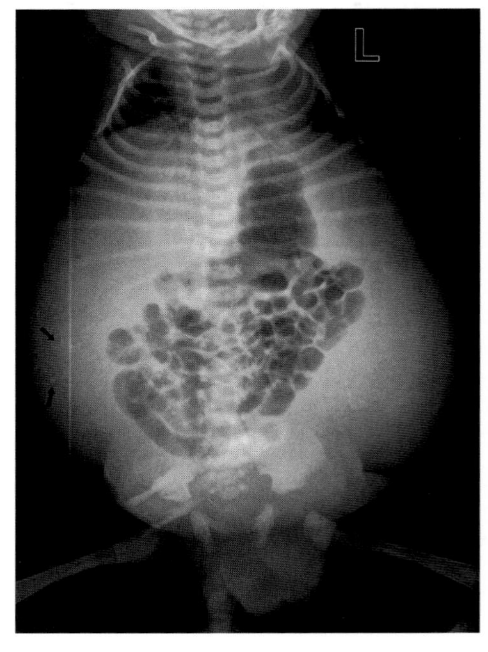

AXR – Showing a massively distended abdomen. Bulging flanks and central bowel loops suggest ascites. Note irregular amorphous intraperitoneal calcifications (*arrows*) in keeping with in utero perforation

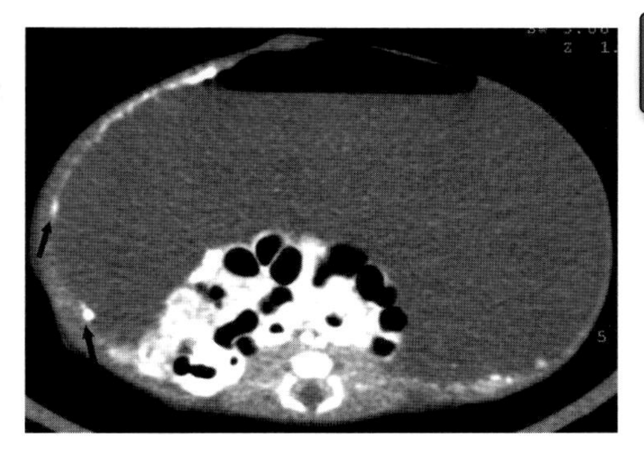

Axial CT – Same patient as in the previous figure, showing meconium ascites causing posterior bowel displacement as well as calcification (*arrows*) in keeping with meconium peritonitis

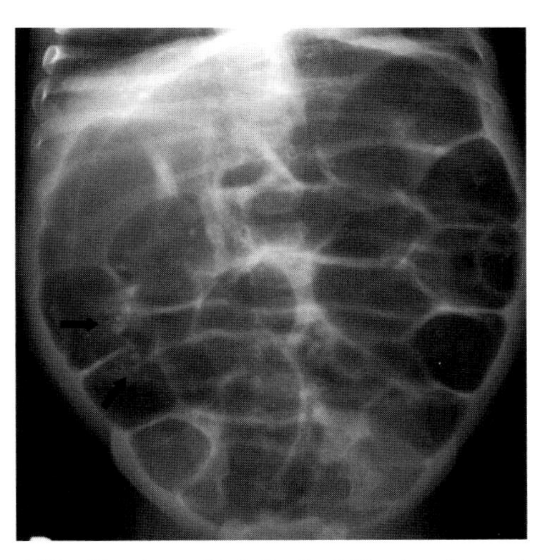

AXR – Showing multiple focal calcifications (*arrows*) throughout the abdomen in a newborn with obstruction. The meconium peritonitis is probably a result of small bowel obstruction (and perforation) due to meconium ileus

Tips

- Associated with ileal atresia and cystic fibrosis.
- Calcification may be the only finding representing a perforation that occurred antenatally, which then sealed without persistent obstruction.
- Calcification disappears with age.

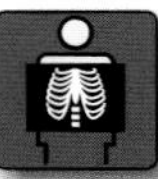

Imaging Options

- Primary: AXR
  Antenatal US
- Back-up: US
  CT/MRI

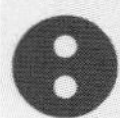

Imaging Findings

AXR

- Scattered amorphous irregular calcification.
- Ascites (central "floating" bowel loops and loss of soft-tissue planes).
- Meconium pseudocysts (sealed off collections that may be calcified and cause mass effect on adjacent bowel).
- Bowel obstruction ± free air (if leak not sealed off postnatally).
- Meconium hydroceles (scrotal enlargement with calcification).

US

- Ascites (complex fluid with increased echogenicity – "Snowstorm appearance")
- Clumped echogenic foci (intraabdominal calcification with acoustic shadowing).
- Pseudocyst (homogenous or heterogenous encysted collection with debris and calcification; thick or thin walled)

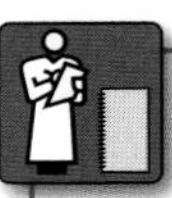

Radiological Differential Diagnosis

- Calcification:
  - Infection (TORCH)
  - Tumours (teratomas, neuroblastomas, hepatoblastomas)
- Ascites:
  - Hydrops
  - Peritonitis
  - Chylous ascites
  - Urine ascites (UPJ or UVJ or PUV)

Meconium Plug, Functional Immaturity Syndrome (Small Left Colon Syndrome)

Surgeon: D. Sidler
Radiologist: D. J. van der Merwe

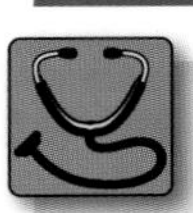

Clinical Insights

- Meconium plug syndrome is a transient form of distal colonic or rectal obstruction in newborns caused by an inspissated, immobile meconium plug (white chalky tip with black body).
- Presents as failure to pass meconium during the first day of life.
- Progressive abdominal distension and vomiting (sometimes bilious).
- Most cases are idiopathic, but has been associated with:
  - Prematurity
  - Hypotonia/hypothyroid
  - Hypermagnesemia
  - Diabetic mother (poorly controlled)
  - Hirschsprung's disease
  - Cystic fibrosis
  - Maternal medication
- Contrast enema can be diagnostic and therapeutic.
- Suction rectal biopsy to exclude the diagnosis of Hirschsprung's disease along with cystic fibrosis screening is warranted in all cases.
- The diagnosis is made after all the above causes are excluded.
- Need for surgery is extremely rare.

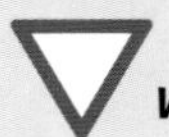

Warning

- Rehydrate before contrast enema

Urgency

- ❑ Emergency
- ☑ Urgent
- ❑ Elective

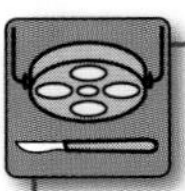

What the Surgeon Needs to Know

- Has the contrast reached above the plug or is there more proximal pathology?

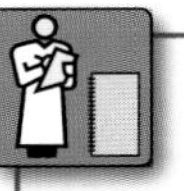

Clinical Differential Diagnosis

- Hirschsprung's disease
- Anorectal malformations
- Cystic fibrosis
- Hypoganglionosis
- Neuronal intestinal dysplasia
- Megacystis–microcolon–intestinal hypoperistalsis syndrome

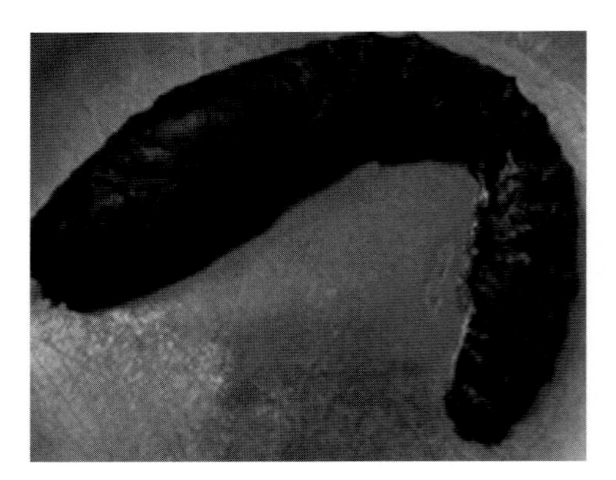

An evacuated meconium plug

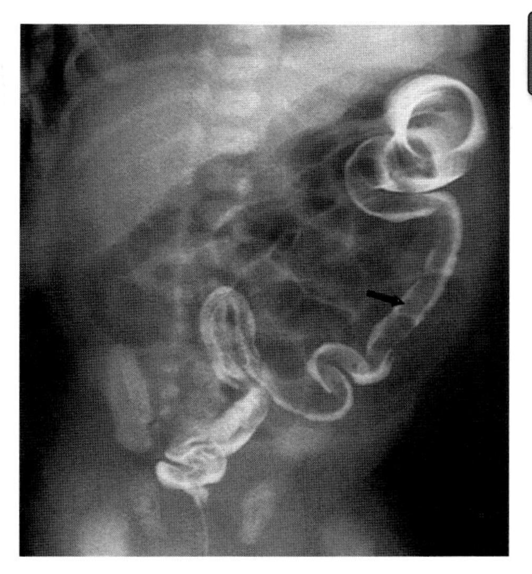

Contrast enema – Contrast is seen outlining the meconium plug seen as a long filling defect (*arrow*)

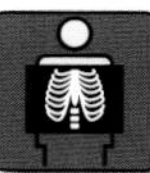

Imaging Options

- Primary: AXR
- Follow-on: Contrast enema

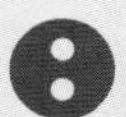

Imaging Findings

AXR

- Multiple dilated loops of bowel suggestive of distal obstruction

Contrast Enema

- Retained meconium seen as a filling defect/plug
- Often associated with a small left colon (transition at splenic flexure)
- No "microcolon" (i.e. it does not involve the whole colon)

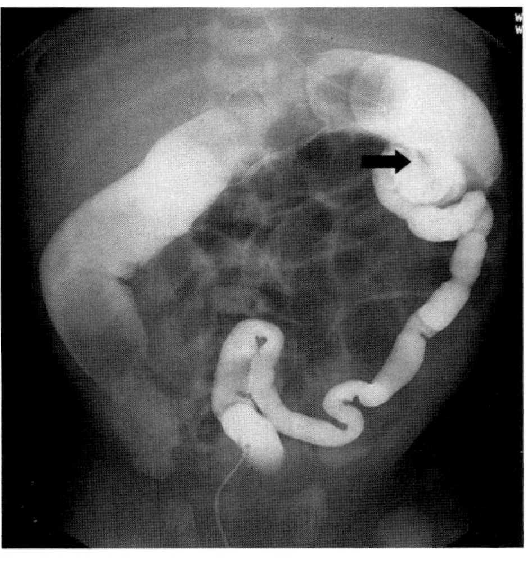

Contrast enema – Contrast demonstrates the caliber change (*arrow*) between the small left colon and the remainder of the colon in a child of a diabetic mother with small left colon and functional immaturity (meconium plug syndrome)

Tips

- Functional immaturity is more common when the mother is diabetic.
- Enema with water-soluble contrast agent, (Do not use a Balloon Catheter).
- Enema often therapeutic.

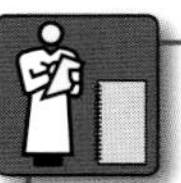

Radiological Differential Diagnosis

- Hirschprung's Disease (symptoms persist after plug passage)
- Ileal atresia (microcolon; dilated loops not opacified)
- Meconium ileus (microcolon; ileal plugs)

Mesoblastic Nephroma

Surgeon: S. Moore
Radiologist: N. Wieselthaler

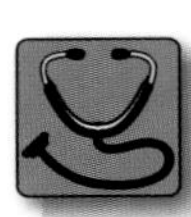

Clinical Insights

- Commonest renal tumour occurring within neonatal period.
- 85% occur in neonate or early infancy.
- Presents as solid renal mass – often diagnosed on antenatal ultrasound.
- There are 2 types:
  - Fibromatous type (< 3 months): Mostly benign.
  - Cellular variety (older child): Has malignant potential and local recurrence (metastases have been reported).
- Related to fibromatosis [Genetic abnormality = chromosome 11 trisomy].
- May have other fibrous masses (e.g. back).
- Treatment is surgical excision.

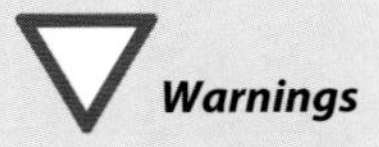

Warnings

- Tumour may produce Renin or prostaglandin.
- May have hypertension or hypercalcaemia.

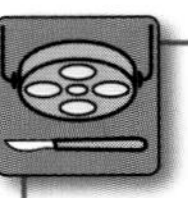

What the Surgeon Needs to Know

- To differentiate from Wilm's tumour

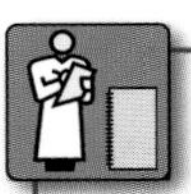

Differential Diagnosis

- Wilm's tumour
- Nephroblastomatosis

Urgency

- ❑ Emergency
- ❑ Urgent
- ☑ Elective

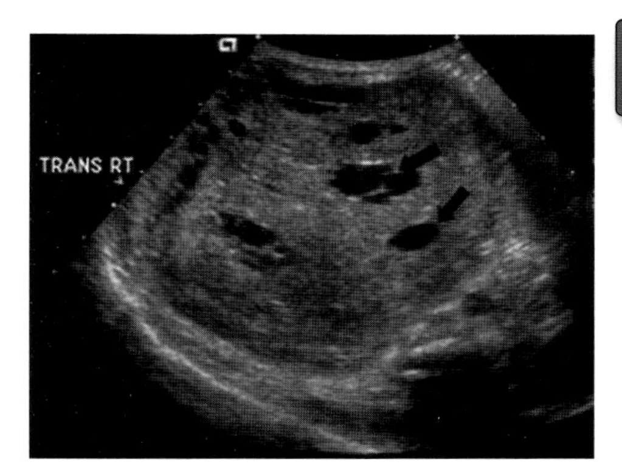

Transverse US – Large inhomogenous solid tumour arising from the right kidney. Cysts are demonstrated (*arrows*) and are common

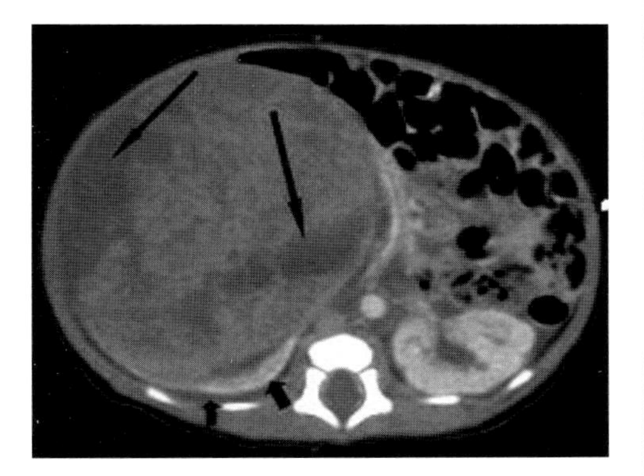

Contrasted CT – Large solid mass arising from the right kidney (note the "claw" sign – *short arrows*) in a neonate. Areas of necrosis are noted as low-density non-enhancing areas (*long arrows*)

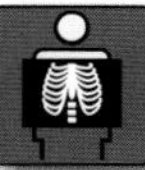

Imaging Options

- Primary: US
- Follow on: CT/MRI

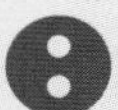

Imaging Findings

- Solid (some are cystic), unilateral renal mass in a foetus/infant < 3 months

US

- Homogenous or heterogenous solid (or cystic) renal mass

CT

- Variable contrast enhancing renal mass

MRI

- T2 hyperintense renal mass

Tips

- Whorled appearance.
- Necrosis, haemorrhage and cysts may occur.
- No calcification.

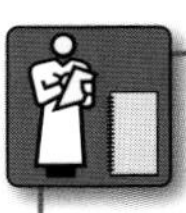

Radiological Differential Diagnosis

Intra-renal

- Wilm's tumour (no imaging differences)

Extra-renal

- Neuroblastoma
- Adrenal haemorrhage

Morgagni Hernia

Surgeon: J. Wilde
Radiologist: B. Khoury

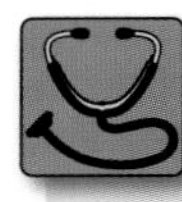

Clinical Insights

- Also referred to as retrosternal hernia, caused by failure of fusion of the costal and sternal diaphragmatic contributions.
- Defect is posterior to the sternum at the site that the internal mammary artery traverses the diaphragm.
- Ninety percent on the right.
- Hernia sac usually present.
- Associated with trisomy 21 in 20%.
- At risk of bowel herniation with consequent GIT or respiratory symptoms.

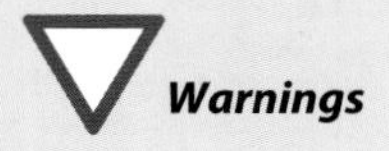

Warnings

- Potential to incarcerate and strangulate and should be repaired soon after diagnosis
- Differentiate from the retrosternal hernia and anatomical constellation of the pentalogy of Cantrell

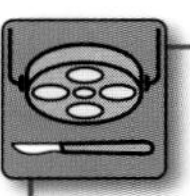

What the Surgeon Needs to Know

- Is this a diaphragmatic defect or a mediastinal mass?
- Where is the diaphragmatic defect?
- What is the thoracic anatomy?
- Are there bowel-related complications such as obstruction or perforation?

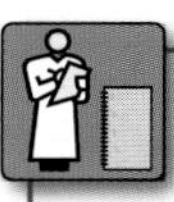

Clinical Differential Diagnosis

- Mediastinal mass
- Hiatus hernia
- Pulmonary malformation (CCAM, sequestration)
- Diaphragmatic hernia in alternate position

Urgency

- ☐ Emergency
- ☐ Urgent
- ☑ Elective

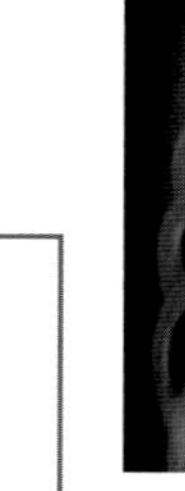

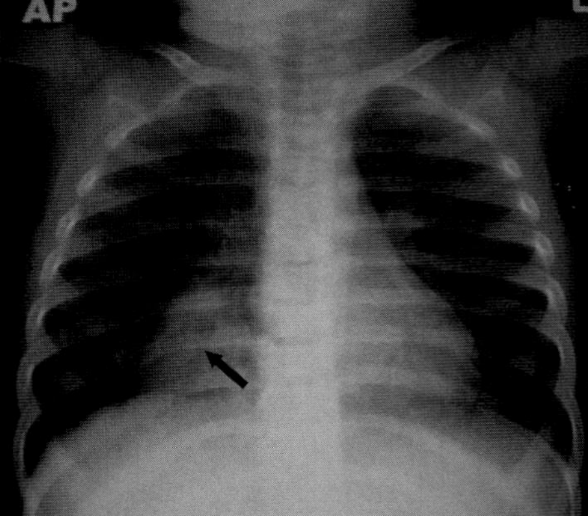

CXR– Demonstrates a right-sided soft-tissue density intra-thoracic mass closely related to the heart (*arrow*) representing a Morgagni hernia

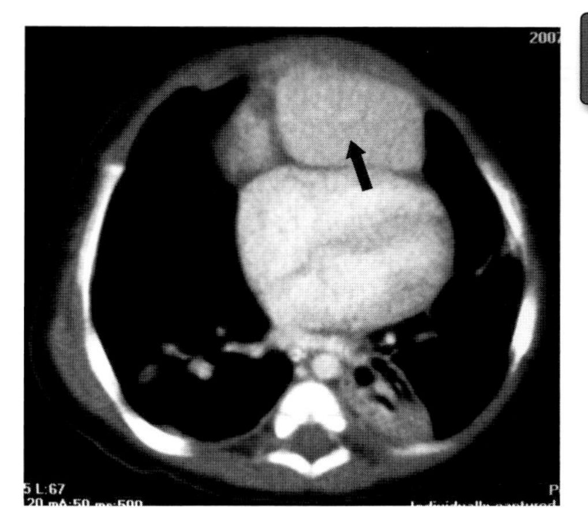

CT – Demonstrates a soft-tissue mass with the characteristics of liver anterior to the heart (*arrow*)

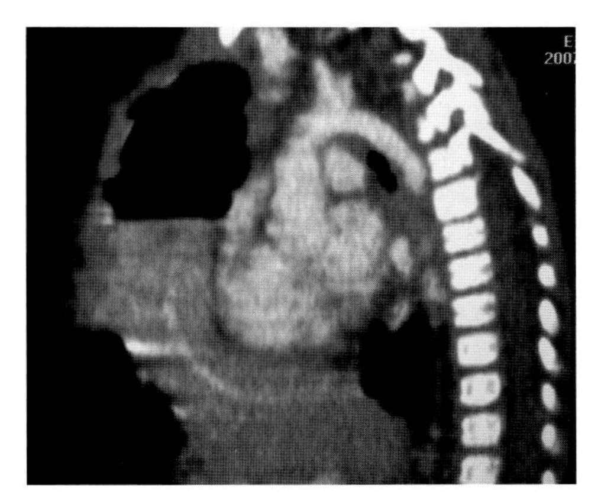

CT sagital reconstruction – Demonstrates that the mass is continuous with liver and represents herniated liver

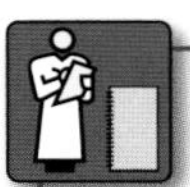

Radiological Differential Diagnosis

- Diaphragmatic hump
- Normal variant
- Pulmonary sequestration
- Bronchogenic cyst
- Enteric duplication cyst
- Neoplasm (pulmonary blastoma/ hepatoblastoma)

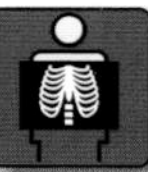

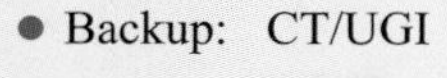

Imaging Options

- Primary: prenatal US, CXR, AXR
- Backup: CT/UGI

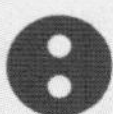

Imaging Findings

Prenatal US

- May be normal or show herniation of colon (or liver) into the right hemi-thorax.
- Typically an anterior hemi-thorax echogenic mass that may extend beyond the heart margin.

CXR/AXR

- May be normal initially as bowel (or liver) may initially be intra-abdominal.
- Opacified right hemi-thorax or localized anteriorly on lateral.
- Lack of aerated ipsilateral lung.
- Under-aerated contralateral lung.
- Mediastinal shift to the left.
- Hepatic flexure may be intrathoracic.
- Right sited hernias may rarely contain liver.

CT

- Usually only required in complex cases when there is a possibility of coexistent congenital lung disease.
- Useful for the evaluation of solid organ herniation, again more common on the right side.
- Define contents of sac.
- Coronal reconstructions elegantly demonstrate diaphragmatic defect with herniated liver, which may have an abnormal superior contour.

UGI

- Not helpful as Morgagni hernia rarely contain foregut structures.
- Enema may confirm hepatic flexure in chest.

Tips

- Thoracic portion of nasogastric tube deviated away from the side of the hernia

Multicystic Dysplastic Kidney (MCDK)

Surgeon: J. Loveland
Radiologist: H. von Bezing

Clinical Insights

- Most common cystic renal mass in the neonate.
- Congenital lesion of kidney secondary to early ureteric obstruction.
- Often asymptomatic requiring no active intervention.
- May present with pain due to progressive enlargement and occasionally hypertension, when nephrectomy may be indicated.
- Most important to differentiate from hydronephrosis.

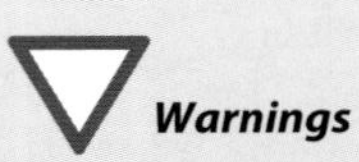

Warnings

- Vesico-ureteric reflux occurs in contra-lateral kidney in up to 30% of the cases.
- Voiding cysto-urethrogram is mandatory.

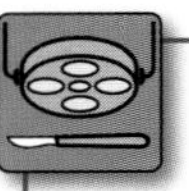

What the Surgeon Needs to Know

- Is it hydronephrosis or a multicystic dysplastic kidney?
- What is the functional status of the contra-lateral kidney?

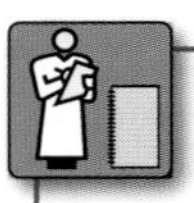

Differential Diagnosis

- Hydronephrosis
- Polycystic kidney disease (autosomal dominant and recessive types)

Urgency

- ☐ Emergency
- ☐ Urgent
- ☑ Elective

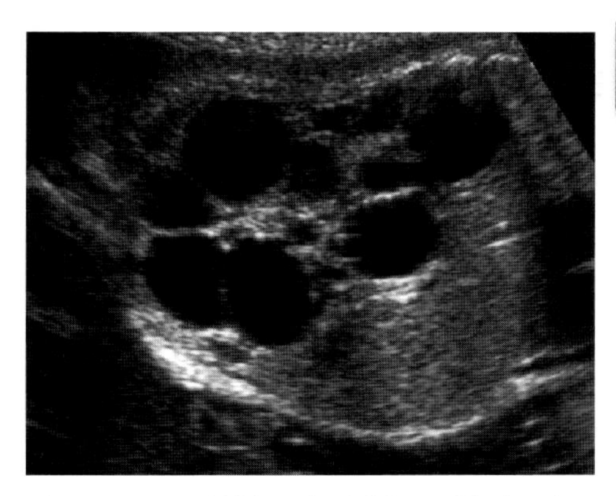

US – No normal kidney is visible, and in its place there are numerous non-communicating cysts and no visible collecting system

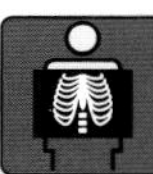

Imaging Options

- Primary: US
- Back-up: DMSA/MAG3 renogram/CT

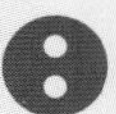

Imaging Findings

- Multiple cysts, various sizes, arranged haphazardly (bunch of grapes).
- Cysts do not connect or communicate with collecting system.
- Echogenic parenchyma if any visible.
- Contra lateral kidney – Hyperplastic.

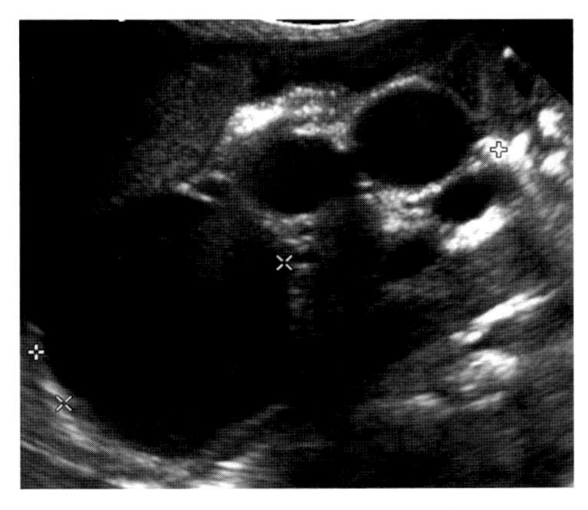

US – Non-communicating renal cysts with some central echogenic parenchyma, which did not show function on DMSA scan

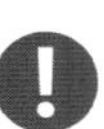

Tips

- One of the dissapearing masses of newborns/fetuses.
- May not be visible or become smaller on follow-up scans.
- Renal dysplasia may be focal in portion of a kidney (often peripheral).
- DMSA/MAG3 show non-function.
- Neoplastic cysts are unusual shapes while MDCK are oval and well defined.

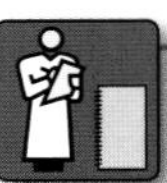

Radiological Differential Diagnosis

- Hydronephrosis
- Polycystic diseases – genetic or syndromal (includes autosomal dominant)
- Wilm's tumour
- Congenital mesoblastic nephroma (seldom cystic but presents in neonate)

Necrotizing Enterocolitis (NEC)

Surgeon: A. Alexander
Radiologist: A. M. du Plessis

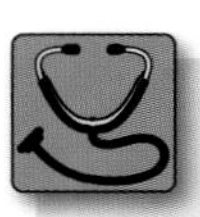

Clinical Insights

- The most common neonatal surgical emergency.
- Unknown aetiology, most likely multifactorial.
- Incidence and severity is inversely proportional to age and weight.
- Affecting 10% of neonates < 1,500 g.
- May occur in term babies:
  - Starts earlier (1–2 days)
  - Often has a pre-disposing cause
- Mortality rate varies according to age and size: 10–50%
- NEC is managed medically initially
- Surgical intervention is required for complications (necrosis, perforation, stricture)

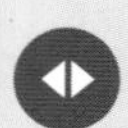

Warning

- Imaging is best done in the ICU as the patients are often too small and sick to move safely

Controversies

- The physiologically stable infant with free air on X-ray may have localized NEC or an isolated perforation. Some of these patients may be managed with peritoneal drains alone.
- The implication of peak flow velocities of mesenteric vessels.

Urgency

- ❑ Emergency
- ☑ Urgent
- ❑ Elective

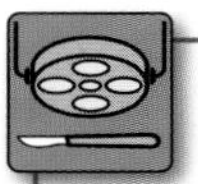

What the Surgeon Needs to Know

- Are there complications of the disease process that will alter management?
  - Free intra-peritoneal air
  - Static loops indicating bowel necrosis
  - Phlegmon/abscess formation
  - Worsening disease on serial X-rays despite best medical care

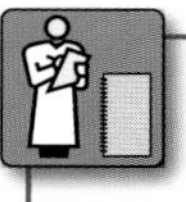

Clinical Differential Diagnosis

- Ileus
- Bowel obstruction
- Hischprung's disease
- Meconeum peritonitis

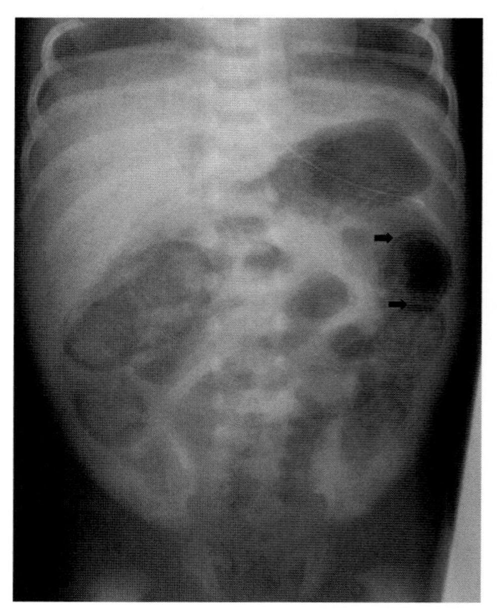

AXR – Curvilinear intramural gas (*arrows*) represents florid NEC

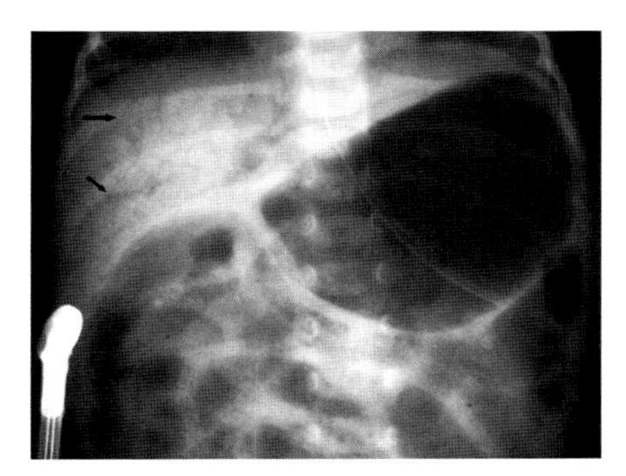

AXR – Identification of portal venous gas (*arrows*) in this patient with subtle pneumatosis suggests the diagnosis NEC in this premature neonate

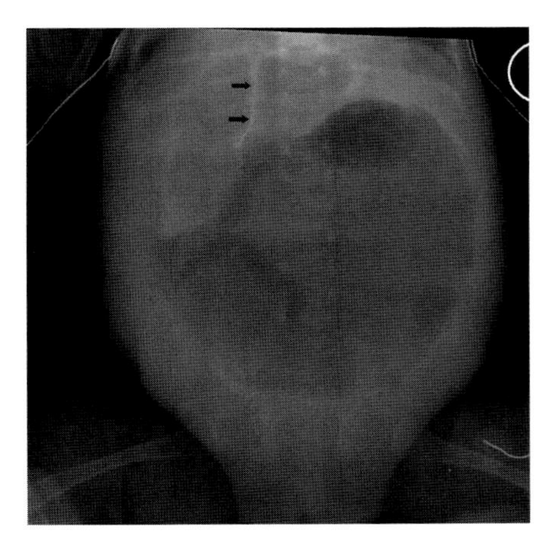

AXR – The free air in this patient has settled under the umbilicus (non-dependent position) and also outlined the falciform ligament (*arrows*), which mimics the tie-up laces of an archaic football accounting for the "foot-ball" sign. Note also how the bowel has decompressed and collapsed

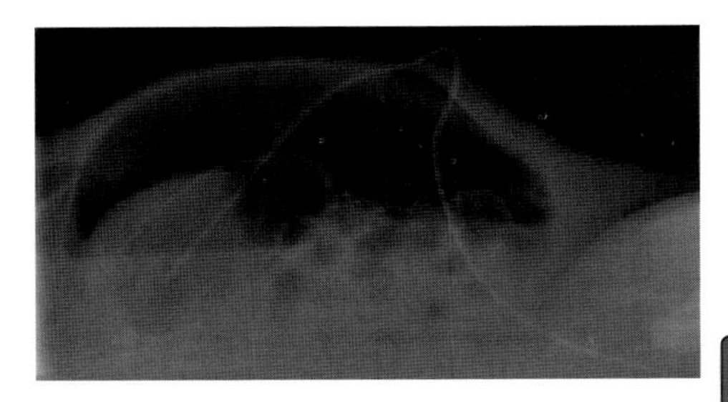

AXR – Horizontal beam lateral is ideal for seeing free air around the edge of the liver, which is now separated from other opaque soft-tissue structures. Rigler's sign identifying the bowel wall is seen anteriorly as further confirmation

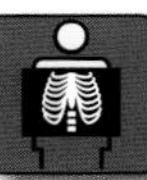

Imaging Options

- Primary: AXR
- Back-up: Horizontal beam lateral X-ray/US

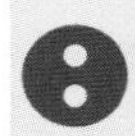

Imaging Findings

AXR

- Focal or diffuse bowel dilatation
- "Fixed" bowel loop on serial films
- Separation of bowel walls (wall thickening or free fluid)
- Pneumatosis, i.e. gas in bowel wall (linear or bubbly)
- Portal venous gas
- Free intra-peritoneal air: Lucent triangles on lateral view; both sides of bowel visible (Rigler's sign); falciform ligament outline (football sign)

US

- Echogenicity/sparkling in bowel walls from intramural gas
- Free fluid (hypoechoic) and free air (echogenic arcs)
- Linear echogenicity in portal venous system

Tips

- Neonates with severe NEC require from 6 to 24-h serial X-rays depending on the condition of the neonate.
- Horizontal beam lateral views are recommended for detecting free air.
- Check chest X-ray for other diagnoses such as lung prematurity.
- The commonest cause of portal venous gas in neonates is related to placement of umbilical vein catheters.

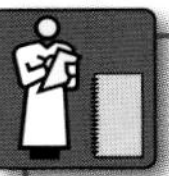

Radiologic Differential Diagnosis

- Non-specific distention/obstruction
- Milk allergy

Nephroblastomatosis

Surgeon: S. Moore
Radiologist: N. Wieselthaler

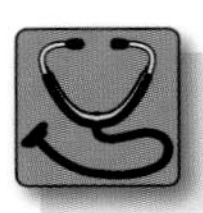

Clinical Insights

- Definition: Persistence of embryonic blastemal tissue beyond 36 weeks of gestational age.
- Two types:
  - Diffuse – Causing generalized enlargement.
  - Multifocal – Causing discrete masses within the parenchyma.
- Pre-malignant condition of kidney (may be a precursor of Wilm's tumour).
- Presents with increase in renal size in neonatal period.
- Reported in association with congenital malformations/syndromes (e.g. Beckwith-Weidemann, aniridia, hemihypertrophy, trisomy 18, hypospadias, undescended testes).
- Occurs in more than 80% of bilateral Wilm's tumours.

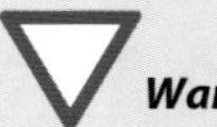

Warnings

- May resemble Wilm's tumour.
- If co-existing with Wilm's tumour on the nephrectomy specimen, residual kidney requires close follow up to pick up metachronous Wilm's tumour early.

Controversy

- Controversy as regards to nature and management

Urgency

- ❑ Emergency
- ❑ Urgent
- ☑ Elective

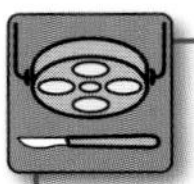

What the Surgeon Needs to Know

- Is nephroblastomatosis present or is it a Wilm's tumour?

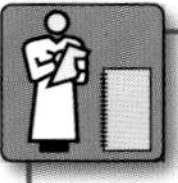

Clinical Differential Diagnosis

- Wilm's tumour
- Mesoblastic nephroma
- Other causes of enlarged kidney

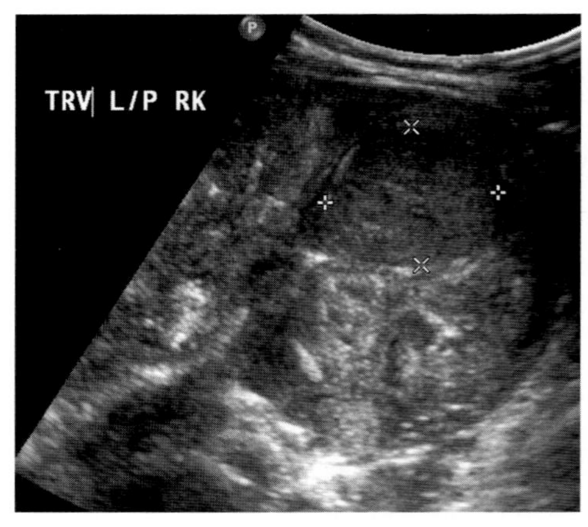

US transverse – Hypoechoic peripheral renal mass (calipers) proven to be nephroblastomatosis

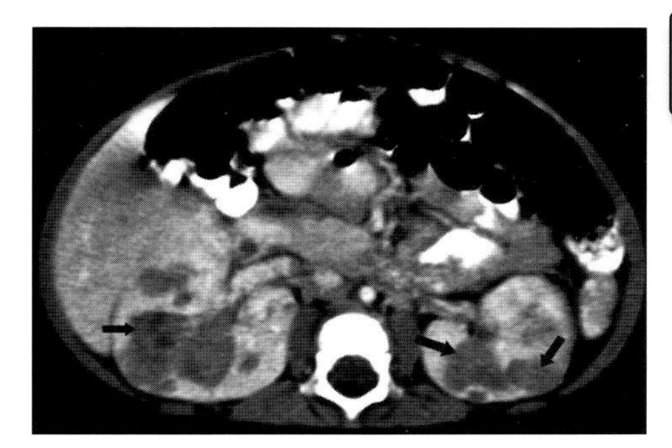

CT with contrast – Bilateral multiple, homogenous, non-enhancing hypodense masses (*arrows*) consistent with bilateral nephroblastomatosis

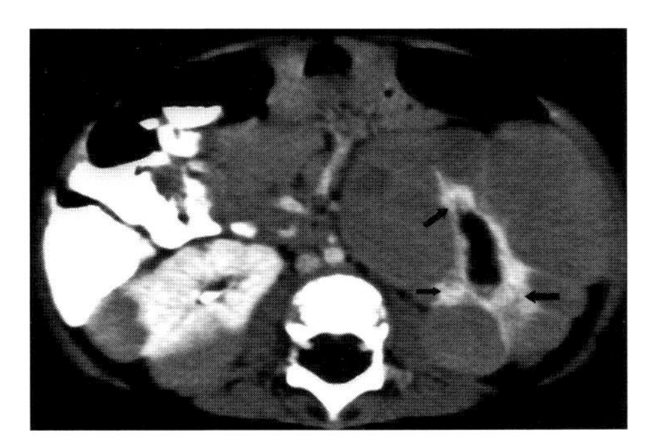

CT with contrast – "multi-focal nephroblastomatosis". On the right there are homogenous non-enhancing peripheral masses. The left kidney is affected disproportionately resulting in the little remaining, normal enhancing parenchyma, looking like "stag antlers" (*arrows*)

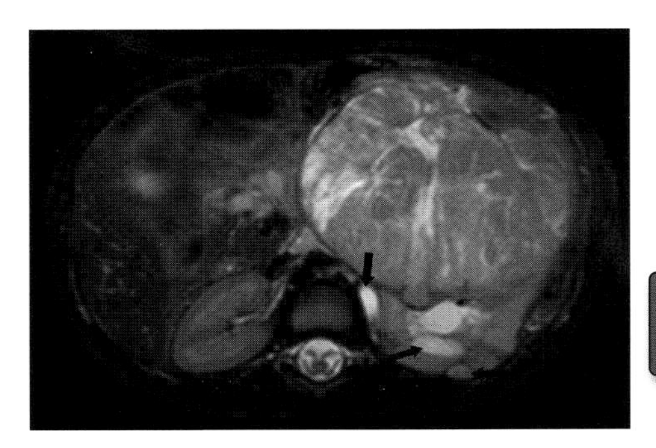

MRI transverse T2-weighted – In addition to the large heterogenous Wilm's tumour anteriorly in the left kidney, there are multiple, predominantly peripheral, flat, homogenous lesions (*arrows*) that represent nephroblastomatosis

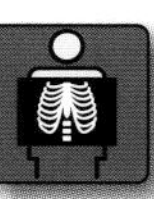

Imaging Options

- Primary: US/CT
- Back-up: MRI

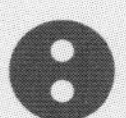

Imaging Findings

US

- Hypoechoic/isoechoic peripheral mass

CT

- Homogenous, hypodense poorly enhancing peripheral nodule
- May be multiple
- "Multifocal nephroblatomatosis": Normal enhancing parenchyma on CT has a "stag-antler" appearance

MRI

- Homogenous, T1 isointense to renal parenchyma, T2 hyperintense

Tips

- Precursor to Wilm's tumour (30–40%).
- Wilm's lesions rounder and heterogenous (nephroblastomatosis often flat, homogenous lesions).
- Most regress spontaneously but need regular monitoring.
- May be associated with syndromes, e.g. Beckwith-Wiedemann.

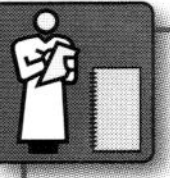

Radiological Differential Diagnosis

- Wilm's tumour
- Lymphoma
- Leukaemia
- Pyelonephritis

Neuroblastoma

Surgeon: S. Moore
Radiologist: N. Wieselthaler

Clinical Insights

- The most common malignant tumour in childhood (with Wilm's tumour).
- Tumour of young (median age: 22 months; 50% <2years).
- Metastatic spread early.
- Ninety percent secrete catecholamines.
- In infancy, some show unique ability to mature.
- Tends to cross midline and surround great vessels.
- May extend through intervertebral foramina and result in spinal cord compression.
- Stage IV S (young age with metastases but not to bone – better prognosis).
- Site:
  - Intra-abdominal 75%
  - Adrenal 50%
  - Thoracic 20%
  - Head and neck <5%
  - Retroperitoneal, paravertebral sympathetic ganglia, pelvic <5%

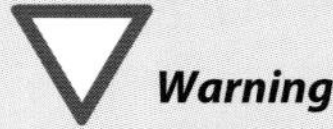

Warning

- May be hormonally active – Hypertension

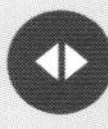

Controversies

- MRI best for intraspinal extension
- Metaiodabenzylguanidine (MIBG) scintigraphy – bone and bone marrow involvement
- Management of the primary in stage IV disease

Urgency

- ❑ Emergency
- ❑ Urgent
- ☑ Elective

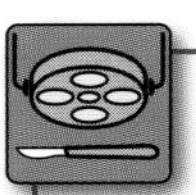

What the Surgeon Needs to Know

- Diagnosis
- Site of the primary
- Presence or absence of local–regional spread
- Secondary mass effect: ureteral obstruction, spinal compression

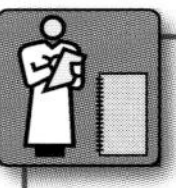

Clinical Differential Diagnosis

- Wilm's tumour
- Rhabdomyosarcoma
- Other retroperitoneal tumours

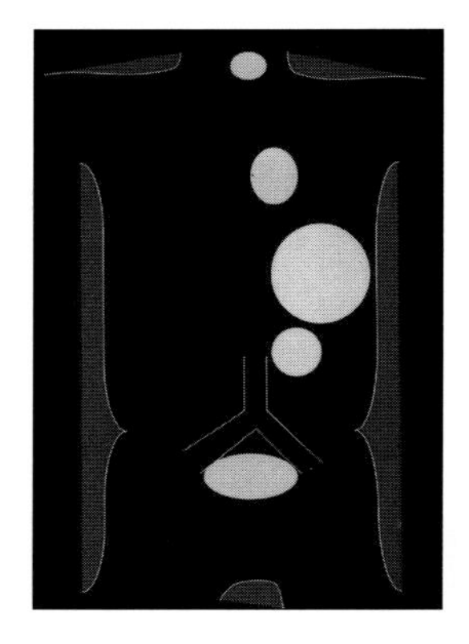

Sites of neuroblastoma in the body

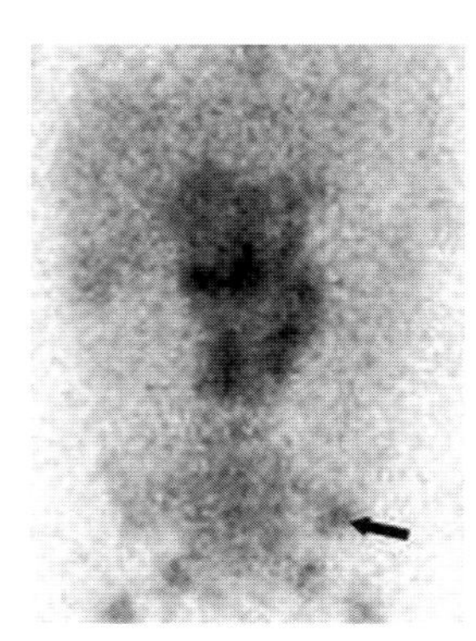

MIBG scan shows uptake in an abdominal neuroblastoma with metastases to the pelvis (*arrow*)

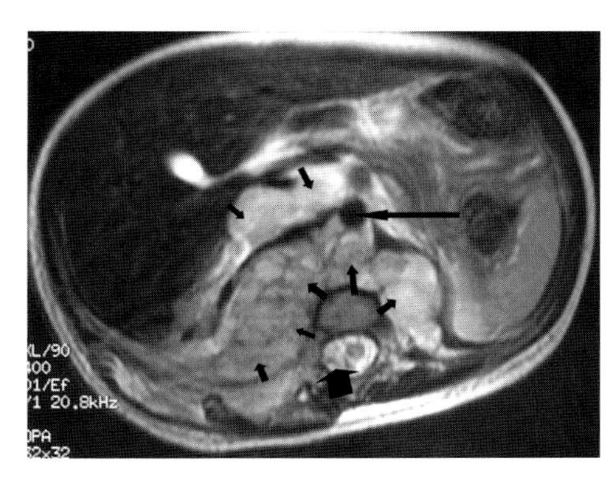

MRI – Axial T2/STIR – Demonstrates a central paraspinal soft-tissue mass that crosses the midline and encases vessels (*short arrows*). Note the aorta "lifted off" the vertebra (*long arrow*) and intraspinal extension from the right (*thick arrow*)

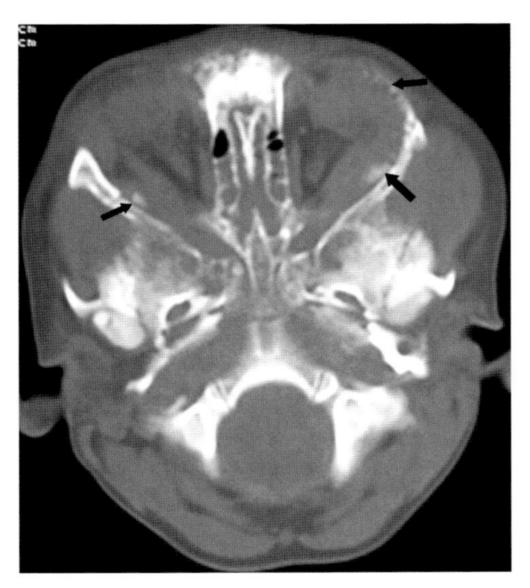

Axial CT of the skull-base demonstrating multifocal neuroblastoma metastases to the orbits with partially calcified soft-tissue masses (*arrows*)

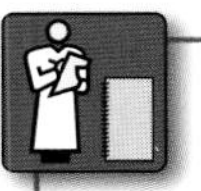

Radiological Differential Diagnosis

- Wilm's Tumour
- Other adrenal masses (adrenal haemorrhage, adrenal carcinoma, phaeochromocytoma)

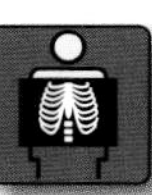

Imaging Options

- Primary: US
- Follow-on: CT/MRI/Nuc Med (MIBG)

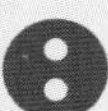

Imaging Findings

- Can arise anywhere along sympathetic chain from the neck to the pelvis
- Usually suprarenal

US

- Mass of varying echogenicity due to necrosis and haemorrhage
- Calcification (often without acoustic shadowing)

CT

- Heterogenous mass ± haemorrhage/necrosis
- Eighty-five percent calcified, invasive growth pattern (i.e. surrounds and encases vessels and extends into spinal canal)

MRI

- High signal on T2
- Best for the assessment of intraspinal extension
- Whole body STIR MRI useful

NM

- MIBG whole body scan and bone scan assess extent and presence of bone metastases

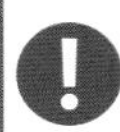

Tips

- Encases organs and vessels (not displaces).
- Aorta lifted off vertebral bodies (normally rests on the vertebral body).
- Mets to bone and liver (and skin in infantile disease).
- Orbital metastases are typical (proptosis is an indication to look for neuroblastoma).
- Thirty percent do not take up MIBG; all receive bone scan in addition.

Non-Accidental Injury (NAI)

Surgeon: A. B. van As
Radiologist: M. Hayes

Clinical Insights

- Significantly under-reported.
- Approximately 5% of all trauma admissions.
- Maintain high index of suspicion when:
  - History and physical findings incongruous
  - Multiple fractures of different ages
  - Metaphyseal fractures
  - Multiple, bilateral, differently aged posterior rib and scapular fractures
  - Multiple and complex skull fractures
  - Spinous process fractures
- All the above fractures are rare and most fractures of abuse are "regular" fractures.
- Skeletal survey indicated for two reasons:
  - Child abuse suspected: Skeletal survey to detect old, other or unusual fractures
  - Child abuse already proven: Skeletal survey to identify clinically missed fractures

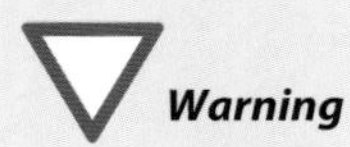

Warning

- Children rarely present with a clear diagnosis

Controversies

- The extent of imaging required for adequately excluding other fractures

Urgency

- ❑ Emergency
- ❑ Urgent
- ☑ Elective

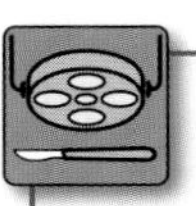

What the Surgeon Needs to Know

- Is there radiological suspicion for child abuse?
- Are there fractures requiring treatment?

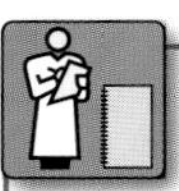

Clinical Differential Diagnosis

- Van Willebrand's disease
- Haemophilia
- Osteogenesis imperfecta
- Scurvy

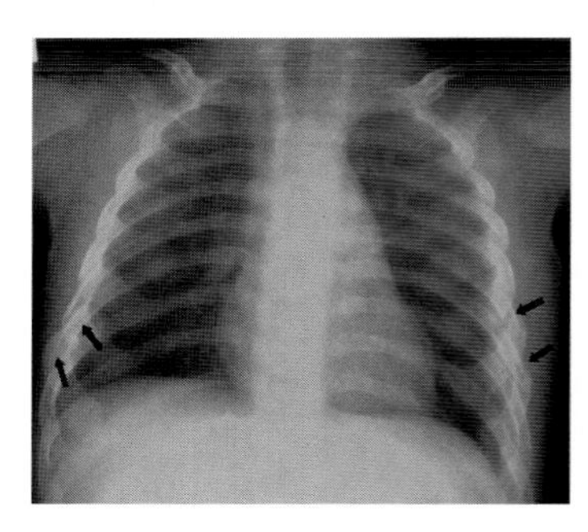

CXR – Demonstrating multiple rib fractures. On the right, there are old fractures with callus sequentially involving ribs 6 and 7 laterally (*arrows*). On the left, there are recent fractures without callus involving ribs 6 and 7 laterally (*arrows*)

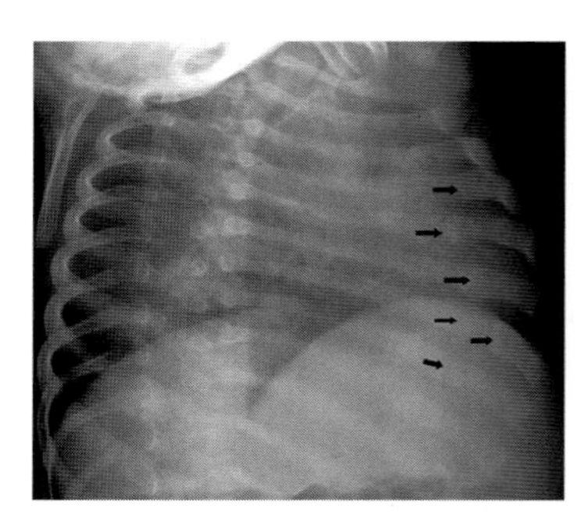

CXR Left-side down oblique – Shows multiple sequential fractures of varying ages of healing involving ribs 4–8 (*arrows*)

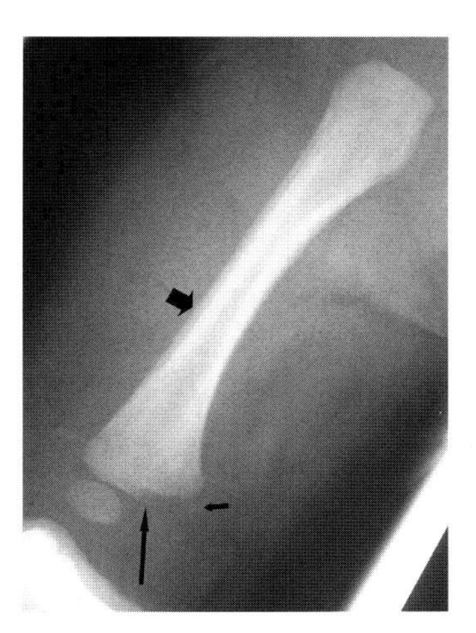

X-ray – Subtle metaphyseal "bucket-handle" fracture (*long arrow*) and corner (*small arrow*) fractures and a perisoteal reaction (*thick arrow*)

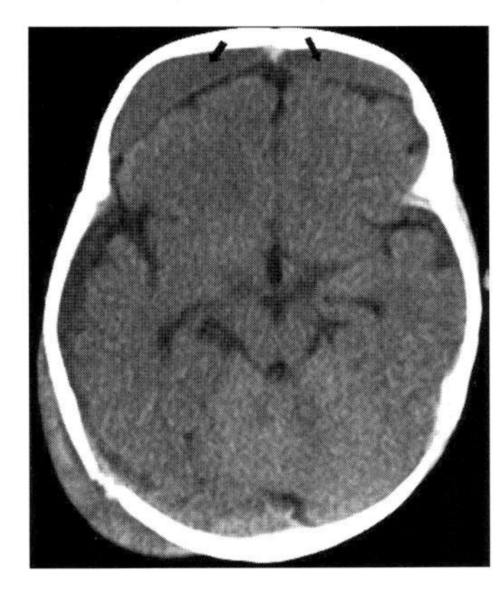

CT non-contrast – Soft-tissue swelling and a dense subdural collection represent acute head injury while "iso-dense" bi-frontal subdural collections (*arrows*) represent subacute head injury

Tips

- Metaphyseal fractures are highly specific.
- Posterior rib fractures, scapula, spinous process fractures highly specific.
- Rib fractures may require repeat films at later stage.
- All patients must have brain imaging.
- MRI must include DWI for cytotoxic oedema.
- Do not let child go home!

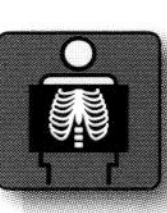

Imaging Options

- Primary: Plain film (skeletal survey)
- Alternate: CT/MRI (brain); LODOX (Statscan)
- Back-up: Bone scan/CT chest and abdomen

Imaging Findings

Skeletal Survey

[Skull X-ray, CXR and oblique, AXR, lateral spine, AP long bones, hands/feet]

- Multiple Fractures – Different ages and sites
- Unusual fractures – E.g. consecutive posterior/lateral ribs
- Metaphyseal corner/bucket-handle fractures
- Exuberant subperiosteal new bone

CT/MRI Brain

- Interhemispheric extra-axial bleeds
- Shear-type brain injuries
- Injuries of different ages
- Subdural/subarachnoid haemorrhage

CT Abdomen/Chest

- Bowel rupture
- Duodenal haematoma
- Liver/spleen/pancreas injury
- Rib and lung injury

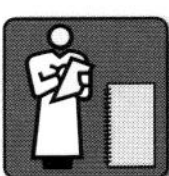

Radiological Differential Diagnosis

- Skeletal dysplasia (osteogenesis imperfecta; spondylometaphyseal; metaphyseal)
- Rickets
- Leukaemia
- Menke Syndrome
- Brain (accidental trauma, bleeding diathesis, subdural empyema)

Oesophageal Atresia

Surgeon: A. Alexander
Radiologist: A. Brandt

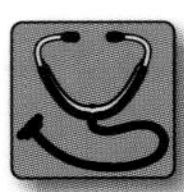

Clinical Insights

- May be detected prenatally:
  - Polyhydramnios
  - Dilated oesophageal pouch
  - Small stomach
- Post-natally the child cannot swallow saliva and drools excessively, frothing its sputum. Feeds are associated with cough, choking and cyanotic episodes.
- Confirmed clinically with the inability to pass a firm nasogastric tube past 10 cm.
- Nearly 40% are associated with other congenital anomalies of the VACTERL syndrome.
- A fistula can exist without an atresia.

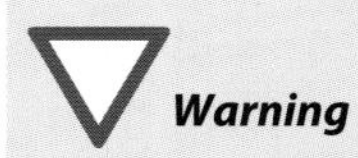

Warning

- These infants can be in extremis as a result of underlying cardiac anomaly, lung hypoplasia, hyaline membrane disease or acquired pneumonia

Urgency

- ❑ Emergency
- ❑ Urgent
- ☑ Elective

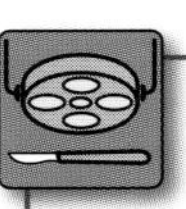

What the Surgeon Needs to Know

- Is this an atresia?
- Is there a tracheo-oesophageal fistula (TOF)?
- Is there a TOF in isolation (without atresia)?
- What is the length of the gap between the proximal atresia and distal oesophagus?
- Are there any underlying congenital abnormalities?

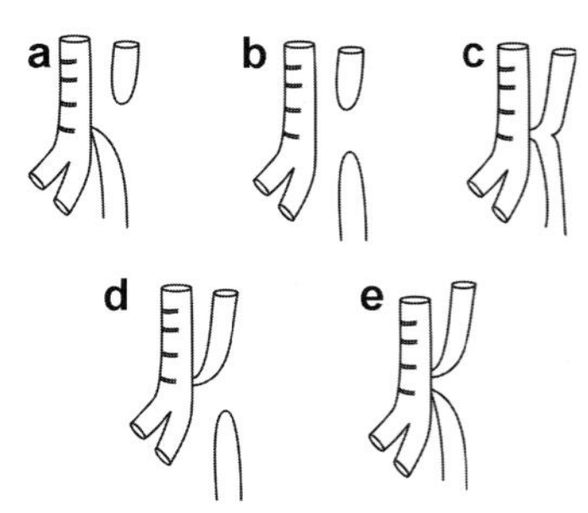

Classification of the spectrum of anomalies and the anatomical relationship with the trachea

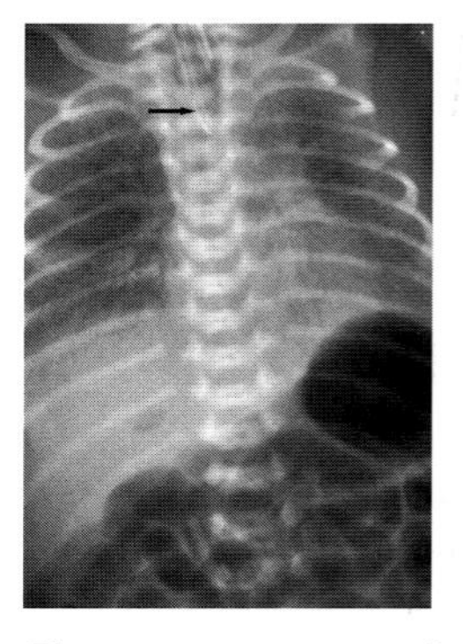

CXR/AXR – The most common type of oesophageal atresia with distal stump tracheo-oesophageal fistula. Dilated oesophagus with Replogel tube in situ (*arrow*) and gas-filled abdomen as a result of the tracheo-oesphageal fistula

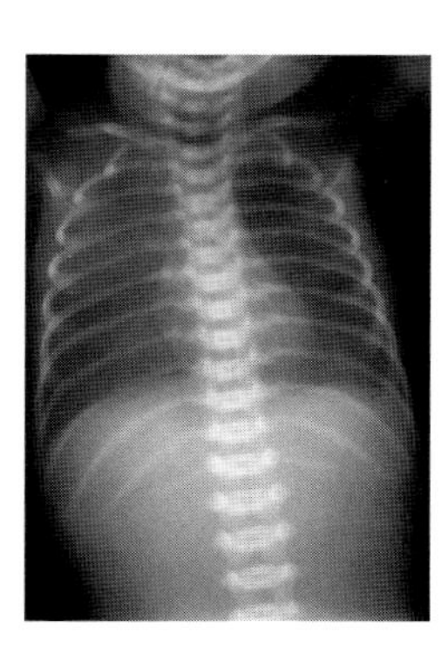

CXR/AXR – Less common type of oesophageal atresia occuring without tracheal fistula. Note the gasless abdomen

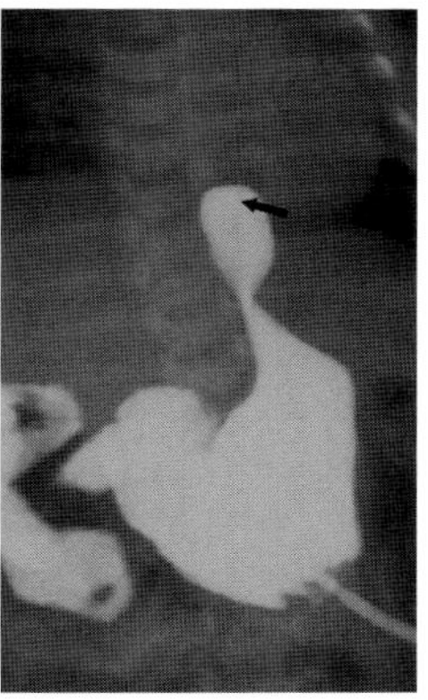

"Gag study" – A gag reflex has been stimulated by manipulating the indwelling tube in the pharynx in an attempt to cause gastro-reflux/vomiting. Reflux of contrast (inserted via gastrostomy) into the distal stump (*arrow*) demonstrates its length

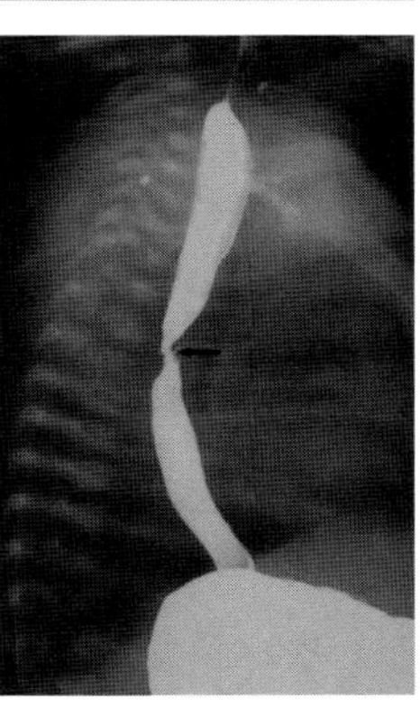

UGI post-repair – After repair there is always a calibre difference at the anastomosis (*arrow*) and a chance of early leakage or of stricture later on

Tips

- Replogel tube is thicker than NGT and lies straight in proximal pouch, containing many side holes for drainage.
- Post-operative check for leak – UGI study with head up 30°, water-souble contrast [not barium] and NGT proximal to anastomotic site.
- Look for other features of VACTREL.

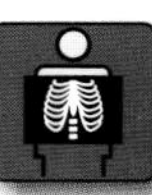

Imaging Options

- Primary: CXR, AXR
- Back-up: Fluoroscopy
- Follow on imaging: Fluoroscopy, U/S.

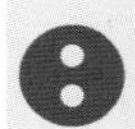

Imaging Findings

CXR

- Air-filled proximal pouch containing Replogel/coiled NGT
- Aspiration pneumonia

AXR

- Gasless abdomen – No distal fistula.
- Gas – filled Bowel – has distal fistula

Fluoroscopy

- Fill proximal pouch with air. Do not use contrast!
- "Gag" study to evaluate length of distal segment. After filling the stomach with contrast via the gastrostomy, the infant is made to gag by manipulating the Replogel/NGT in the pharynx. This is intended to cause gastro-oesophageal reflux/vomiting, thereby demonstrating the length of the distal stump.

UGI

- Post-op contrast swallow to check for leaks, stricture, reflux

US

- Establish side of aortic arch; surgical approach is on the opposite side

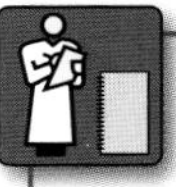

Radiological Differential Diagnosis

- Can be mimicked by pharyngeal perforation (forceful NGT placement) on plain film.

Oesophageal Caustic Stricture

Surgeon: A. Numanoglu
Radiologist: R. George

Clinical Insights

- Stricture formation takes 10–14 days following the caustic ingestion.
- May involve pharynx, entire oesophagus and antrum.
- Gastro-oesophageal reflux is common.
- Repeated studies may be required to asses the response to dilatations.
- Oesophageal perforation is an uncommon but serious complication following dilatation.
- Oesophageal replacement for extensive scarring or failed dilatation can be done with colonic interposition or gastric pull-up.

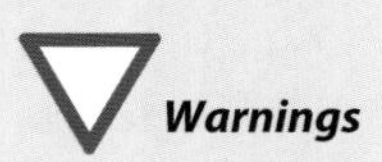

Warnings

- Aspiration can occur during the study.
- Tracheo-bronchial fistula may develop after dilatation.

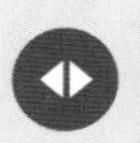

Controversy

- Nil

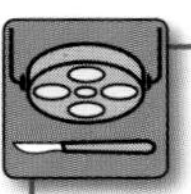

What the Surgeon Needs to Know

- Is there a single, multiple or diffuse strictures?
- Position, degree and length of the stricture/s.
- Is there a leak if performed immediately after the dilatation?
- Gastro-esophageal reflux?
- Colonic interposition:
  - Passage of contrast to the stomach?
  - Is there any redundancy?
  - Is there any obstruction/stenosis?

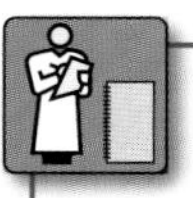

Differential Diagnosis

- Gastro-oesophageal reflux strictures

Urgency

- ☐ Emergency
- ☐ Urgent
- ☑ Elective

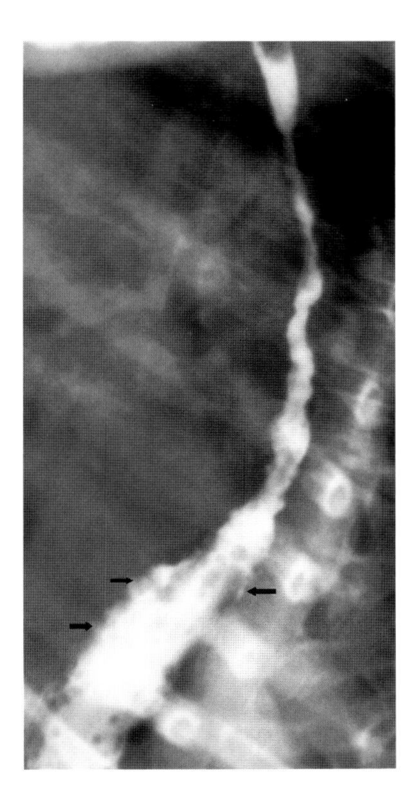

Lateral view UGI – Long-segment stricture of oesophagus with ulcerations (*arrows*) due to corrosives

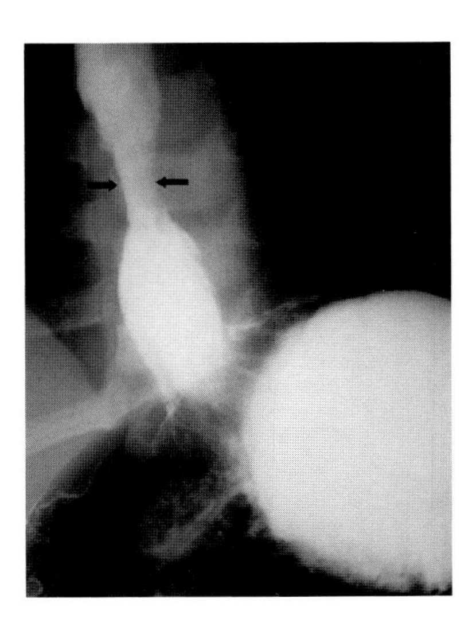

AP view UGI – Short stricture of distal oesophagus (*arrows*) a few centimeters above the gastro-oesophageal junction related to reflux

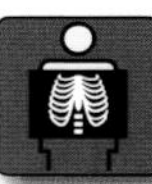

Imaging Options

- Primary: UGI
- Back up: CXR/CT
- Intervention: Fluoroscopic guided balloon dilation

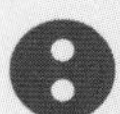

Imaging Findings

- UGI: Corrosive oesophagitis:
  - Dilated boggy oesophagus with ulcerations initially.
  - Long segment strictures at 1–3 months (multiple random smooth tapered strictures).
- CXR – Mediastinal widening, pneumomediastinum, pleural effusions with acute perforation after corrosive ingestion
- CT – for diagnosing mediastinitis

Tips

- Use water-soluble contrast in acute cases/ when aspiration/fistula/leak likely
- For corrosive strictures also evaluate pylorus
- Mid oesophageal – more likely due to surgery for tracheo – oesophageal fistula
- Lower oesophageal – more likely due to Reflux disease, prolonged nasogastric intubation
- Remember infection e.g., HIV

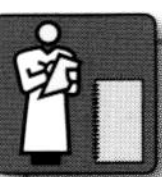

Radiological Differential Diagnosis

- Other causes of stricture
- Normal ring A and B
- Gastro-oesophageal junction in hiatus hernia
- Cricopharyngeus spasm
- Oesophageal web

Ovarian Cyst

Surgeon: D. Sidler
Radiologist: A. Maydell

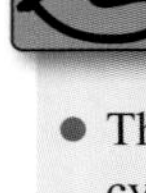

Clinical Insights

- There are two peak periods for ovarian cysts, the first year of life and at the time of menarche.
- In utero, ovarian cysts develop under the influence of maternal, placental and fetal hormones.
- The majority of ovarian cysts are benign, either functional (follicular) or neoplastic (teratoma).
- Enlarged ovaries become susceptible to torsion.
- The diagnostic workup depends on the presenting symptoms, the size of the cyst and the age of the child.
- In most infants the diagnosis is made by ante-natal ultrasound.
- The most common presenting symptom in the older child is abdominal pain.

Warnings

- A simple cyst must be differentiated from a complex one (cystic and solid areas). Complex cysts rouse suspicion of neoplasia.
- Sudden acute onset of pain needs urgent investigation for a possible ovarian torsion.

Controversy

- In infants, the size of cyst determines surgical intervention (>5 cm).

Urgency

- ❑ Emergency
- ☑ Urgent
- ❑ Elective

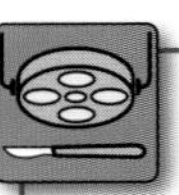

What the Surgeon Needs to Know

- Non-resolving ovarian cysts need surgical referral.
- Is the cyst simple or complex? Simple cysts over 5 cm in diameter can be aspirated; complex cysts should be excised (laparascopically or open).

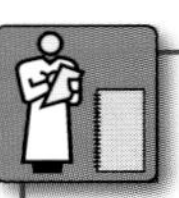

Clinical Differential Diagnosis

- Ovarian torsion
- Teratoma, germ cell tumour (dysgerminoma)
- Duplication cyst
- Appendicitis
- Mesenteric cysts

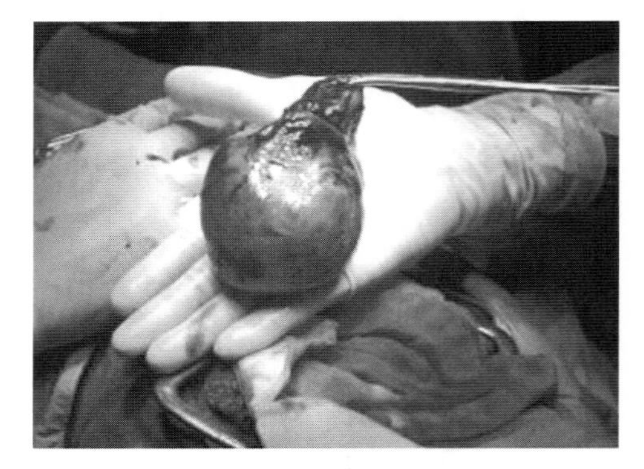

An ovarian cyst removed after torsion; histology – benign teratoma

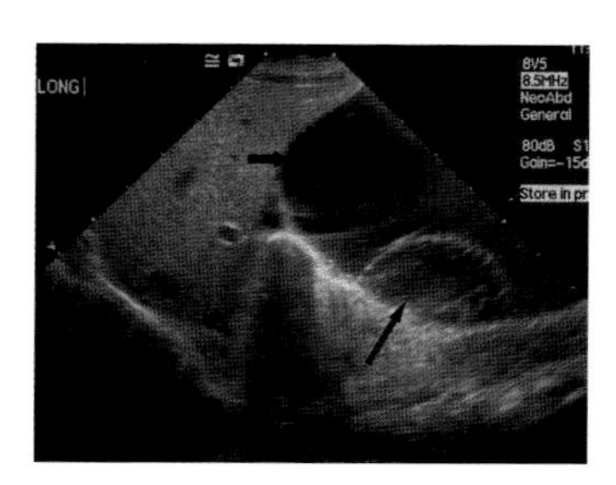

US longitudinal – Demonstrating a large ovarian cyst (*short arrow*) in a neonate extending up to the level of the liver. The cyst has a complex internal content and a cyst within cyst appearance (*long arrow*) [Image courtesy Dr. Kieran McHugh]

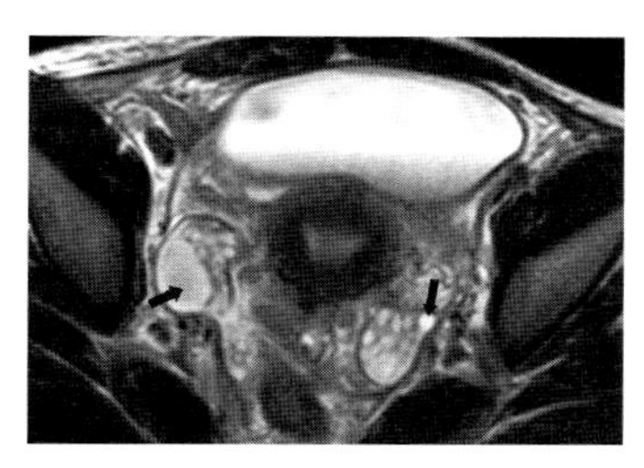

MRI T2 – Bilateral follicular cysts seen as high signal (*arrows*)

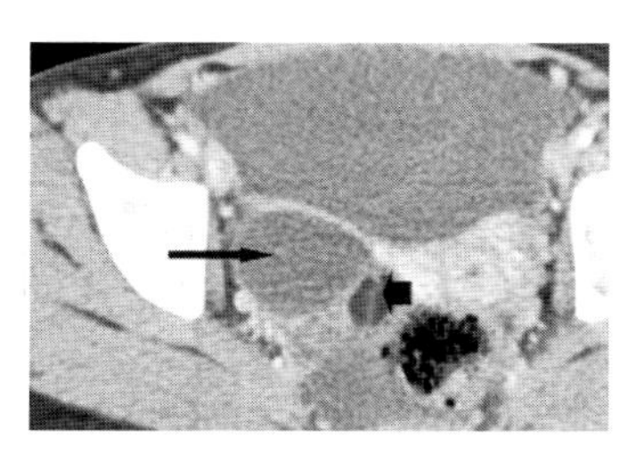

CT demonstrates a right ovarian cystic mass (*long arrow*) with a fatty component (*short arrow*) in keeping with a teratoma

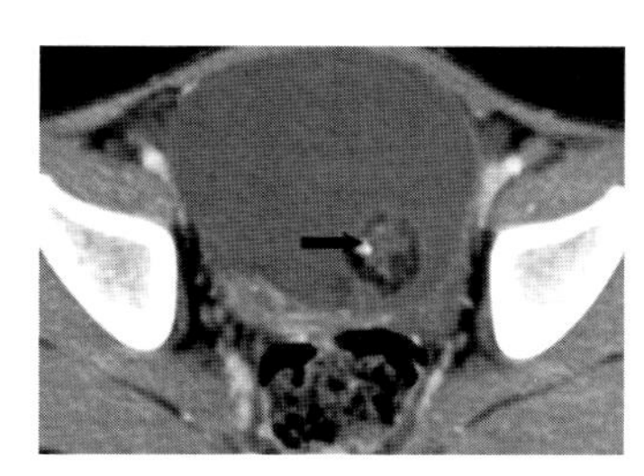

CT demonstrates a parametrial cystic mass with fat and calcium in keeping with a mature teratoma (*arrow*)

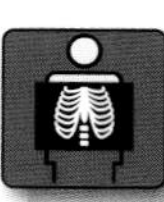

Imaging Options

- Primary: US and Doppler
- Back-up: MRI/CT

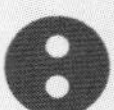

Imaging Findings

- Simple cysts (most likely benign): Unilocular, uniform thin wall around single cavity, no internal echoes.
- Complex cysts (benign/malignant): Multilocular, irregular thick wall, internal echoes.
- US signs of malignancy – Liver metastases, ascites, lymphadenopathy.
- Doppler US – Tumour vessels have higher flow/increased vascularity.
- MRI – Demonstrates structure of origin, mural nodules, presence of fat and extent of pelvic involvement.
- CT – Demonstrates fat and calcium.

Tips

- Follicular cysts < 1 cm common in neonates (often bilateral large cysts).
- Bilateral cysts found in association with cystic fibrosis, Mc Cune Albright and endocrinopathies.
- When large (>2 cm) simple cysts should be monitored for involution.
- Complex cysts and cysts greater than 2 cm require further imaging with CT or MRI.

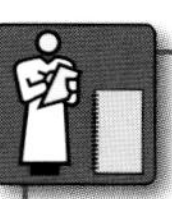

Radiological Differential Diagnosis

- Enteric duplication cyst/omental cyst/mesenteric cyst
- Ovarian torsion
- Pelvic inflammatory disease
- Appendicitis/appendix abscess
- Neoplasm (benign and malignant ovarian)/(neuroblastoma, lymphoma, leukaemia)

Pancreatitis (Acute)

Surgeon: C . Davies
Radiologist: J. W. Lotz

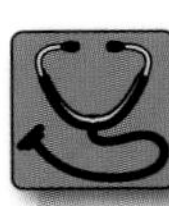

Clinical Insights

- Pancreatitis is rare in children.
- Presentation is with abdominal pain, tenderness, guarding and peritonism.
- The causes are:
  - Trauma
  - Congenital abnormalities (choledochal cysts, pancreatico-biliary malunion)
  - Hyperlipidaemia
  - Drug induced (steroids, antiretrovirals, chemotherapy)
  - Viral infections (mumps)
  - Ascaris infestation
  - Gallstones
  - Idiopathic
  - Familial

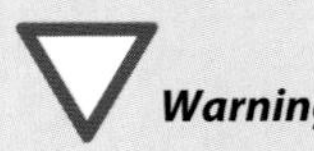

Warning

- These children can be extremely sick and imaging should take place after adequate resuscitation only.

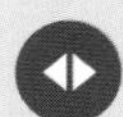

Controversies

- CT scans should be reserved for the diagnosis of trauma, acute haemorrhagic pancreatitis, complicated pancreatitis and where diagnostic doubt exists.
- Demonstrating duct anatomy with MRCP.
- Pancreatic duct divisum and pancreatitis.

Urgency

- ❑ Emergency
- ❑ Urgent
- ☑ Elective

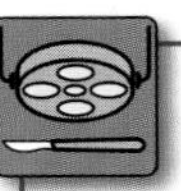

What the Surgeon Needs to Know

- Is this pancreatitis?
- Is there an underlying cause?
- Are there complications (pseudocyst, ascites, pleural effusion, abscess)?
- Is there any discrete mass noted in the parenchyma?

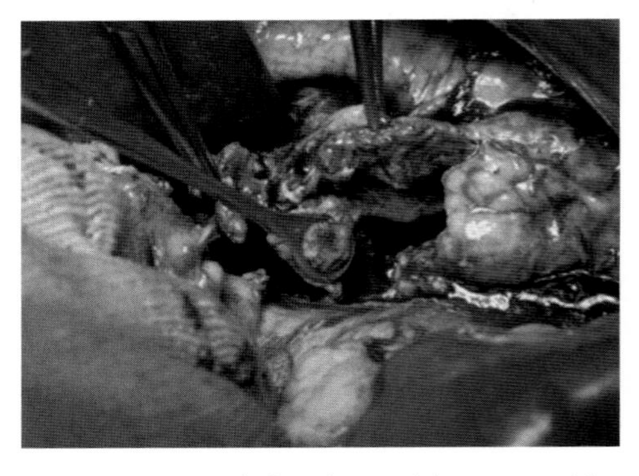

Necrosectomy: An infected necrotizing pancreatitis

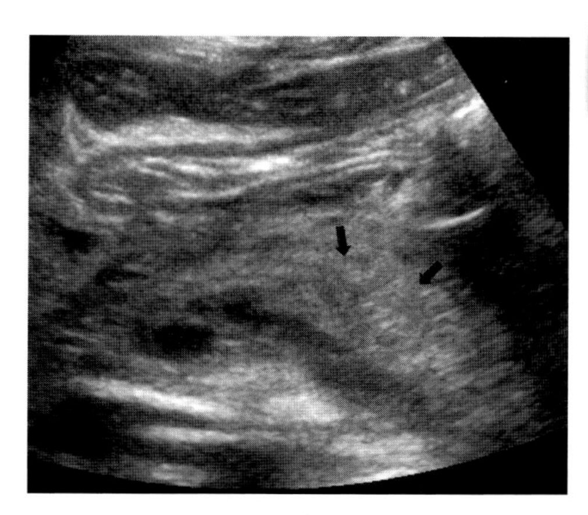

US transverse – Through the epigastrium showing an enlarged echogenic pancreas (*arrows*)

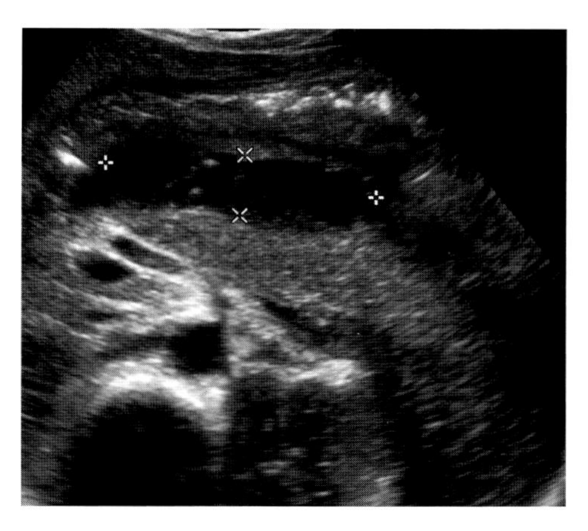

US transverse – Demonstrates cystic collections (calipers) representing pseudocysts anterior to the neck and head regions of the pancreas

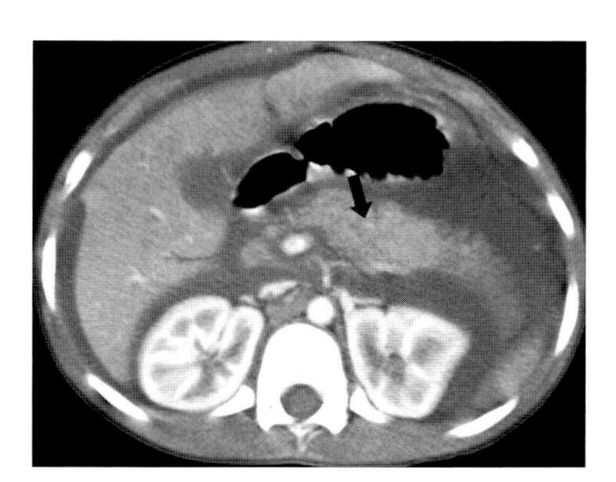

CT axial post-contrast – Showing an oedematous pancreas (*arrow*) and ascites

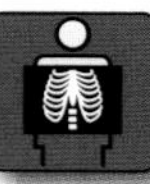

Imaging Options

- Primary: Ultrasound/AXR
- Back-up: CT/MRI (MRCP)

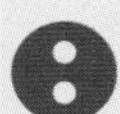

Imaging Findings

US

- Can be normal.
- Enlarged echogenic or hypoechoic pancreas with irregular margins.
- Dilated main pancreatic and common bile ducts.
- Peri-pancreatic fluid collection and pleural effusion.
- Calcifications may be seen in recurrent hereditary pancreatitis and CF.

CT

- Only for complicated pancreatitis and pre-operative
- Normal size or large pancreas
- Intra-/extra-pancreatic fluid collection/ pseudocyst
- Dilated pancreatic duct
- Calcification if recurrent

MRI/MRCP

- MRCP to define ducts and assess for obstructive pathology

Tips

- Perform imaging against the background of biochemical profile (elevated serum amylase)

Parotid Mass

Surgeon: O. Basson
Radiologist: A. Maydell

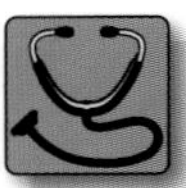

Clinical Insights

- In children, causes are multiple, commonest being mumps.
- A common feature of HIV infection in areas of high prevalence.
- Recurrent parotitis of childhood is far less common.
- Suppurative parotitis usually arises from lymph nodes within parotid.
- The facial nerve is at risk during parotid abscess drainage.
- Parotid tumours are rare in children but have a high incidence of malignancy.
- Parotid is a common site for vascular abnormalities including hemangiomas, vascular malformations and cystic hygroma.

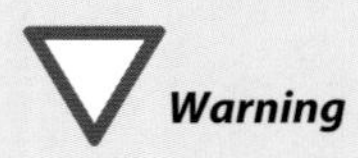

Warning

- HIV precautions may be needed.

Controversy

- Is sialography useful in children? MR sialography precludes need to cannulate duct.

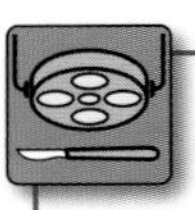

What the Surgeon Needs to Know

- Can features suggestive of HIV infection be identified?
- Can a calculus be identified?
- Is the ductal system dilated?
- If mass present, is it:
  - In superficial or deep lobe?
  - Solid or cystic?
  - Single or multiple?

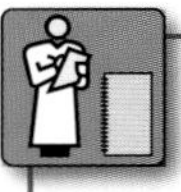

Clinical Differential Diagnosis

- Mumps
- Pseudomegaly, e.g. hypertrophy of masseter
- HIV-related parotid cysts
- Juvenile recurrent parotitis
- Parotitis
- Sialectasis
- Tumour including infantile hemangioma
- Hamartoma
- Vascular malformation

Urgency

- ❑ Emergency
- ❑ Urgent
- ☑ Elective

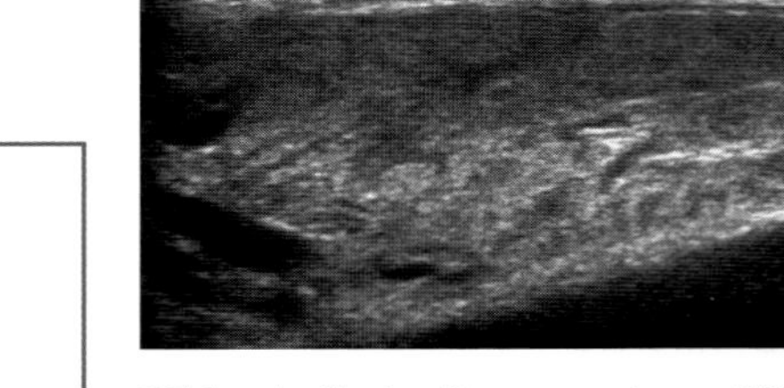

US longitudinal – Demonstrating a diffusely echogenic and enlarged parotid in a child with inflammatory parotitis

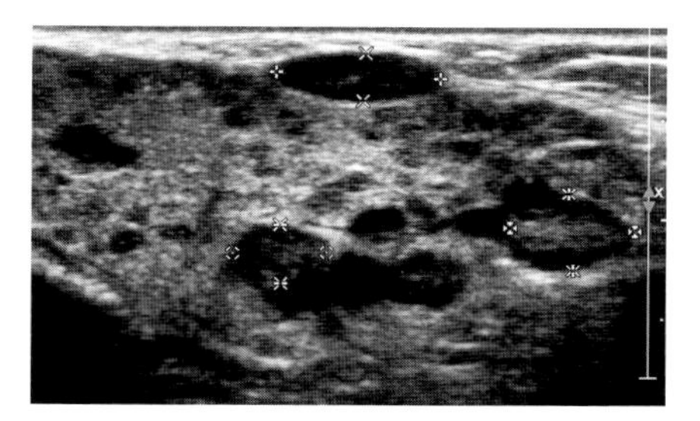

US longitudinal – In a child with bilaterally painless enlarged parotids demonstrates multiple parotid cysts (calipers) compatible with the patient's positive HIV status

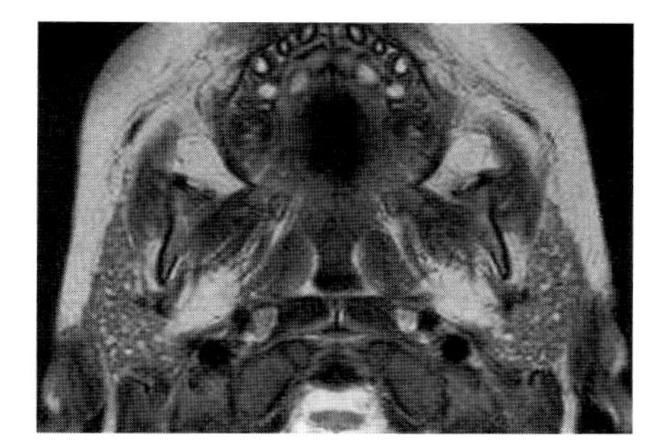

MRI axial T2 – Demonstrating bilateral enlarged parotid glands with multiple cysts in a HIV-positive child, in keeping with lymphoepithelial disease

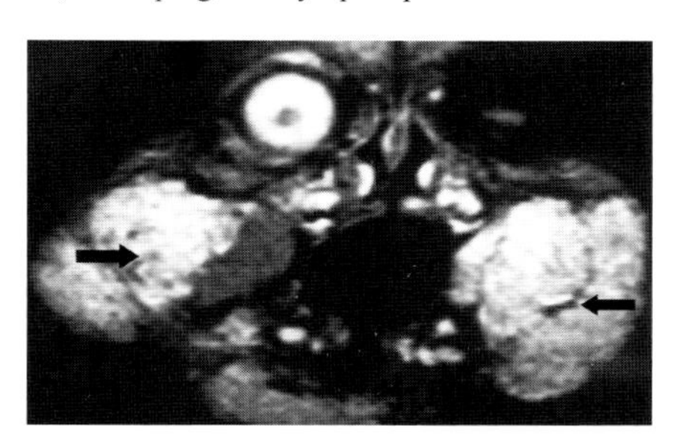

MRI coronal T2 – Bilateral massively enlarged parotid glands showing high signal and multiple flow voids, in keeping with hemangiomas (*arrows*)

Tips

- Identify whether uni or bi-lateral disease (HIV and viral parotitis often bilateral)
- CT and coronal reformat helpful to evaluate relation to external auditory canal
- MRI for deep extensions, sinus tracts and facial nerve involvement

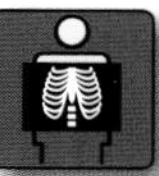

Imaging Options

- Primary: US
- Back-up: CT/MRI
- Follow on: Sialography for stricture or sialectasis

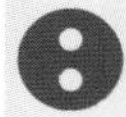

Imaging Findings

US

- Diffuse: Exclude diffuse inflammation from focal mass
- Cystic: Exclude abscess (tender) with pyrexia and HIV lymphoepithelial cysts
- Calcifications: Exclude calculus disease

Doppler

- Identify/exclude vascular density and peak flow of hemangioma
- Identify non-flow related cystic spaces of cystic hygroma

CT/MRI

- Focal nature of mass or total involvement/destruction of gland
- Enhancing heterogenous pattern in neoplasms
- Cystic, solid or mixed patterns occur in different varieties of mass
- Central necrosis in malignant neoplasms
- Extent, involvement of facial nerve, vascular structures, base of skull/foramina and pterygopalatine fossa

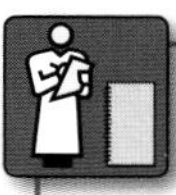

Radiological Differential Diagnosis

- Infective: mumps, TB, bacterial suppurative sialoadenitis
- HIV-associated lymphoepithelial disease
- Sarcoidosis, Sjögren disease
- Benign: hemangioma, lymphangioma, pleomorphic adenoma
- Malignant: rhabdomyosarcoma, mucoepidermoid carcinoma, lymphoma, leukemia

Pelviureteric Junction (PUJ) Obstruction

Surgeon: J. Lazarus
Radiologist: H. von Bezing

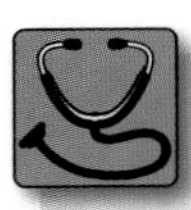

Clinical Insights

- Congenital PUJ obstruction is the most common cause of upper urinary tract obstruction seen on ultrasound in children.
- Congenital hydronephrosis may be benign and resolves in 75% of cases. The rest are truly obstructed and cause progressive renal damage if not corrected.
- MAG-3 or DTPA diuretic renogram can identify the obstructed PUJ and defines the differential renal function. Truly obstructed renal units will display a decline in function over time.
- Indications for surgery include:
  - Pain, infections and stones
  - Deteriorating US findings
  - A differential function of <40% or progressive declining function

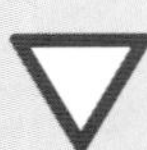

Warnings and  *Controversies*

- The diuretic renogram should be correlated with the ultrasound findings.
- The renogram is typically delayed until 4 weeks of age to allow renal maturation.

Urgency

- ❑ Emergency
- ❑ Urgent
- ☑ Elective

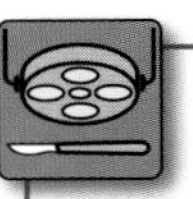

What the Surgeon Needs to Know

- Accurate determination of the AP pelvic diameter
- Is there preservation of cortex
- Presence of a dilated ipsilateral ureter
- Structure of contralateral kidney
- Bladder size, wall thickness and residual volumes

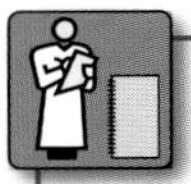

Clinical Differential Diagnosis

- Non-obstructing hydronephrosis
- Hydroureteronephrosis (where the ureter was missed on sonar)
- Multicystic dysplastic kidney

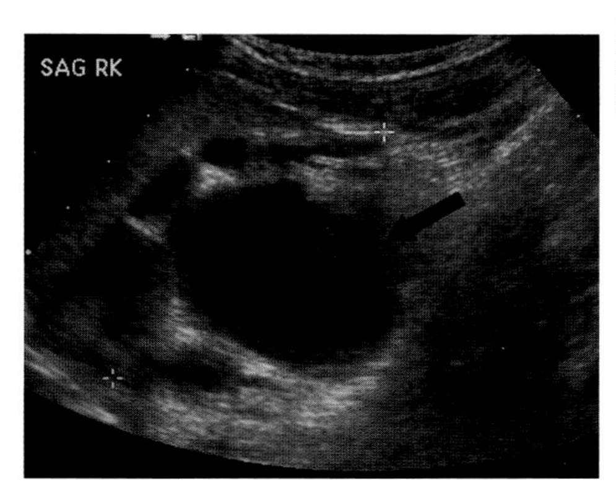

US longitudinal – Demonstrates dilated calyces and a dilated renal pelvis (*arrow*) consistent with a PUJ obstruction [courtesy Doug Jamieson]

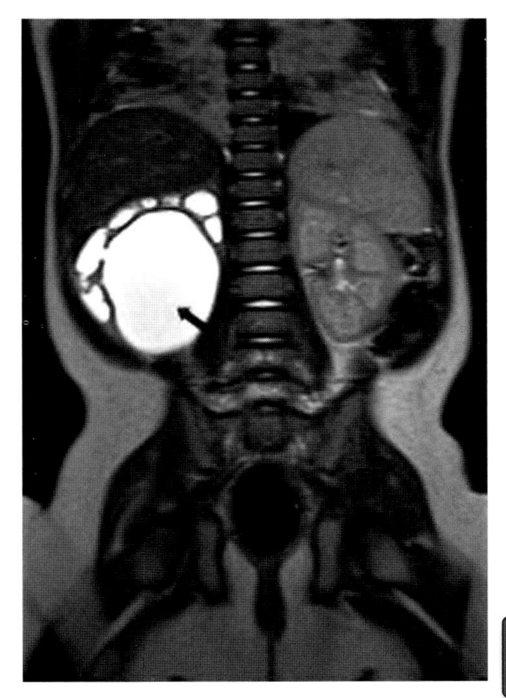

MRI coronal T2 – Demonstrates a massively dilated left renal pelvis (*arrow*) without any ureteric dilation in keeping with a PUJ [courtesy Doug Jamieson]

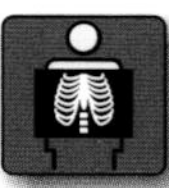

Imaging Options

- Primary: US
- Back-up: Nuc Med (MAG 3 renogram)/ MCUG (to exclude PUV and VUR)/MRI/MRU

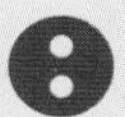

Imaging Findings

US

- Calyces and renal pelvis dilated but no distal ureter seen.
- No evidence dilated ureter, ureterocoele, bladder or posterior urethral dilatation.

Nuc Med

- Mag 3 demonstrates an obstruction and a level at the pelvi-ureteric junction.

MRI/MRUrogram

- Replaces IVP for demonstrating anatomy (heavily weighted T2 – thick slab).
- Time-resolved contrast-enhanced MRI can also demonstrate obstruction.

Tips

- AP renal pelvis measurement on transverse US is used as the standard and for follow-up.
- <1 cm = normal, 1–2 cm = grey area, >2 cm = abnormal.
- Ultrasound cannot prove an obstruction – Mag 3 renogram is used for this.

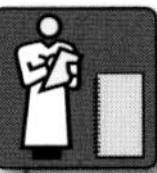

Radiological Differential Diagnosis

- Hydronephrosis of other etiologies
- Megacalycosis or congenital megacalyces
- MDCK (no communication between pelvis and calyces)

Posterior Urethral Valve (PUV)

Surgeon: J. Lazarus
Radiologist: H. von Bezing

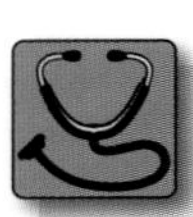

Clinical Insights

- PUV is a congenital obstructing membrane in the posterior male urethra.
- PUV has a spectrum of severity with the most complicated cases presenting with:
  - Neonatal renal insufficiency
  - Pulmonary hypoplasia
  - Early death
- 25% of paediatric renal transplant recipients have a background of PUV.
- MCUG forms the cornerstone of diagnosis:
  - A dilated posterior urethra, typically with a ratio of 5:1 in comparison with the anterior urethra.
  - A trabeculated, small-volume bladder with diverticula.
  - Vesico-ureteric reflux.
  - A hypertrophied bladder neck.
- Passage of a urethral catheter is the initial treatment; valve ablation follows once the child is stable.
- Lifelong clinical and radiological follow up is required.

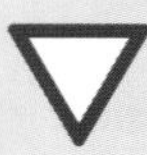

Warnings and  *Controversies*

- As a result of newborn oliguria, ante-natal hydronephrosis may transiently improve and a repeat sonar is recommended in these cases.
- Hydronephrosis may persist after successful valve ablation.
- Incontinence in an older boy should prompt evaluation to exclude PUV.

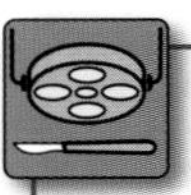

What the Surgeon Needs to Know

- Degree of residual hydronephrosis on follow-up
- Renal growth on follow-up
- Features of dysplasia
- Bladder wall thickness
- Post-micturition residual volume

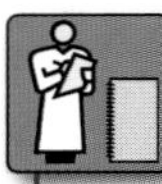

Clinical Differential Diagnosis

- Neuropathic bladder
- Bilateral refluxing or obstructed megaureters
- Urethral stricture
- Prune belly syndrome

Urgency

- ☐ Emergency
- ☐ Urgent
- ☑ Elective

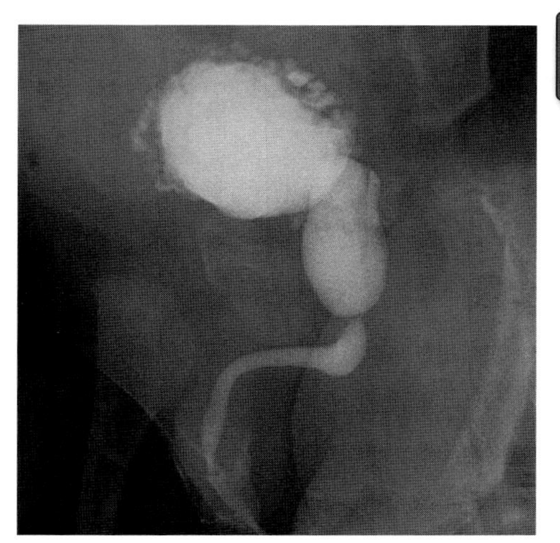

MCUG – A thick-walled trabeculated bladder is present and is the result of posterior urethral valve. The valve is best recognised by the calibre difference between the posterior and anterior urethra

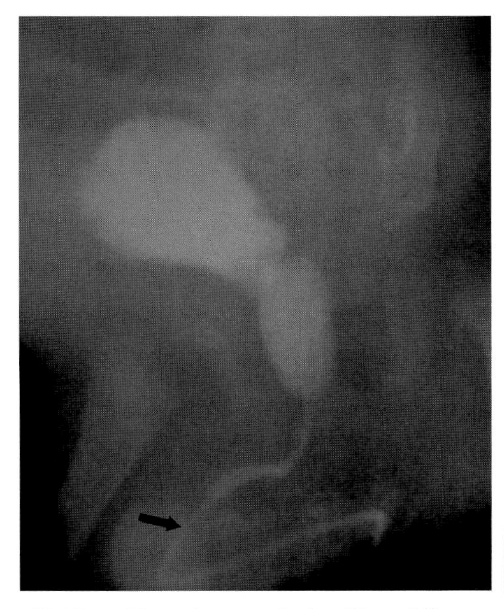

MCUG – There is a marked calibre difference between the posterior and anterior urethra even while the catheter (*arrow*) is in position in keeping with PUV

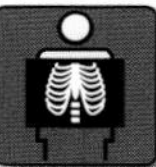

Imaging Options

- Primary: MCUG, US

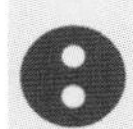

Imaging Findings

MCUG

- Variation of severity.
- Calibre change in urethra. More severe show ratio of posterior:anterior 6:1 (normal is 3:1).
- Valve tissue may not be seen.
- Bladder wall thick with trabeculations/ sacculations/diverticula.
- VUR and reflux into utricle.

US

- Enlarged thick-walled bladder.
- Hydronephrosis, hydro-ureter (Uni- or Bilateral).
- Peri-renal urinoma may occur.
- "Keyhole" dilated posterior urethra.

Tips

- Catheter need not be removed during MCUG.
- Calibre ratio of posterior:anterior urethra may not return to normal after surgery and may remain at 4:1.

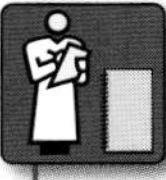

Radiological Differential Diagnosis

- Anterior urethral valves – Different site
- Voiding dysfunction
- Cecoureterocele
- Urethral stricture
- Non-obstructive "ring" in posterior urethra

Ranula (Plunging Ranula)

Surgeon: O. Basson
Radiologists: P. janse van Rensburg, L. janse van Renbu

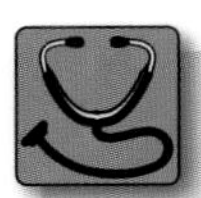

Clinical Insights

- Name arises from appearance of the soft belly of a frog.
- Usually occur in floor of mouth
- A mucocoele of a minor salivary gland or from the sublingual gland; epithelial lined.
- May arise in an obstructed submandibular duct.
- May progress deeply around the mylohyoid muscle into the neck as a mucus extravasation without epithelial lining – plunging ranula.
- Usually clinically obvious, and imaging only required if diagnosis in doubt.

Warning

- If late presentation or if infected, may force tongue upwards and backwards to cause airway obstruction.

Controversy

- Which is the gland of origin?

Urgency

- ❑ Emergency
- ❑ Urgent
- ☑ Elective

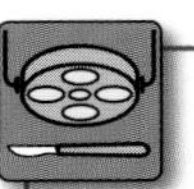

What the Surgeon Needs to Know

- Is this an isolated cystic swelling or a cystic portion of other pathology?
- Is there a calculus present?
- Is the submandibular gland involved – Pathology in this gland in children may be malignant.

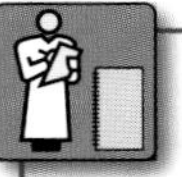

Clinical Differential Diagnosis

- Cystic hygroma
- Teratoma/hamartoma

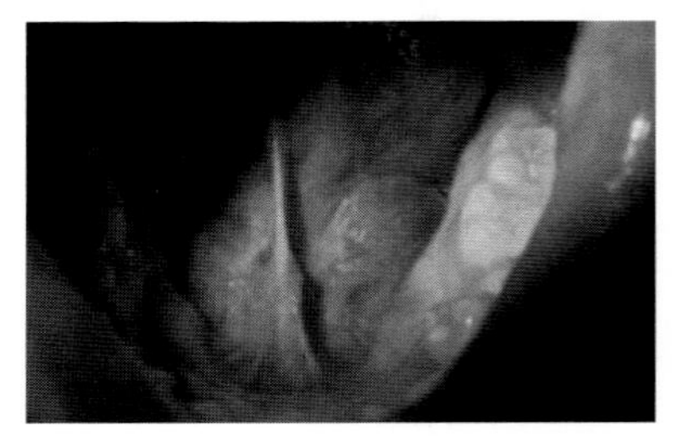

Swelling in the left side of the floor of the mouth in a patient with a ranula

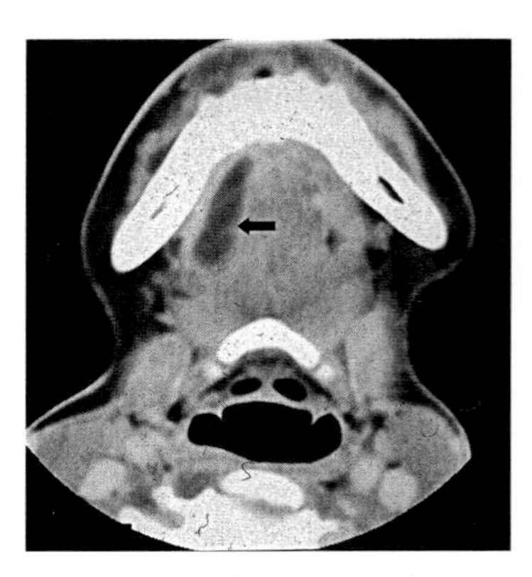

Contrast-enhanced axial CT – Low density mass in right sublingual space at the origin of the ranula (*arrow*) with mild wall enhancement

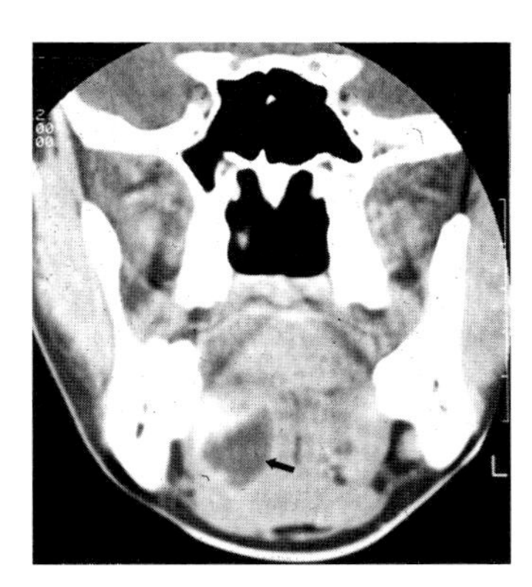

Contrast-enhanced coronal CT – Demonstration of the sublingual position of the ranula (*arrow*)

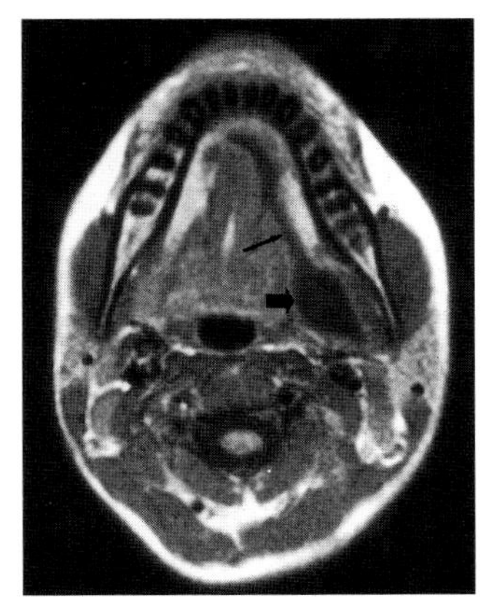

Axial T1-weighted MRI – Left-sided comet shaped plunging ranula with the tail in the sublingual space (*thin arrow*) and the head in the submandibular space (*thick arrow*).

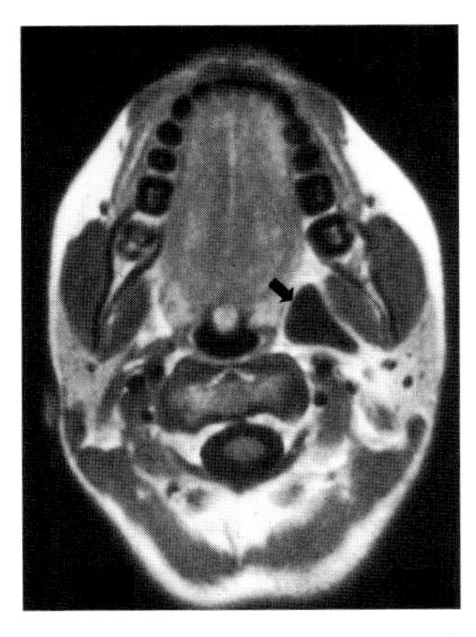

Axial T1-weighted enhanced MRI – Wall enhancement and extension of the left-sided ranula (*arrow*) into the parapharyngeal space

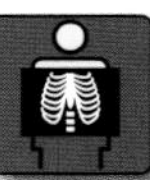

Imaging Options

- Primary: CT
- Alternative: MRI

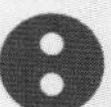

Imaging Findings

CT/MRI

- Thin-walled, well-defined low-density mass (CT low, T1 low, T2 high)
- Comet shaped
- Originates from sublingual space ("tail")
- Extends into submandibular space forming a pseudocyst ("head")
- May involve inferior parapharyngeal space
- Wall may enhance

Tips

- May plunge anteriorly to submandibular gland or cross midline
- Infected lesion exhibits distention and thicker wall
- Multiplanar imaging useful to evaluate transspatial extension

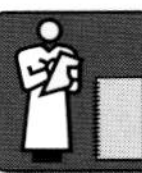

Radiological Differential Diagnosis

- Simple ranula (sublingual retention cyst)
- Dermoid
- Second branchial cleft cyst
- Lymphangioma
- Suppurative lymph node
- Abscess

Renal Calculi

Surgeon: A. Alexander
Radiologist: S. Cader

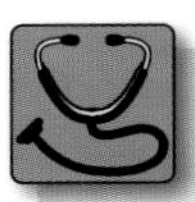

Clinical Insights

- Nephrolithiasis is relatively uncommon in the paediatric population.
- Calculi are an indicator of metabolic dysfunction, anatomical abnormalities or infection.
- The majority of paediatric calculi are calcium stones.
- Younger children:
  - Present atypically with urosepsis, haematuria or abdominal pain
  - Have a larger stone burden, most often involving the kidney
  - Neonatal stone disease is often iatrogenic (lasix)
- Older children:
  - Tend to present with ureteric stones and have a higher rate of spontaneous passage
- Uncomplicated small (<5 mm) stones tend to pass spontaneously and are best treated with hydration and analgesia.

Warnings

- Sepsis in the presence of an obstructing renal stone is a surgical/radiological emergency.
- Obstruction and stones in a solitary kidney is a urological emergency.
- Urate stones are not visible on X-ray.

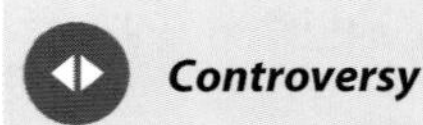

Controversy

- Shock wave lithotrypsy vs. percutaneous nephrolithotrypsy vs. endourology as the best modality for stone management

Urgency

- ❑ Emergency
- ❑ Urgent
- ☑ Elective (unless septic)

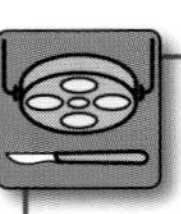

What the Surgeon Needs to Know

- Number of calculi?
- Position (spontaneous passage more likely in lower ureter)?
- Size (<5 mm more likely to pass)?
- Is there an underlying anatomical abnormality?
  - Uretero-pelvic junction obstruction
  - Ureteric strictures
  - Nephrocalcinosis
  - Calycael diverticulum
  - Medullary sponge kidney
- Osteopaenia (which may indicate abnormal calcium homeostasis)?

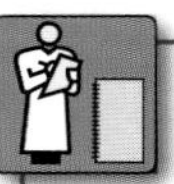

Clinical Differential Diagnosis

- Nephrocalcinosis
- Deflux injection bleb at the ureteric orifice
- Calcified ureteric polyp

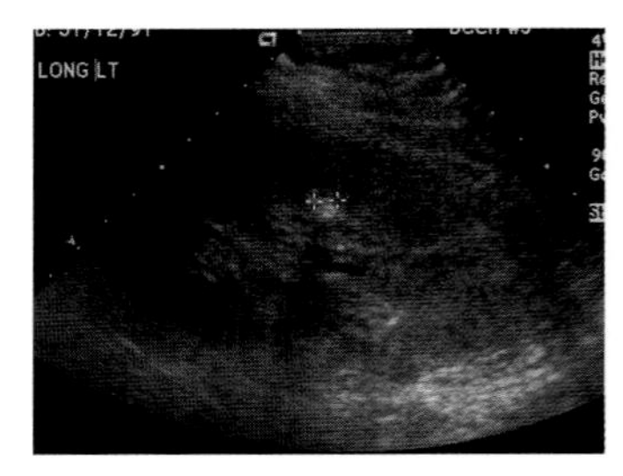

US – Showing an echogenic caculus with posterior acoustic shadowing (*arrow*) [courtesy Doug Jamieson]

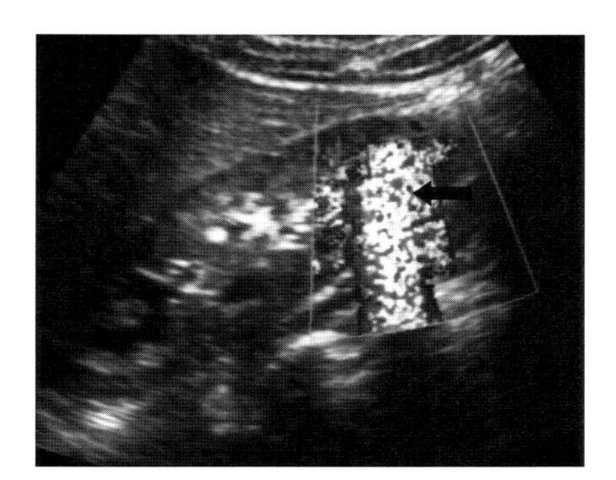

US – Demonstrating the "twinkling sign" (*arrow*) of color Doppler

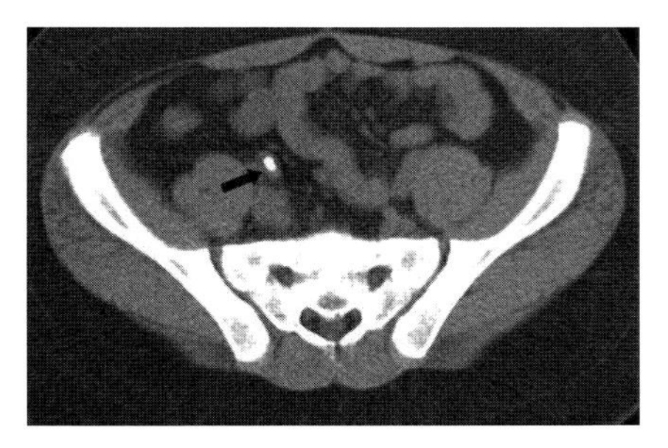

CT – Non-contrast technique demonstrating a right ureteric calculus (*arrow*)

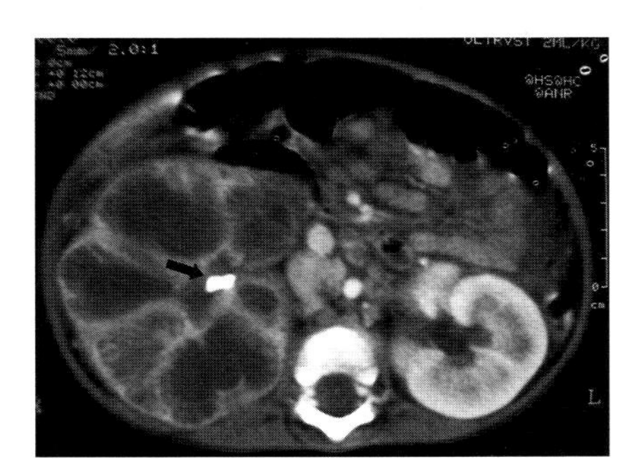

Contrasted CT performed to define a renal mass demonstrates an enlarged kidney with areas of low density and a (staghorn) calculus (*arrow*) in keeping with xanthogranulomatous pyelonephritis

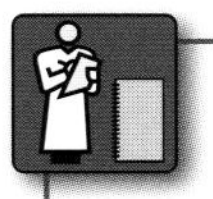

Radiological Differential Diagnosis

- Nephrocalcinosis
- Calcification in a neoplasm

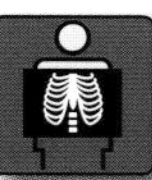

Imaging Options

- Primary: AXR, US
- Secondary: CT, IVP

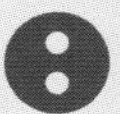

Imaging Findings

AXR

- Visible if radioopaque (may be radiolucent).
- May be seen in the renal areas, in the ureters (over transverse processes of L2–L5 vertebra) or in the bladder.
- May fill the pelvicaliceal system and form a staghorn configuration.

US

- Echogenic foci with acoustic shadowing posterior to calculi
- Good for detecting secondary hydronephrosis and hydroureter

CT (Non-Contrast Technique)

- Visualized as high density
- Better than IVP
- High radiation dose – Reserved for ureteric calculi and those not seen on US

IVP

- Not recommended
- If causing obstruction may have increasingly dense nephrogram with renal enlargement and/or delayed pyelogram with dilatation of collecting system/ureter

Tips

- The "twinkling" sign can be used to confirm a calculus when there is no acoustic shadowing. A positive sign is when color Doppler demonstrates distinct sparkles in the region expected to show the acoustic shadow.
- Xanthogranulomatous pyelonephritis presents as a renal mass, but a clue to differentiating this from other masses is the presence of a stag-horn calculus at the renal pelvis.

Renal Ectopia (Crossed Fused Ectopia/Pelvic Kidney)

Surgeon: A. Alexander
Radiologists: H. von Bezing, J. Naidu

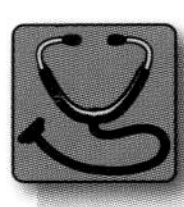

Clinical Insights

- This term describes a kidney not in its normal position – Either lying contralateral to its ureteric bladder insertion (crossed) or ipsilateral (pelvic and other positions).
- Often noted incidentally but crossed varieties especially can present with obstruction, infection, as an abdominal mass and rarely with hypertension.
- "Fused ectopia" is by far the most common (85%) of the crossed variety.
- It is not always easy to confirm the presence of fusion in crossed renal ectopia.
- "Crossed fused ectopia" has been classified based on:
  - Position of the crossed kidney in relation to the normal kidney
  - Rotation of both kidneys (the ectopic one is most often malrotated)
  - Degree of fusion
  - Orientation of the crossed kidney and the fused complex
- Associated abnormalities include:
  - Skeletal, ano-rectal and genital abnormalities
  - The ureter of the crossed kidney can be ectopic
  - Vesico-ureteric reflux is common

Warnings

- Consider pelvic kidney as a cause of a palpated pelvic mass
- Consider renal ectopia in a unilateral kidney
- Confirm the reason for presentation: obstruction, infection

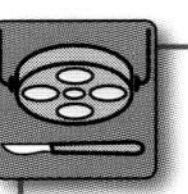

What the Surgeon Needs to Know

- Are there associated urogenital abnormalities, especially reflux?
- Are there renal scars, calculi or Wilm's tumour?
- Are there associated systemic abnormalities?

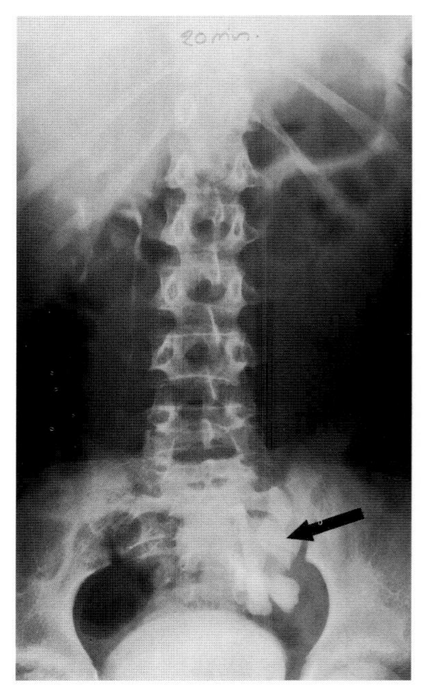

IVU – Demonstrates the dilated calyceal system of an ectopic left kidney in the left pelvis (*arrow*)

Urgency

- ☐ Emergency
- ☐ Urgent
- ☑ Elective

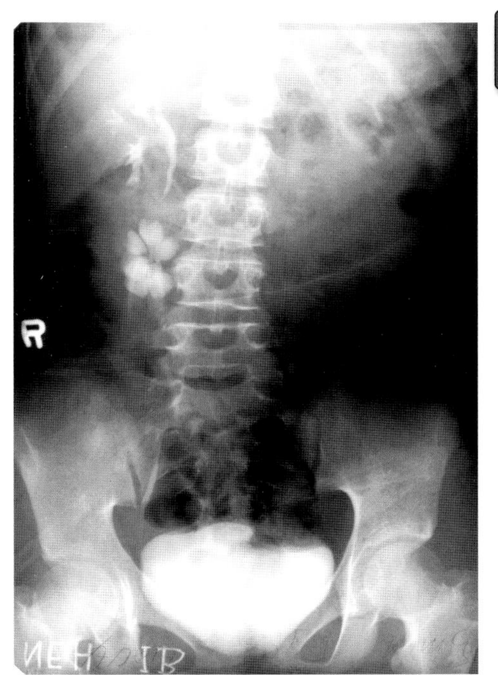

IVU – Demonstrates crossed fused ectopia with no visible system on the left

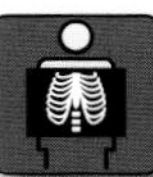

Imaging Options

- Primary: US
- Back-up/Alternative: Nuc Med, IVU, MRI, CT

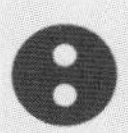

Imaging Findings

US

- Normal renal tissue in abnormal location
- No kidney in the flank with a "Lying down" adrenal sign/"pancake" adrenal (a flat ipsilateral adrenal)
- Ectopic kidney: "Mass" in the pelvis (kidney often multicystic/hydronephrotic)
- Normal/enlarged contralateral kidney
- Crossed fused kidneys: fused kidneys, one of which is rotated and inferior.

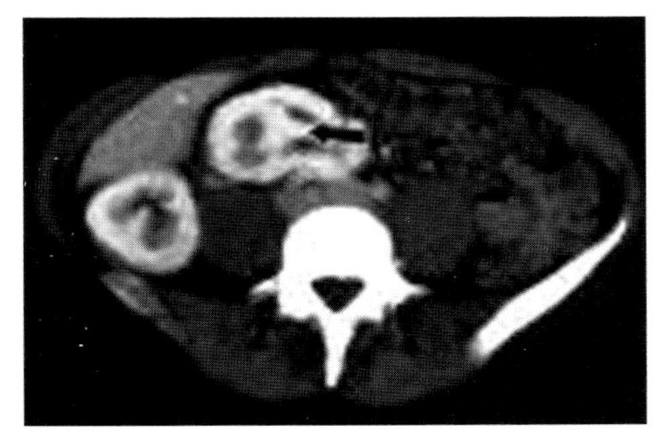

CT – Demonstrates the crossed position of the left kidney (*arrow*) seen separately from the right kidney but to the right of the midline

Tips (Associations)

- Renal agenesis
- Genital anomalies
- Cardiac and skeletal anomalies
- VACTERL

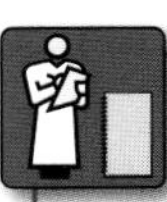

Radiological Differential Diagnosis

- Unilateral renal agenesis
- Any "mass" typical for ectopic location – desmoid, omental cake
- Intussusception (Pseudokidney sign)

Retropharyngeal Abscess (Pre-vertebral abscess)

Surgeon: O. Basson
Radiologists: P. Janse van Rensburg, L. Janse van Rensburg

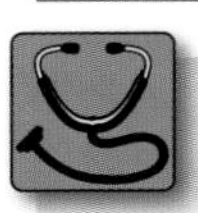

Clinical Insights

- Majority occur in children under the age of 4 because retropharyngeal nodes drain infected tonsils, teeth, sinuses or pharynx.
- Child is toxic, drools and may have stertor and even stridor if the larynx is compressed.

Warnings

- These infants may have severe airway compromise.
- If airway is compromised, child must be assessed by an ENT before imaging – Emergency drainage may be necessary.
- Widening of retropharyngeal space is frequently an "artefact" due to flexion or crying.

Urgency

- [x] Emergency
- [ ] Urgent
- [ ] Elective

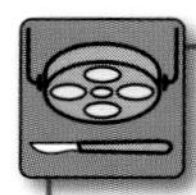

What the Surgeon Needs to Know

- Is retropharyngeal space widened? If so, then CT is needed to identify the presence of abscess and determine intra-thoracic extension.

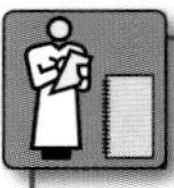

Clinical Differential Diagnosis

- Laryngotracheobronchitis
- Acute epiglottitis
- Quinsy

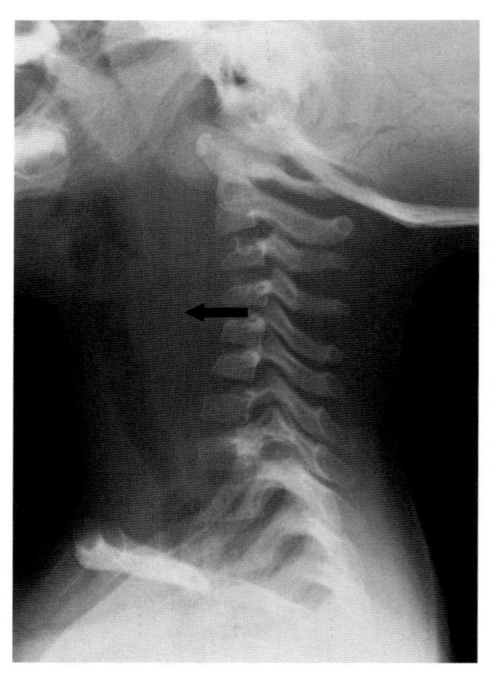

X-ray lateral neck – Severe widening of the retropharyngeal soft tissue (*arrow*) and loss of cervical lordosis

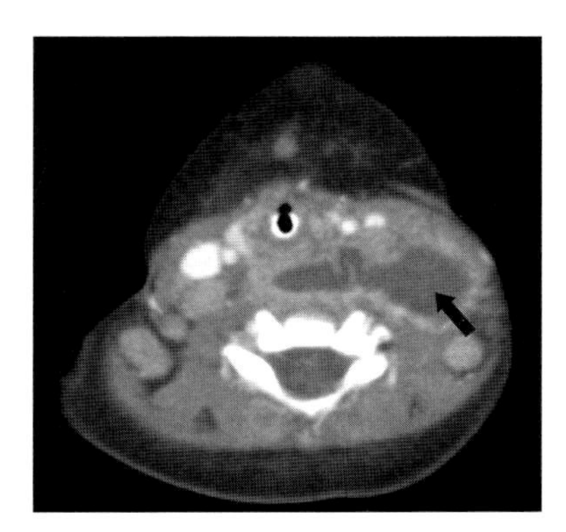

CT post-contrast – Ring enhancement of a retropharyngeal abscess extending to the left of the midline (*arrow*). Note mass effect on the adjacent vessels [courtesy Doug Jamieson]

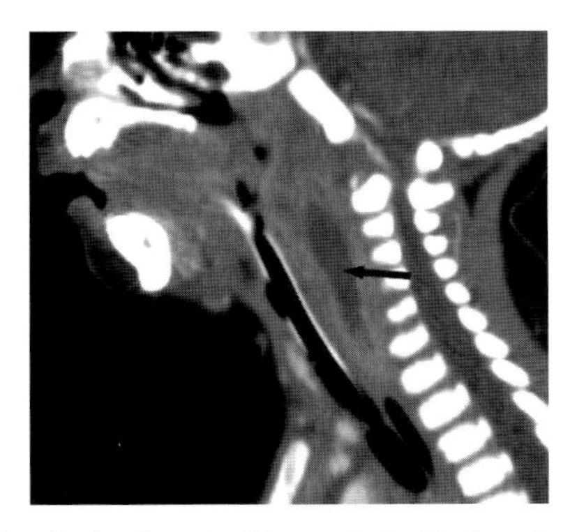

CT sagittal reformat – Demonstrates the low density retropharyngeal abscess extending cranio-caudally (*arrow*) [courtesy Doug Jamieson]

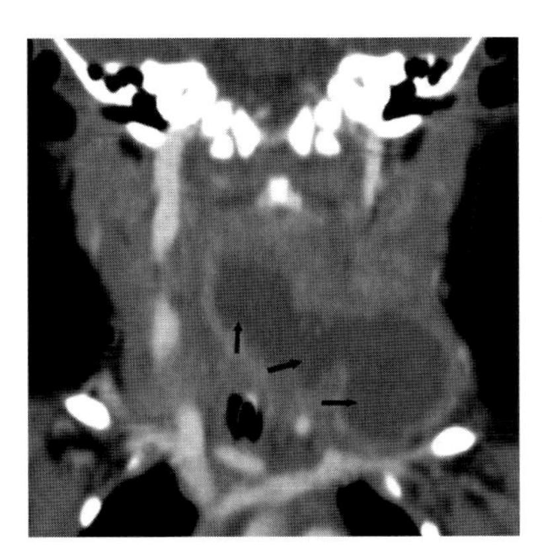

CT coronal reformat demonstrates the irregular margins, low density content and ring enhancement associated with a retropharyngeal abscess (*arrows*) [courtesy Doug Jamieson]

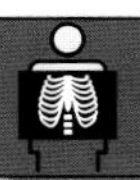

Imaging Options

- Primary: Lateral neck X-ray
- Follow-on: CT

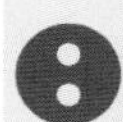

Imaging Findings

Lateral Neck X-Ray

- Widening of the pre-vertebral soft tissue
- Loss of cervical lordosis
- Gas in pre-vertebral soft tissue is diagnostic (not to be confused with swallowed air)

CT

- Low attenuation area expanding retropharyngeal space ± ring enhancement
- Mass effect on adjacent structures
- Complications: mediastinitis, vascular or airway compromise

Tips

- Perform X-ray neck in extension during inspiration (flexion and crying mimics abscess)
- Adenitis, cellulitis and abscess are a continuum
- Scan from skull base to carina ('danger space' extends this far)

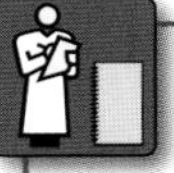

Radiological Differential Diagnosis

- Pseudothickening of retropharyngeal soft tissue (technical)
- Suppurative adenitis (±oedema)
- Reactive adenopathy
- Lymphatic malformation
- Upper respiratory tract infection: epiglotitis, laryngotracheobronchitis
- Neoplasm

A B C D E F G H I J K L M N O P Q R S T U V W X Y Z

Rhabdomyosarcoma

Surgeon: S. Moore
Radiologist: P. J. Greyling

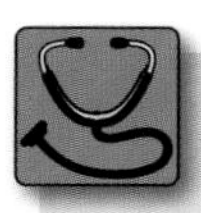

Clinical Insights

- Tumour of embryonic muscle
- 5% of malignant tumours in children
- 60% of soft-tissue tumours in children
- Occurs at any site, any time
- 66% less than 10 years of age
- Two peak occurrences:
  - 2–6 years – Mostly head and neck and genito-urinary
  - 15–19 years – Extremities, trunk, male genital system
- Site-specific signs and symptoms
- May present as asymptomatic mass
- Hidden location often delays presentation
- Generalized – fever, anorexia, weight loss, pain
- Prognosis related to age, site, tissue type and stage

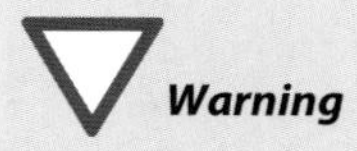

- Syndromic associations:
  - Neurofibromatosis
  - Li-Fraumeni
  - Beckwith-Wiedemann

Urgency

- ❑ Emergency
- ❑ Urgent
- ☑ Elective

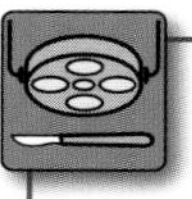

What the Surgeon Needs to Know

- Site-specific diagnostic features
- Extent of spread

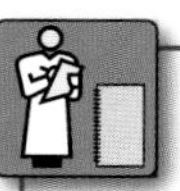

Clinical Differential Diagnosis

- Neuroblastoma
- Lymphoma/leukaemia
- PNET (primitive neuroectodermal tumour)
- Wilm's tumour
- Other small blue cell tumours

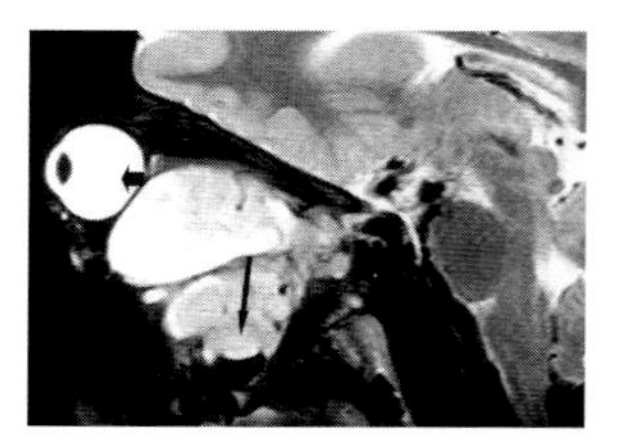

MRI sagittal oblique STIR – A mass has displaced the globe (*short arrow*) and optic nerve superiorly has expanded the orbit and destroyed the orbital floor and extended into the maxillary sinus and the alveolar bone (*long arrow*)

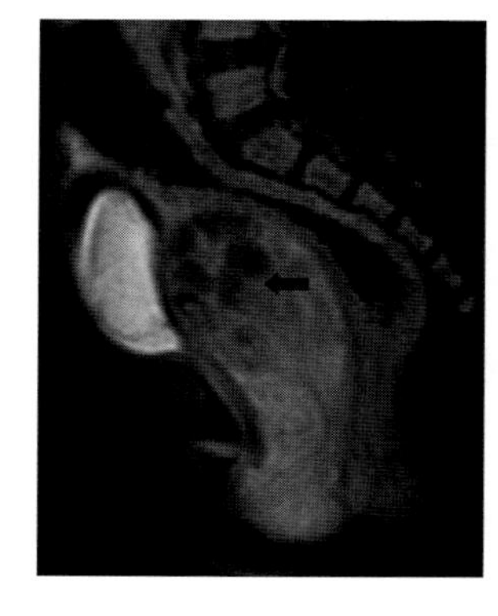

MRI sagittal STIR – Of the pelvis demonstrates a vaginal mass (*arrow*) representing a rhabdomyosarcoma

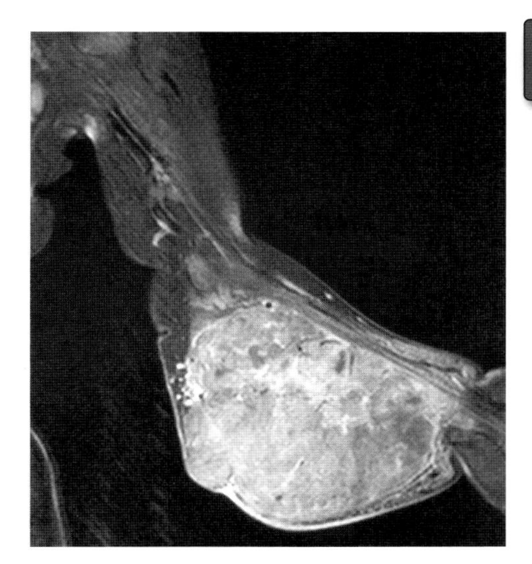

MRI STIR – Of the upper limb in a 4- month-old boy with a rhabdomyosarcoma of the right fore arm demonstrating an inhomogeneous, fairly well-encapsulated mass

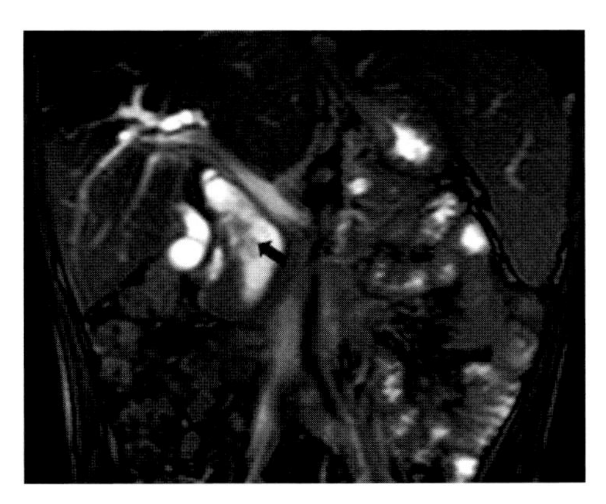

MRI coronal heavily T2 weighted – Demonstrates a mass arising from the biliary tree (*arrow*), which in a child is most likely to be a rhabdomyosarcoma

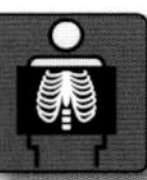

Imaging Options

- Primary: MRI
- Follow-on: CT/US/Nuc Med (bone scan)

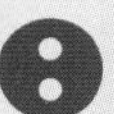

Imaging Findings

- Genitourinary
  [Boys: bladder, prostate and para-testicular]
  [Girls: vulva/vagina (infancy), cervix (reproductive years)]
- Extremities
- Head and neck (orbit)

US

- Heterogeneous echogenicity ± hypoechoic areas (cystic)
- Hyperemic on flow Doppler

CT

- Heterogeneous mass
- Variable contrast enhancement
- Local invasion
- Liver metastases

MRI

- Iso/hypointense on T1
- Hyperintense on T2
- Heterogeneous enhancement
- Local invasion
- Liver metastases

Tips

- MRI: Assess meningeal extension, intraspinal extension and orbital involvement.
- Site matters for diagnosis, therapy and prognosis.

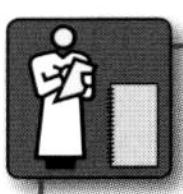

Radiological Differential Diagnosis

- Head and Neck – lymphoma, neuroblastoma, infection
- Abdominopelvic – neuroblastoma, lymphoma, sacrocoocygeal teratoma
- Limb – Ewing's sarcoma, fibromatosis, synovial sarcoma, infection

Sacrococcygeal Teratoma

Surgeon: I. Simango
Radiologist: N. Wieselthaler

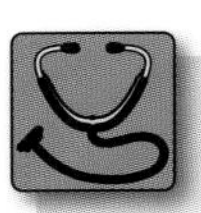

Clinical Insights

- Germ cell tumours account for 3% of neoplasms in children and adolescents.
- Teratoma: Tumour derived from at least 2 of the 3 germ cell layers.
- The commonest type of extra-gonadal germ cell tumour.
- 3–4 times more common in girls.
- Apparent at birth in most cases.
- Less than 10% malignant at birth.
- By 6 months, 40– 80% are malignant.
- Beyond 1year, >80% are malignant.
- Associated anomalies in 20% of cases.
- Aim of surgery: Complete excision including the coccyx.
- Altman classification:
  - Type i – (47%) predominantly external (A)
  - Type ii – (35%) seen externally but significant intra-pelvic component (B)
  - Type iii – (8%) primarily pelvic/ abdominal but is apparent external (C)
  - Type iv – (10%) purely pelvic; no external component (D)

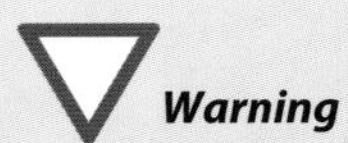

- The coccyx must be removed at surgery to avoid recurrence.

Urgency

- ❑ Emergency
- ❑ Urgent
- ☑ Elective

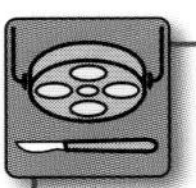

What the Surgeon Needs to Know

- Staging.
- Vascularity – Median sacral artery is the primary vessel of supply.
- Local recurrence.
- Complications: hydronphrosis, neurogenic bladder and bowel obstruction.

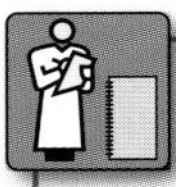

Clinical Differential Diagnosis

- Lipomyelomeningocoele
- Myelomeningocoele
- Dermoid cyst
- Currarino triad

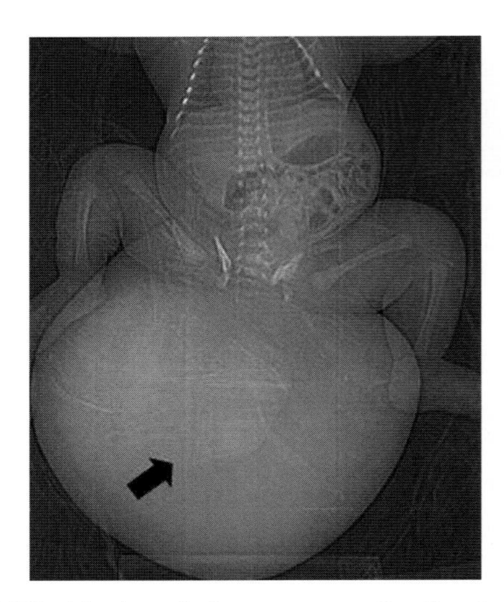

AXR – Massive soft-tissue mass extending from buttock/lower pelvis (*arrow*) in a neonate consistent with a sacrococcygeal teratoma (SCT)

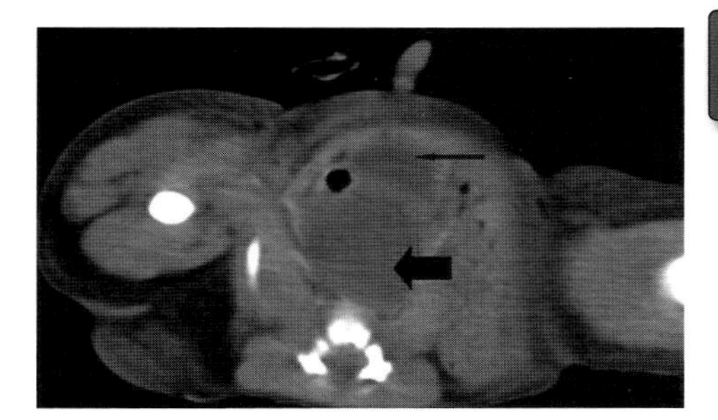

CT – Pre-sacral cystic mass (*thick arrow*) consistent with a SCT. Note the bladder (*thin arrow*) anterior to the mass

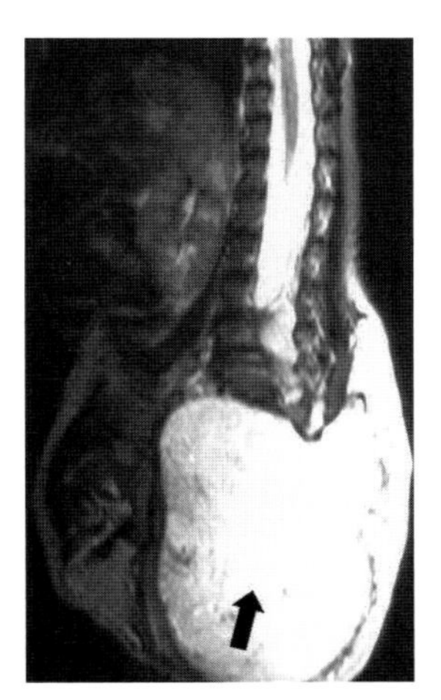

MRI T2 sagittal – A large hyper-intense sacral mass is shown (*arrow*) consistent with a SCT

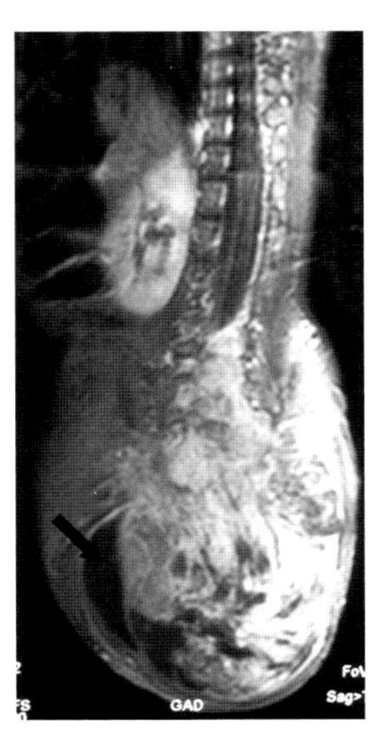

MRI T1 sagittal with gadolinium – Note the variable contrast enhancement of the large SCT with a cystic component (*arrow*)

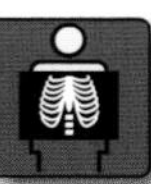

Imaging Options

- Primary: MRI
- Back-up: CT
- Default: (AXR)

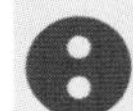

Imaging Findings

CT/MRI

- Large soft-tissue mass that grows around coccyx
- Solid/cystic/mixed
- Mixed signal intensity/density depending on tissue component
- Variable contrast enhancement
- Frequently contain calcification

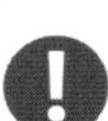

Tips

- May be purely extrapelvic, intrapelvic or a combination.
- Enhancement does not predict malignancy.
- CT/MRI used to define extent/guide surgery.

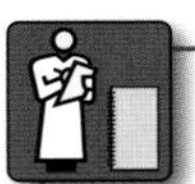

Radiological Differential Diagnosis

- Exophytic rhabdomyosarcoma
- Myelomeningocoele (particularly anterior meningocoele)

Scrotal Mass (See Sects. Torsion Testis and Epidydimo-Orchitis for "Acute Scrotum")

Surgeon: A. Alexander
Radiologist: A. Bagadia

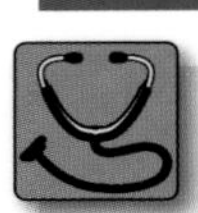

Clinical Insights

- A scrotal mass in a child is more likely to be benign than malignant.
- Masses may arise from the testicle, epididymis, cord structures or paratesticular tissue.
- A history of trauma often accompanies the discovery of the mass.
- Neoplasms are usually painless and non-tender (orchioblastoma, teratoma, yolk sac tumour, Leydig cell tumour).
- Incidence of tumours is bimodal; 12–18 months and puberty.
- 65–85% of all paediatric testicular tumours are of germ cell origin.
- Higher incidence of tumour (seminoma) in undescended testis

Warnings

- May present as hydrocoele and prevent adequate clinical palpation of testis; therefore, exclude masses in tense hydrocoeles.
- May cause precocious puberty if hormonally active (leydig cell).

Controversy

- Natural history of microcalcification (carcinoma in situ) remains uncertain in the prepubertal testis

Urgency

- ❑ Emergency
- ❑ Urgent
- ☑ Elective

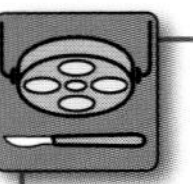

What the Surgeon Needs to Know

- Is it solid or cystic?
- What is the structure of origin?
- What is the status of the contra-lateral scrotum?
- What is the status of draining lymphnodes?

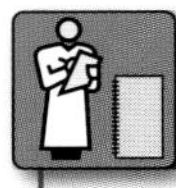

Clinical Differential Diagnosis

- Solid – Tumour or inflammation
- Cystic – Hydrocoele or epidydimal cyst
- Testicular:
  - Orchitis
  - Germ cell tumours
  - Non-germ cell tumours
  - Lymphoma
- Cord structures:
  - Torsion of epididymis
  - Epididymal cyst
  - Encysted hydrocoele
  - Cystic dysplasia of rete testis
- Paratesticular tissue:
  - Rhabdomyosarcoma

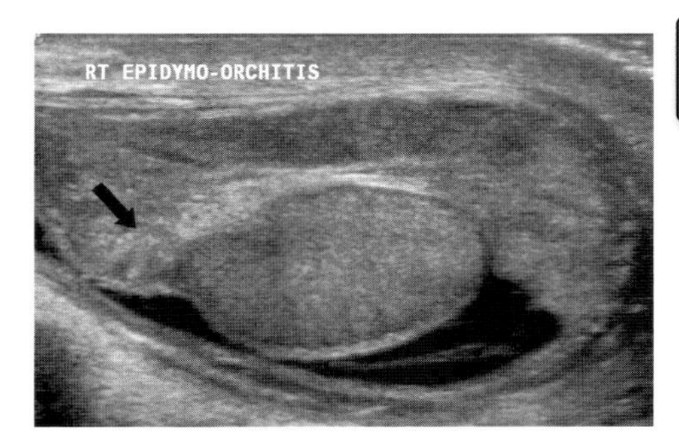

US – Showing an extratesticular mass (*arrow*), which was acutely tender and swollen clinically and proved to be hypervascular (not shown) on Doppler examination, consistent with epidydimo-orchitis

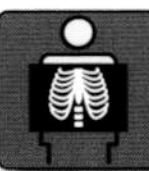

Imaging Options

- Primary: US
- Follow on: CT (intra-abdominal staging)
  PET (residual tumour/tumour response)

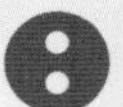

Imaging Findings

US

- Extratesticular:
  - Mass adjacent to testis
- Intratesticular:
  - Irregular, lobulated, well-defined hypo-echoic or complex
  - Variable vascularity on Doppler examination
  - Cystic areas, calcification ± fibrosis – Suggest teratoma/teratocarcinoma
  - Poorly marginated tumour with invasion of tunica and testicular contour distortion – Suggests embryonal cell Ca
  - Haemorrhage ± focal necrosis – Suggests choriocarcinoma

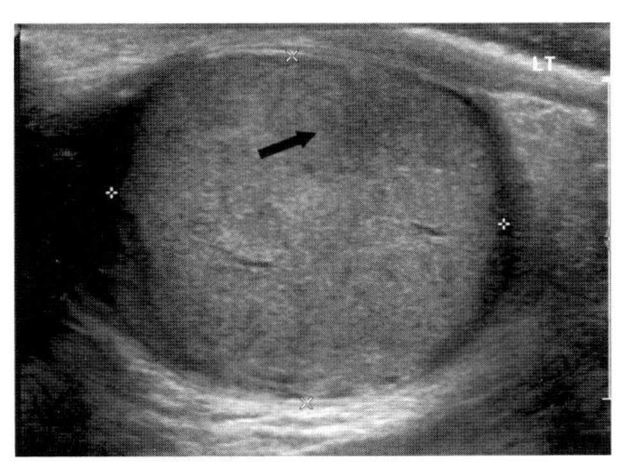

US – Hyopoechoic, ill-defined area anteriorly (*arrow*) representing a testicular neoplasm

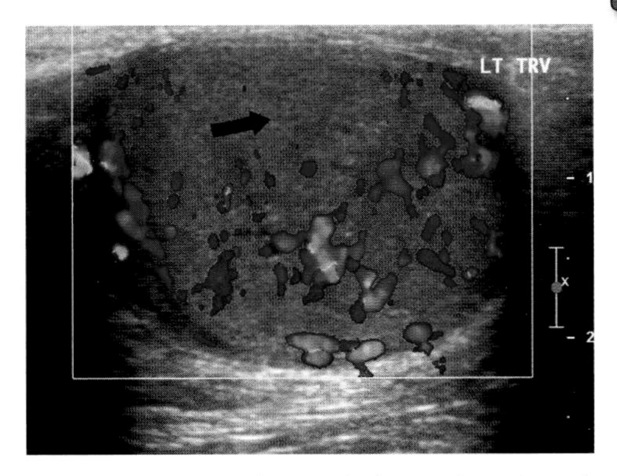

US – A hypovascular intratesticular neoplasm (*arrow*)

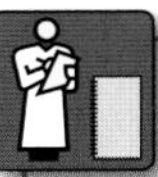

Radiological Differential Diagnosis

- Extratesticular
  - Rhabdomyosarcoma
  - Epidydimo-orchitis
  - Inguinal/scrotal hernia
- Intratesticular
  - Epidydimo-orchitis
  - Haematoma – subacute
  - Epidermoid cyst
  - Testicular granuloma (TB)
  - Lymphoma/leukaemia
  - Focal infarct

Sequestration Pulmonary (Sequestrated Segment)

Surgeon: A. Brooks
Radiologist: T. Kilborn

Clinical Insights

- Defined as a segment or lobe of non-functioning lung tissue with no communication to the normal tracheobronchial tree and with arterial blood supply from a systemic vessel.
- May be extralobar (separate from normal lung; own visceral pleura) or intralobar (within normal lung parenchyma).
- Antenatal diagnosis possible between 16–24 weeks.
- Mostly an incidental finding, but may present with repeated chest infections.
- The diagnosis should be considered in children and young adults with recurrent left lower lobe pneumonia.
- May be a cause of haemoptysis.
- Treated with segmental resection or lobectomy.

Warnings

- The systemic arterial supply may arise from the abdominal aorta and may result in life-threatening bleeding at surgery if not recognized.
- Antenatal sonographic differentiation between sequestration and CCAM may be difficult.
- Extralobar sequestration may also occur in the mediastinum, within or beneath diaphragm and may have a connection with the foregut.

Controversy

- Angiography is seldom necessary (as long as one is aware of the possibility of the infradiaphragmatic origin of the systemic arterial blood supply and other imaging modalities are used).

Urgency

- ☐ Emergency
- ☐ Urgent
- ☑ Elective

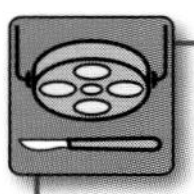

What the Surgeon Needs to Know

- The origin of the arterial supply.
- The pulmonary venous return should be clearly identified because of the association of anomalous venous drainage of a lobe or lobes of the right lung to the inferior vena cava below the diaphragm (Scimitar syndrome).

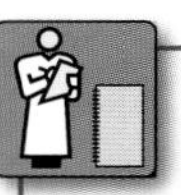

Clinical Differential Diagnosis

- Congenital cystic adenomatoid malformation (CCAM)
- Bronchiectasis

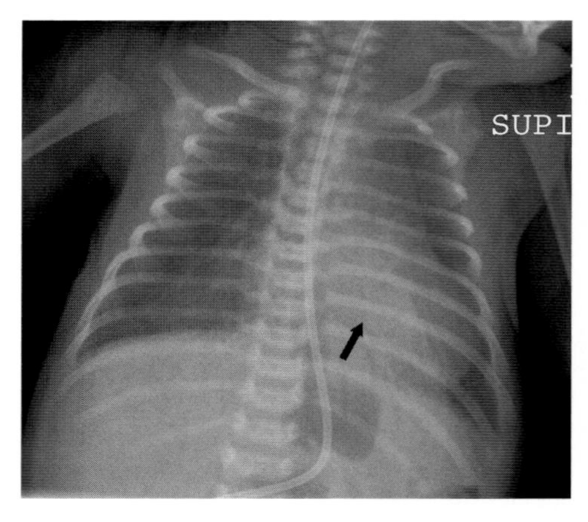

CXR AP – Left lower lobe wedge-shaped opacification (*arrow*) in an infant with recurrent chest infections

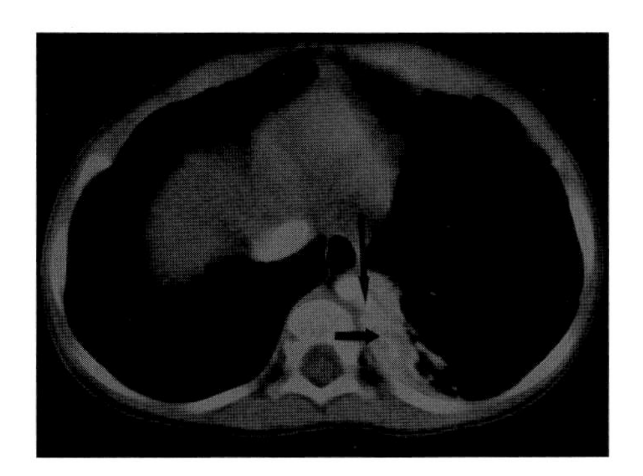

CT post-contrast – Left sequestration seen as posterior wedge shaped area of density (*small arrow*). Arterial supply is from the descending aorta (*long arrow*)

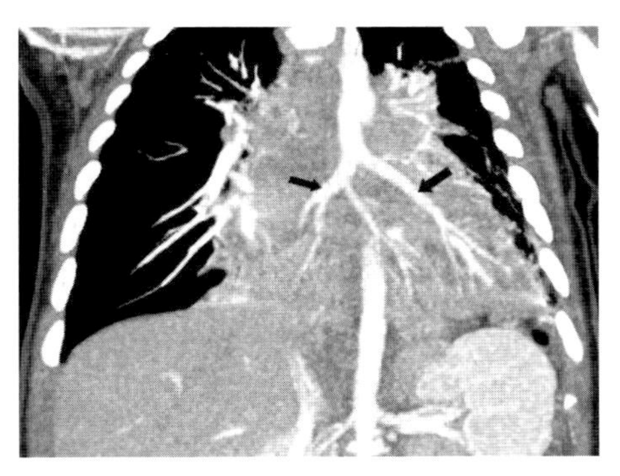

CT coronal reformat (same infant as in the earlier figure) – Demonstrates large bilateral systemic feeding vessels from aorta (*arrows*)

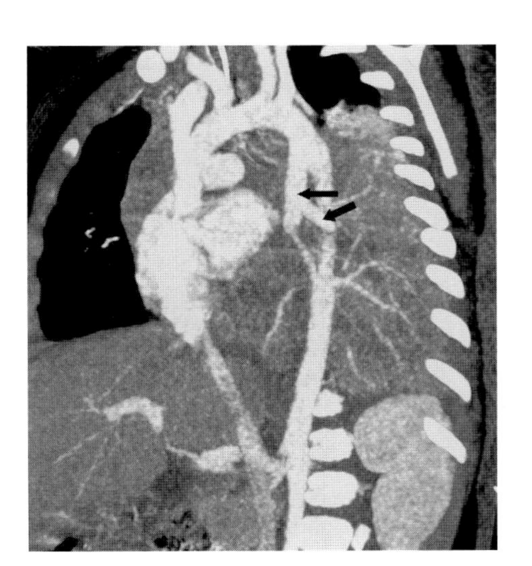

CT sagittal oblique reformat – Large systemic feeding vessel to a sequestration (*arrows*)

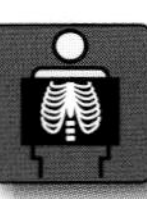

Imaging Options

- Primary: CXR
- Follow on: CT
- Back- up: US, angiography

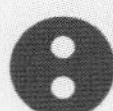

Imaging Findings

- Persistent lower lobe opacity on sequential radiographs (L > R).
- CT in arterial phase shows systemic artery arising from aorta and feeding sequestration. Sequestration appears as an area of pulmonary opacification.
- CT can also define venous drainage.
- If sequestration contains air consider infection but mixed lesions with CCAM also contain air.

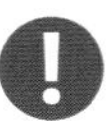

Tips

- If diagnosis is suspected, need to document systemic supply – multislice CT angiogram with multiplanar reformats is the most useful imaging modality as it also allows interrogation of the adjacent parenchyma.
- Need to image from arch to renal arteries as systemic supply may be subdiaphragmatic.

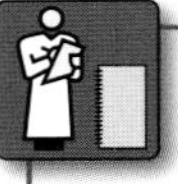

Radiological Differential Diagnosis

- Chronic pneumonia (no systemic supply)
- Aspirated foreign body/chronic bronchial obstruction

Sternomastoid Pseudotumour (Fibromatosis Colli)

Surgeon: A. Darani
Radiologist: T. Kilborn

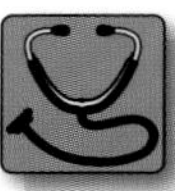

Clinical Insights

- Cause unknown – Often related to forceps or breech delivery.
- Due to fibrous replacement of muscle bundle causing a palpable mass.
- 0.4% of births, present at approximately 2–3 weeks post-partum.
- Usually present with anterolateral neck mass.
- Torticollis may be present – Head is rotated opposite to the involved side with lateral flexion to the affected side.
- Right sided in 60%, bilateral in 2–8%.
- Spontaneous resolution by 6 months of age in 50–70%, 10% persist >12 months.
- Management is conservative with physiotherapy.
- Sternocleidomastoid release indicated if limited head rotation still present at 12–15 months.
- Associated with concomitant hip dysplasia.

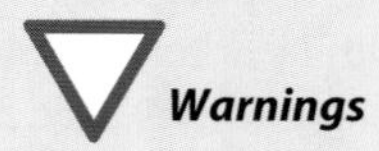

Warnings

- Risk of facial hemihypoplasia, plagiocephaly or postural compensation if persistent
- Needs physiotherapy after surgical division of the muscle and neck fascia

Urgency

- ☐ Emergency
- ☐ Urgent
- ☑ Elective

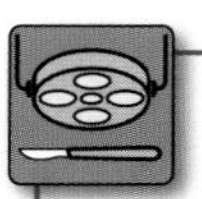

What the Surgeon Needs to Know

- Is the mass related to the sternocleidomastoid?

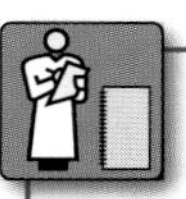

Clinical Differential Diagnosis

- Cervical hemivertebra
- Posterior fossa tumour
- Atlantoaxial subluxation
- Retropharyngeal abscess, lymphadenitis
- Ocular torticollis (squint)
- Rhabdomyosarcoma

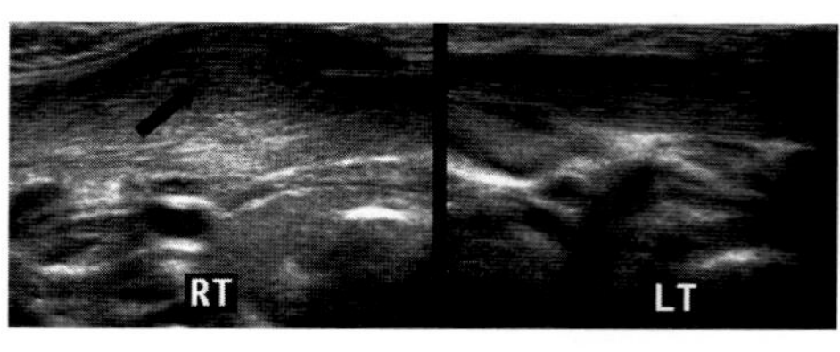

US longitudinal – Showing fusiform enlargement of the right sternocleidomastoid muscle (*arrow*) when compared with the normal muscle on the left. Note slight increase in echotexture and lack of extension outside the muscle

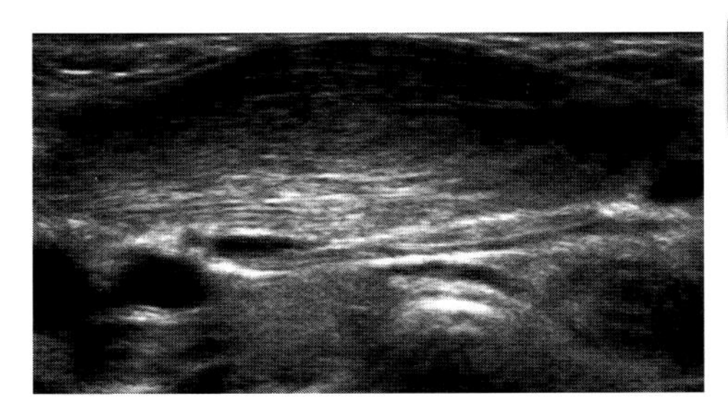

US longitudinal – Zoomed appearance of the sterno-mastoid pseudotumour

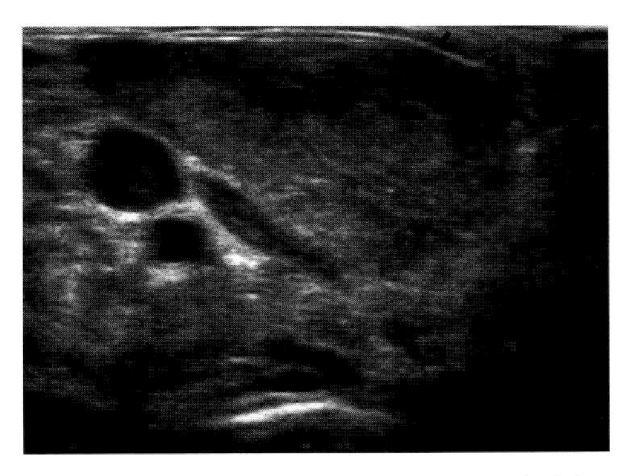

US transverse – Demonstrating the convex bulging of the sternomastoid with preservation of fascial planes (*arrows*)

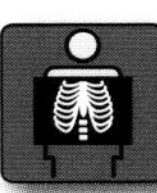

Imaging Options

- Primary: Ultrasound
- Secondary: MRI
- Back-up: X-Ray, CT

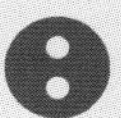

Imaging Findings

US

- Focal or diffuse enlargement of the sternocleidomastoid muscle.
- Can be hypo-, hyper- or iso-echoic to normal muscle.
- 10% can have calcification demonstrating posterior acoustic shadowing.
- No extra-muscular involvement, respects fascial planes.

MRI

- T1 – Hypo/isointense to normal muscle.
- T2 – Variable signal intensity; hypointense areas represent evolving fibrosis otherwise hyper/isointense to normal muscle.

CT

- Isodense/calcified enlarged muscle
- Defines bony anatomy for diagnosing other causes of torticollis

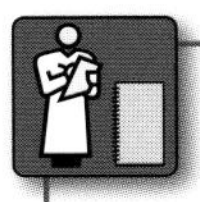

Radiological Differential Diagnosis

- Neuroblastoma – calcified, has bony erosion and intraspinal extension.
- Rhabdomyosarcoma – invasive, vascular.
- Lymphoma – lobulated adenopathy.
- Branchial cleft anomaly – cystic.
- Cervical thymus – Echogenicity similar to and continuity with mediastinal thymus.
- Cervical teratoma – Heterogeneous, usually large with cysts and calcification.
- Spinal fusion abnormality presenting with torticollis – hemi- or fused vertebrae, bony bar, omovertebral bone.

Tips

- US is the best imaging modality; compare with contralateral side.
- Perform MRI if atypical on US.
- May need X-ray ± CT if suspect bone abnormality or erosion.

Takayasu's Arteritis

Surgeon: C. Davies
Radiologist: S. Przybojewski

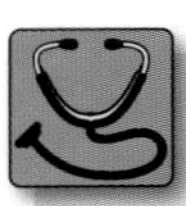

Clinical Insights

- A chronic inflammatory disease of the large arteries:
  - 20% will have monophasic disease without relapse
  - 50% of the remaining 80% will enter remission on immune suppressants
  - It causes stenosis, occlusions or aneurysms in the aorta and its major branches
- Clinically it manifests as:
  - Aorta – Claudication
  - Renal – Hypertension
  - Pulmonary – Pulmonary hypertension
  - Coronaries – Myocardial ischaemia

Controversy

- Causal relationship with TB; 90% have active TB or strongly positive Mantoux

Urgency

- ❑ Emergency
- ❑ Urgent
- ☑ Elective

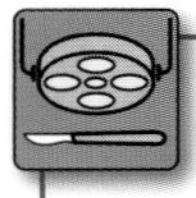

What the Surgeon Needs to Know

- What vessels are involved? (Particularly with regard to kidney perfusion)

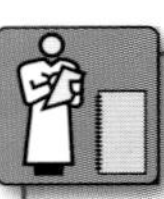

Clinical Differential Diagnosis

- Congenital stenosis
- Other infective causes of aortitis (TB, giant cell)
- Fibromuscular dysplasia

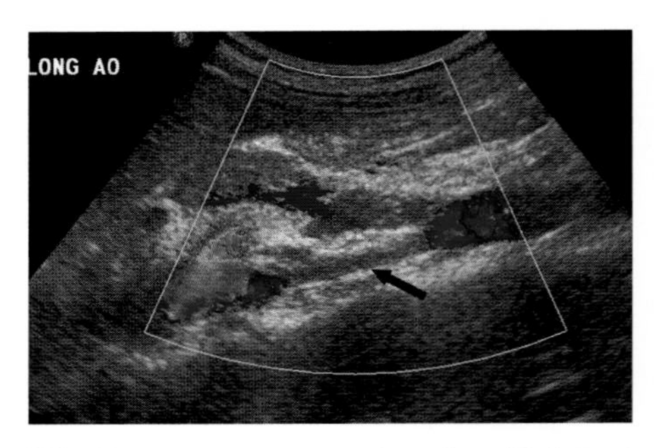

US – Demonstrates a stenosis at the mid abdominal aorta (*arrow*) with no visible flow on colour Doppler imaging

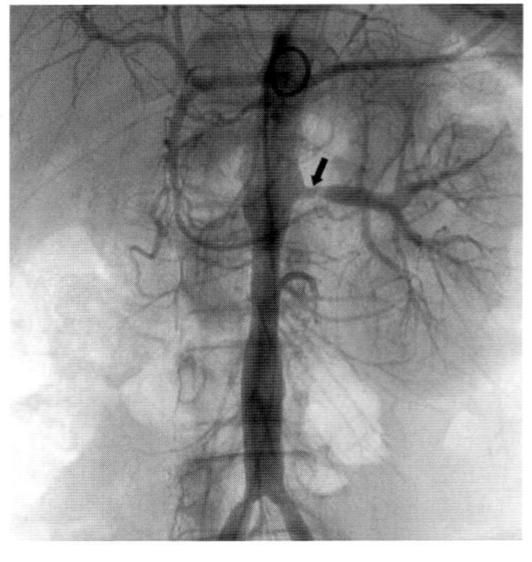

Angiography – Demonstrates alternating levels of fusiform dilation and narrowing involving the abdominal aorta and iliac vessels. The right renal artery is completely occluded and the left demonstrates narrowing at the origin (*arrow*), which feeds off an anuerysmal portion of the aorta

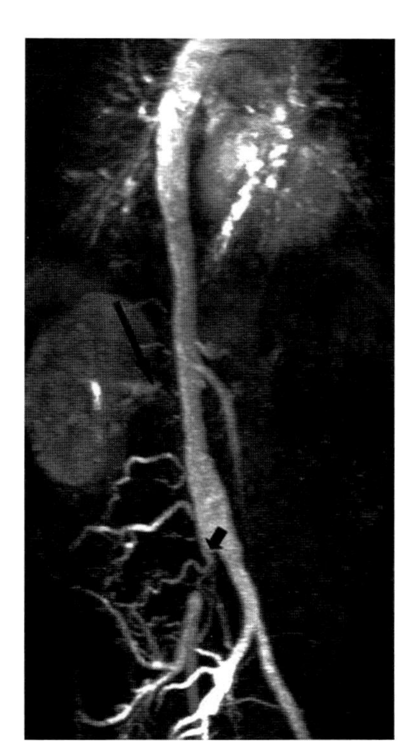

MRA – Demonstrates absence of the left renal artery, severe stenosis of the right renal artery (*long arrow*) and concentric narrowing of the mid thoraco-abdominal aorta. There is also complete stenosis of the right common iliac artery (*short arrow*)

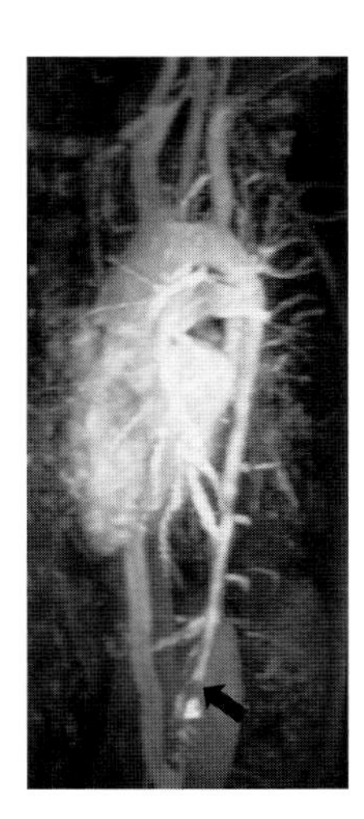

MRA – Demonstrates cutoff of the abdominal aorta (*arrow*) below the celiac trunk

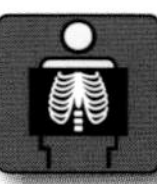

Imaging Options

- Primary: US
- Follow-on: CTA; MRA/MRI
- Follow-up: Angiography

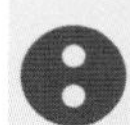

Imaging Findings

US

- Irregularity of aorta with areas of stenosis and saccular dilation.
- Doppler shows occlusion and stenoses as evidenced by dampened flow.

CT/MRI (MRA)

- Aortic stenoses, fusiform/saccular aneurysms
- Pulmonary trunk dilatation, "pruned" pulmonary arteries
- Arterial wall thickening, calcification, enhancement (MRI)
- Irregular stenoses/occlusions at origins of major aortic branches

Angiography

- Irregularity of aorta ("corrugated" appearance) with stenoses/occlusion of origins of major branch vessels

Tips

- Medium to large vessel involvement
- Acute phase: Vessel wall enhancement on MRI
- Chronic phase: Aortic and branch vessel narrowing/occlusion
- Involvement of pulmonary arteries virtually diagnostic

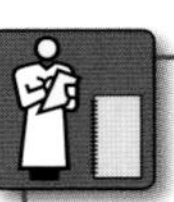

Radiological Differential Diagnosis

- Fibromuscular dysplasia
- TB "mycotic" aneurysm
- Syphilitic aortitis

Thymic Mass/Cyst

Surgeon: M. Arnold
Radiologist: T. Kilborn

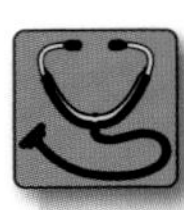

Clinical Insights

- A rare cause of a soft non-tender swelling in the anterior triangle of neck/ mediastinum
- Along path of thymopharyngeal duct from angle of mandible to thoracic inlet:
  - Ectopic thymic tissue
  - Undescended thymus
  - Cervical cysts (uni- or multilocular)
- Deep to or anterior to sternocleidomastoid muscle
- Fifty percent extend into thoracic cavity
- Infants and young children affected
- If very large, may compress other structures
- Associated with myaesthenia gravis

Warning

- Distinguish benign lesions from malignancy

Controversy

- Benign thymic masses need not be excised; unclear repercussions on immune function if it is the only functioning thymic tissue.
- Surgical excision of cervical cysts is recommended. Their aetiology is uncertain.

Urgency

❑ Emergency
❑ Urgent
☑ Elective

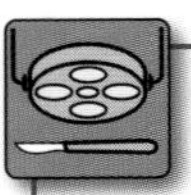

What the Surgeon Needs to Know

- Anatomical relations of important vascular and nervous structures in neck.
- Is there mediastinal thymic tissue in the case of ectopic cervical thymic mass?

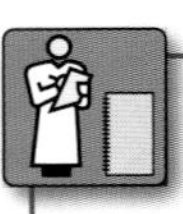

Clinical Differential Diagnosis

- Abscess
- Second branchial cleft remnant
- Ectopic thyroid or salivary tissue
- Primary malignancy (thyroid, parathyroid, salivary gland, carotid body tumour, lymphoma)
- Reactive or metastatic lymph node
- Lymphatic or vascular malformation

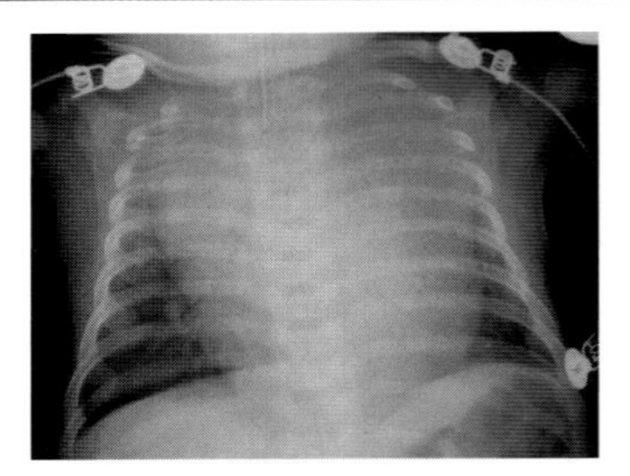

CXR – Enlarged thymus with tracheal compression, requiring intubation

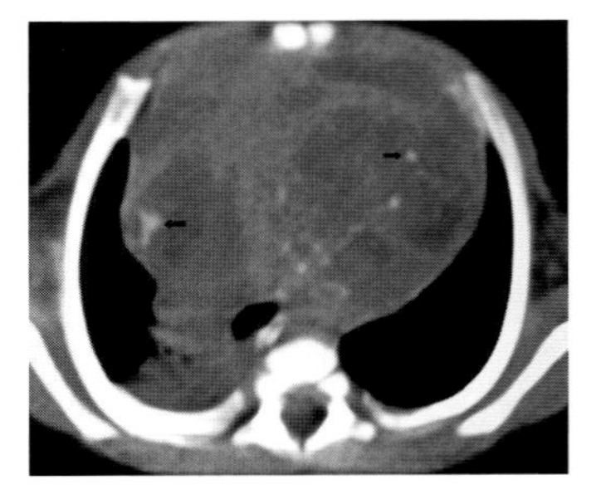

CT non-contrast – Inhomogeneous anterior mediastinal mass containing fat and calcium (*arrows*) consistent with a teratoma

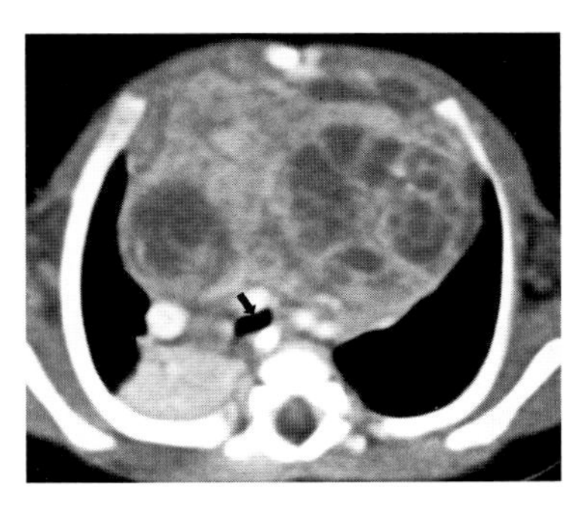

CT post-contrast – Inhomogeneous enhancement of biopsy proven thymic teratoma. Note the compression of the trachea (*arrow*)

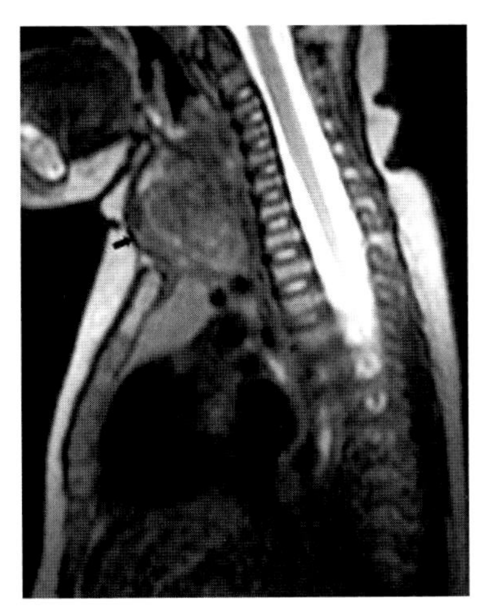

MRI Sagittal T2 – An inhomogeneous mass involving the superior part of the thymus (*arrow*) and lying in the superior mediastinum as demonstrated. There is tracheal compression (A normal thymus does not compress or displace structures)

Tips

- Ultrasound should be performed through the suprasternal notch with a linear probe in infants and curvilinear probe in older children.
- Anterior mediastinal nodes as in PTB usually have cleavage planes and ring or "ghost" enhancement on CT.
- Thymoma is rare in young children. Thymic lymphoma is more likely.

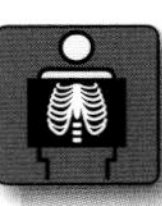

Imaging Options

- Primary: CXR, US
- Follow on: CT/MRI

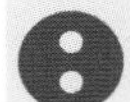

Imaging Findings

CXR

- A normal thymus on X-ray does not displace or compress structures. Instead it is molded, e.g. against the ribs giving the wave sign. It is somewhat see-through (vessels are seen through it) and often has a characteristic shape of a yachting sail ("spinaker sail sign").
- On CXR an abnormal thymus will show a wide mediastinum with displacement of mediastinal structures. Look for calcification suggesting teratoma or LCH.

US

- A normal thymus is readily seen on ultrasound as an anterior mediastinal structure containing septae. It moves with respiration and does not displace or compress vessels.
- A simple thymic cyst will typically be anechoic.
- On US a thymic mass is heterogeneous and displaces/compresses normal structures.

CT

- CT is best for showing calcification.
- CT shows inhomogeneous contrast enhancement, fat and calcium in teratomas; calcification and cysts in LCH.

MRI

- MRI STIR shows the thymus as a homogeneous high signal structure.

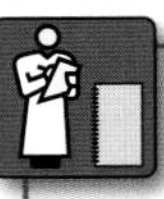

Radiological Differential Diagnosis

- Normal thymus
- Thymic cyst
- Teratoma
- Thymoma
- LCH

Thyroglossal Cyst

Surgeon: H. Peens-Hough
Radiologist: T. Kilborn

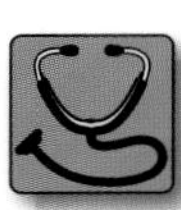

Clinical Insights

- Equal prevalence in boys and girls.
- Most commonly presents at 2–10 years of age.
- Cystic mass in the midline of the neck, anywhere from the base of the tongue to thyroid isthmus, (Can be slightly off-midline – usually to the left).
- Moves up with protrusion of the tongue.

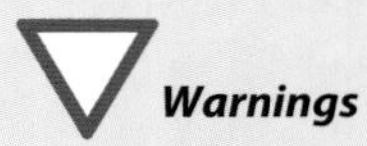

Warnings

- Risk for developing papillary carcinoma and chronic infection.
- The thyroglossal cyst must be removed with the central portion of the hyoid bone to prevent recurrence (Sistrunk's procedure).

Urgency

- ❑ Emergency
- ❑ Urgent
- ☑ Elective

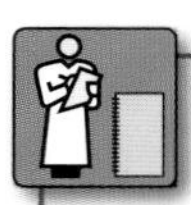

Clinical Differential Diagnosis

- Dermoid cysts
- Lingual thyroid
- Branchial cysts
- Lymph nodes

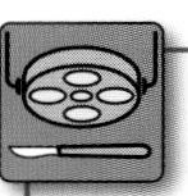

What the Surgeon Needs to Know

- Is the mass exclusively cystic?

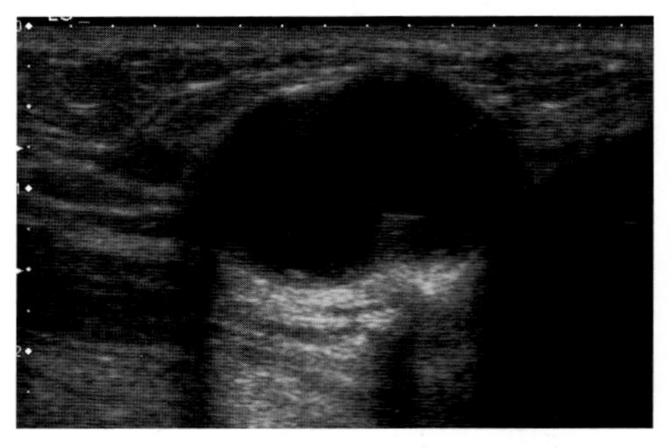

US – Showing anechoic midline cyst just above the level of the hyoid bone

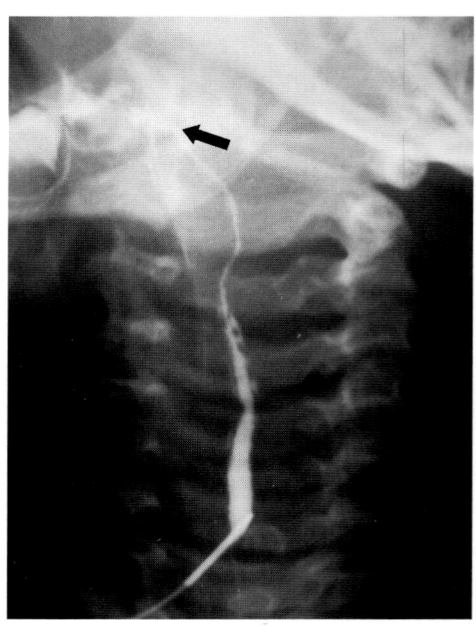

Sinogram – Contrast outlining patent thyroglossal duct extending to the base of the tongue (*arrow*)

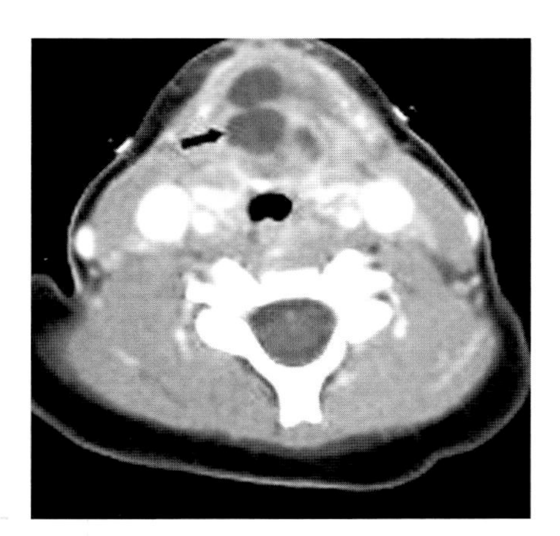

CT axial post-contrast – Showing peripheral enhancement and septation of midline neck cyst (*arrow*) in keeping with an infected thyroglossal duct cyst

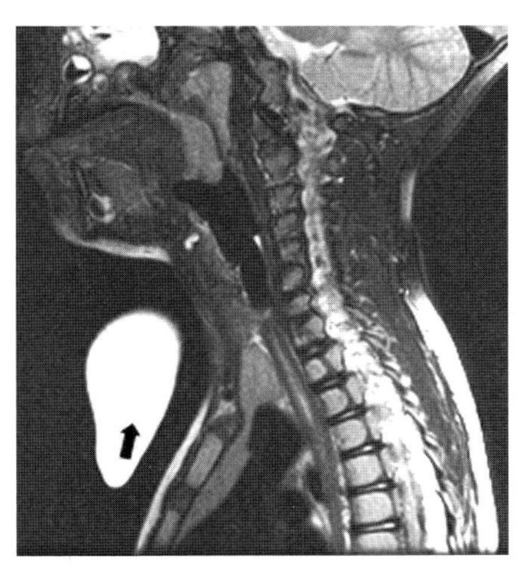

MRI Sagittal T2 – Demonstrates a high signal midline cystic mass (*arrow*) in keeping with a thyroglossal cyst

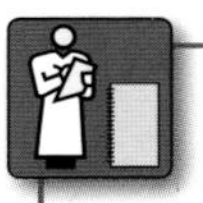

Radiological Differential Diagnosis

- Lingual/sublingual thyroid (appears solid)
- Lymphadenopathy (non-cystic unless necrotic)
- Dermoid (contains fat on CT/MR)
- Obstructed laryngocoele
- Branchial cyst (paramedian)

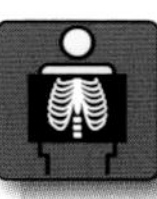

Imaging Options

- Primary: US
- Follow-on: CT/MRI
- Back-up: Fluoroscopy (sonogram)/Nuc Med

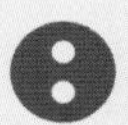

Imaging Findings

US

- Ultrasound confirms normal thyroid and shows midline anechoic neck mass occurring anywhere from base of tongue to suprasternal notch, usually closely related to hyoid.
- Twenty-five percent are off midline but occur near the thyroid cartilage.
- Internal echoes on ultrasound if contains proteinaceous material or infected.

CT/MRI

- Only needed if
  - Cyst is suprahyoid
  - Diagnosis is in question
  - Mass is infected
  - Concern about carcinoma
- MRI
  - T1 hypo/T2 hyperintense
  - Non-enhancing unless infected
- CT
  - Hypodense, occasionally septated
  - Non-enhancing unless infected

Sinogram

- May be necessary to identify thyroglossal duct tract.

Tips

- US can be used to confirm if cyst is related to the hyoid – It will move when tongue is protruded.
- <1% associated with carcinoma, but if solid eccentric mass seen in relation to cyst, this needs to be considered.

Thyroid Neoplasm

Surgeon: D. Sidler
Radiologist: T. Kilborn

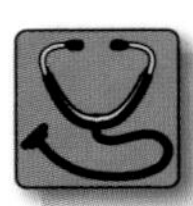

Clinical Insights

- Thyroid masses have to be investigated fully to differentiate malignant from benign disease, including fine-needle aspiration biopsy (FNAB).
- No attempts should be made to differentiate follicular adenoma from carcinoma by FNAB, since capsular and vascular invasion can only be determined on an excised specimen.
- The physical examination persistence of the nodule, progressive growth and cosmetic appearance are the main indications for surgery.
- Medullary thyroid carcinoma has a strong genetic component: MEN II A and B and familial thyroid cancer syndrome.

Warnings

- FNAB, US and Nuc Med should not replace clinical judgement or suspicion as the most important determinants in management.
- Children with MEN II A and B should have prophylactic early thyroidectomies (5 and 1 year respectively).

Controversy

- Since malignancy can occasionally be a cystic or a hot nodule, ultrasound and radionuclide scanning are of limited utility.

Urgency

- ❑ Emergency
- ❑ Urgent
- ☑ Elective

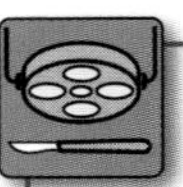

What the Surgeon Needs to Know

- Presence of cervical lymphadenopathy

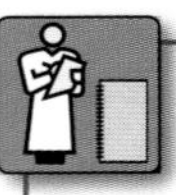

Clinical Differential Diagnosis

- Thyroiditis
- Goiter
- Thyroid adenoma/carcinoma
- Thyroglossal cyst
- Teratoma
- Lymph node
- Sebaceous cyst

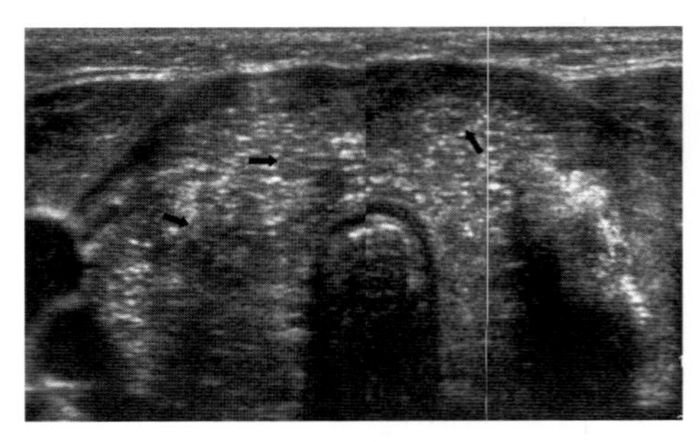

US transverse – The thyroid shows enlargement, inhomogeneity (*arrows*) and calcification bilaterally in keeping with thyroid carcinoma (papillary)

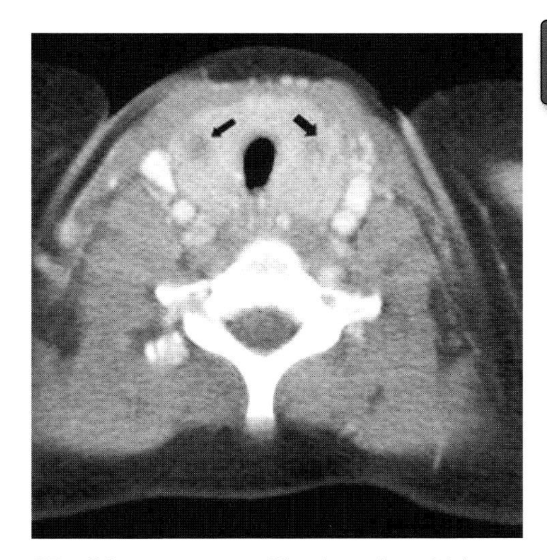

CT axial post-contrast – Showing enlarged inhomogeneously enhancing thyroid (*arrows*) and bilateral cervical lymph nodes

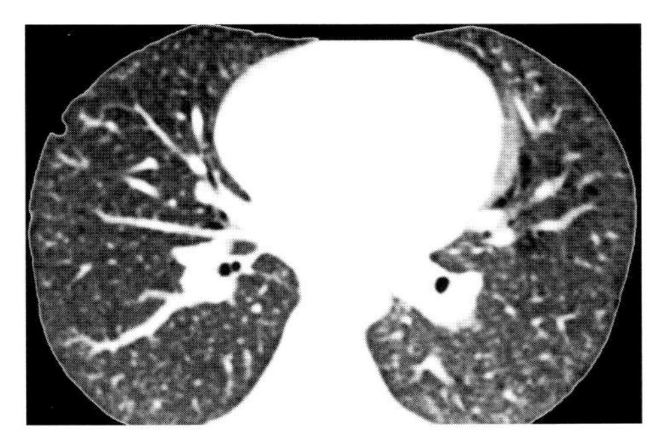

CT axial – In the same patient as in the earlier figure, showing multiple (showers) lung metastases

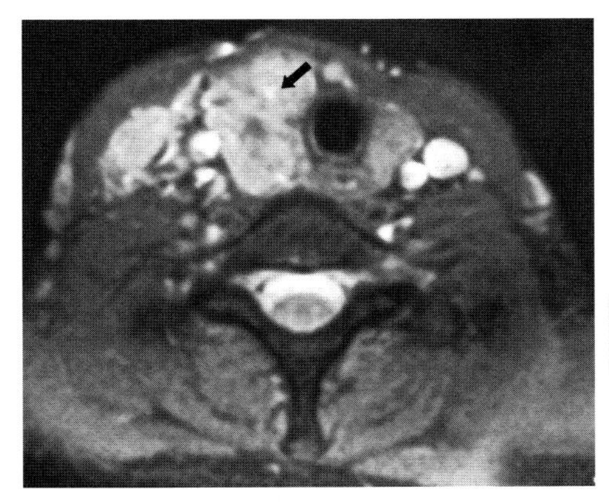

MRI T2 weighted – Demonstrates a right lobe high signal mass (*arrow*) in keeping with carcinoma

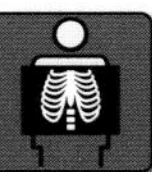

Imaging Options

- Primary: US
- Back-up: Nuclear medicine
- Follow on: CT/MRI

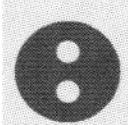

Imaging Findings

US

- Demonstrates a mass that may be solid or cystic, single or multifocal.
- Usually hypoechoic but may have calcification (hyperechogenicity).

Nuclear Medicine

- Tc99m or I123.
- Any thyroid nodule that takes up isotope must be presumed malignant.
- Bone metastases are rare in children, but can be identified on bone scan.

CT/MRI

- Contrast-enhanced CT is necessary for staging
- Assess degree of lymphadenopathy
- Assess for lung metastases

Tips

- Non-contrast CT may show normal thyroid as hyperdense due to normal iodine content and the mass as a hypodense lesion.

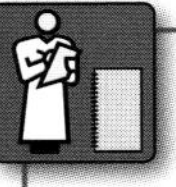

Radiological Differential Diagnosis

- Thyroiditis (diffusely enlarged gland)
- Thyroid adenoma (uncommon)
- Thyroglossal cyst (extrathyroid)

Tonsillar Abscess (Quinsy)

Surgeon: O. Basson
Radiologist: T. Kilborn

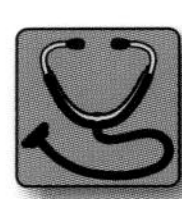

Clinical Insights

- Abscess between tonsillar capsule and superior constrictor muscle.
- May arise spontaneously, or as a complication of tonsillitis.
- Usually unilateral.
- Presenting features include sore throat, dysphagia, drooling, trismus, "hot-potato" voice.
- Surprisingly less common in children (the commonest age-group for tonsillitis) than in adolescents and young adults.

Warning

- May progress into parapharyngeal space or cause laryngeal oedema – Airway is then at risk.

Controversy

- Imaging is rarely necessary, unless there is a need to distinguish from a parapharyngeal abscess

Urgency

- ❑ Emergency
- ☑ Urgent
- ❑ Elective

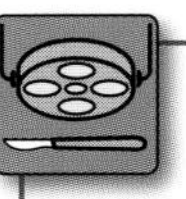

What the Surgeon Needs to Know

- Is there an abscess?

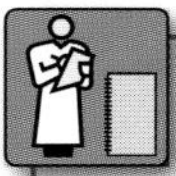

Clinical Differential Diagnosis

- Peritonsillar cellulitis
- Parapharyngeal mass
- Asymmetry in patient with tonsillitis
- Neoplasia (lymphoma)

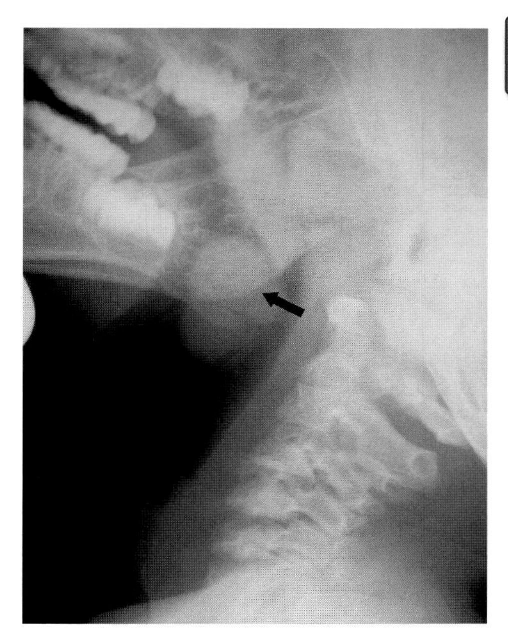

X-ray – Lateral "soft tissue" view of neck showing enlarged tonsils (*arrow*)

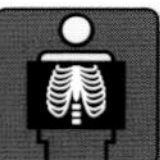

Imaging Options

- Primary: X-ray (lateral "soft tissue" neck)
- Follow-on: CT

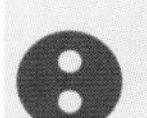

Imaging Findings

Lateral Neck Radiograph

- Enlarged palatine tonsils appear as a soft-tissue mass overlying the posterior inferior soft palate.

CT

- Indicated if suspecting spreading cellulitis or abscess.
- Contrast-enhanced CT will show the abscess as a rim enhancing area of low density usually involving retropharynx/prevertebral soft tissue.

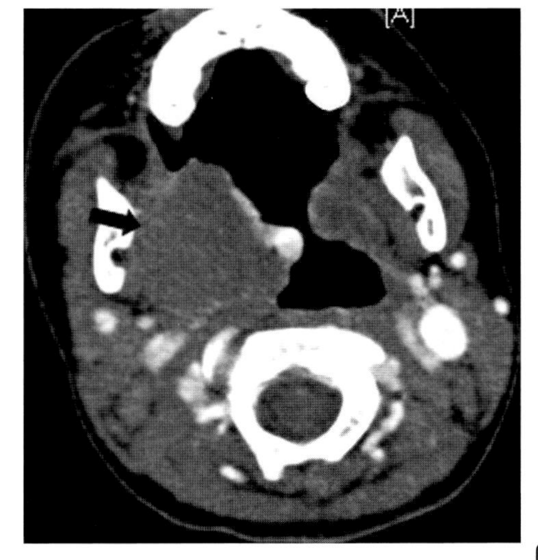

CT axial post-contrast – right-sided parapharyngeal low density, ring-enhancing tonsillar abscess (*arrow*) and a swollen left palatine tonsil

Tips

- Acute tonsillitis does not require imaging.

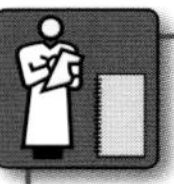

Radiological Differential Diagnosis

- Retropharyngeal abscess
- Lymphoma

Torsion Testis

Surgeon: A. Alexander
Radiologist: A. Bagadia

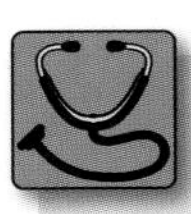

Clinical Insights

- Presents as an acute scrotum (sudden onset of pain)
- Bimodal incidence:
  - Under three
  - Onset of puberty
- May be extra-vaginal (uniquely neonatal) or intra-vaginal

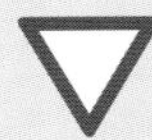

Warning

- If not immediately available, imaging should not delay surgical exploration.

Controversies

- Role of Doppler ultrasound in excluding torsion testis as a cause for acute scrotum.
- A missed neonatal torsion need not undergo orchiectomy.
- In missed neonatal torsion, the contralateral testis is at risk and should be pexied as an emergency.

Urgency

- [x] Emergency
- [ ] Urgent
- [ ] Elective

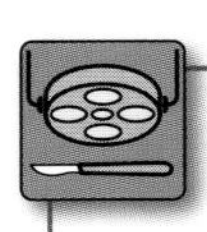

What the Surgeon Needs to Know

- Is there arterial perfusion in the parenchyma of the testis?

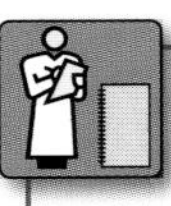

Clinical Differential Diagnosis

- Epididymo-orchitis
- Appendix testis/epididymis torsion
- Acute hydrocoele
- Incarcerated inguinal hernia
- Tumour
- Idiopathic scrotal oedema

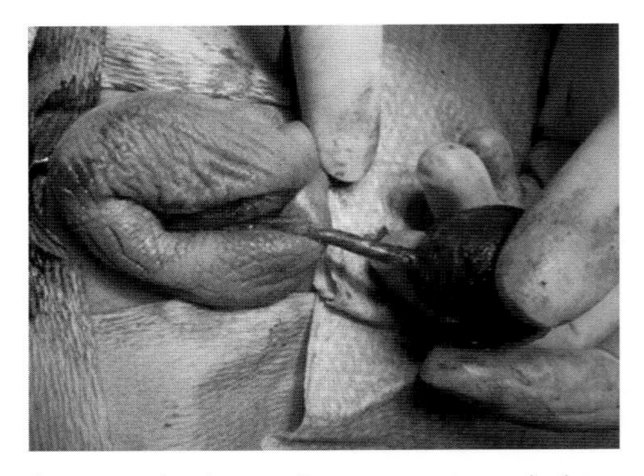

Intra-operative image of an acute extra-vaginal torsion in a neonate

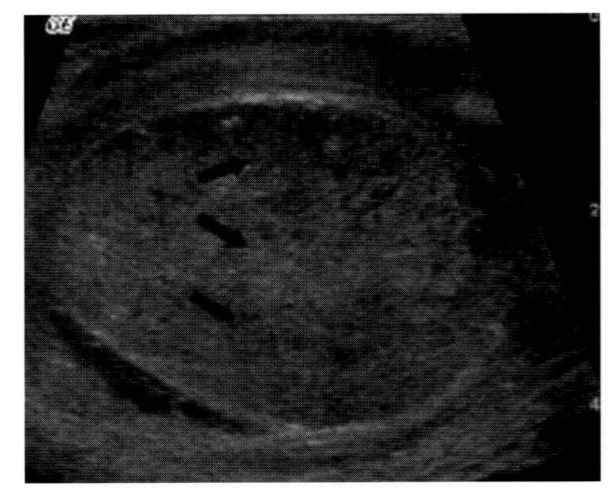

US longitudinal – Demonstrates a heterogenous echopattern (*arrows*) in the large (swollen) left testis

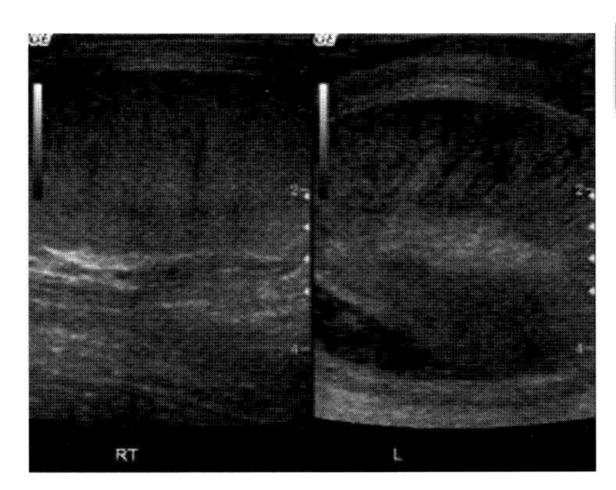

US transverse – Compares the two testes and demonstrates normal homogenous echotexture and rete testis on the right (*RT*) with an enlarged torted left testis showing a heterogenous echopattern (*L*)

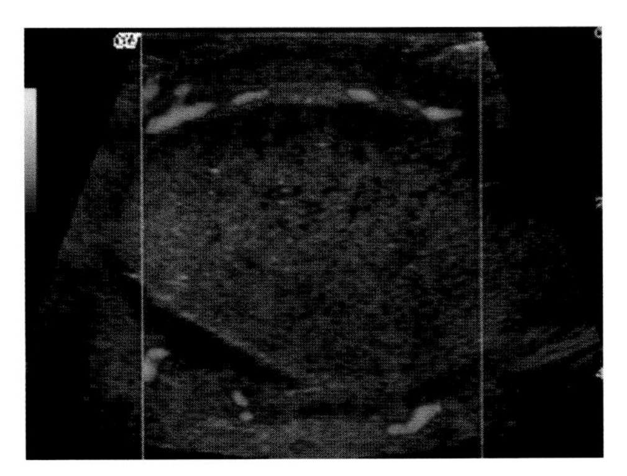

US Doppler – Of abnormal left testis shows no central parenchymal flow and excessive peripheral flow

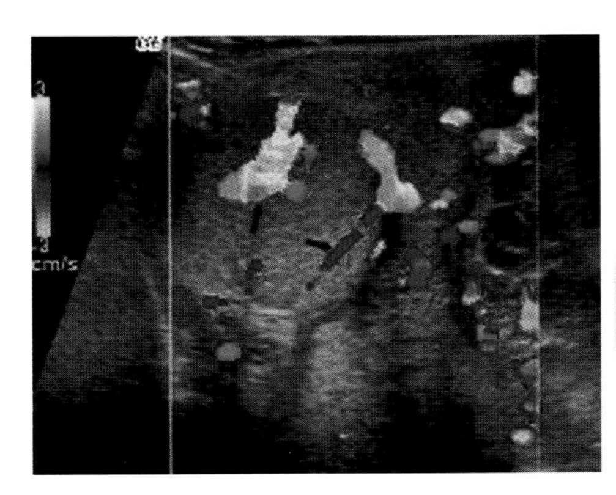

US Doppler – Normal right testis in the same patient as in the earlier figure with central testicular flow (*arrows*)

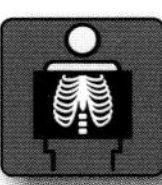

Imaging Options

- Primary: No imaging; US
- Back up: Nuc Med

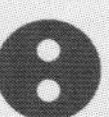

Imaging Findings

- Many institutions explore all "acute scrotums" and advocate "no imaging."

US

- Acute phase:
  - May be normal
  - Swollen epididymis/appendix testis: hyper- or hypo-echoic with reflective rim
  - Enlarged swollen heterogeneous or variably reduced echogenicity of testis
  - Spiral twist of spermatic cord causing a "torsion knot" or "whirlpool" pattern
  - Reactive hydrocoele
  - Colour Doppler – May be normal; absent/decreased flow within testis; increased vascularity in swollen peri-testicular tissue
- Chronic phase:
  - Small atrophied hypo-echoic testis
  - Enlarged echogenic epididymis

Imaging Tip

- Colour Doppler must be optimised to detect slow flow
- Power Doppler useful in neonates/infants
- Compare with contra-lateral normal testis

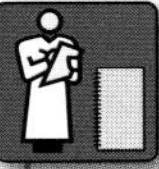

Radiological Differential Diagnosis

- Torsion of appendix testis or testicular appendage
- Acute epididymo-orchitis
- Testicular trauma
- Testicular tumour

Trauma Abdomen

Surgeon: A. B. van As
Radiologist: S. Theron

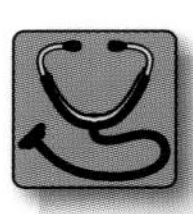

Clinical Insights

- The most common cause is a motor vehicle accident.
- 80% pedestrian, 20% (unrestrained) passengers.
- The vast majority (90%) are polytrauma patients.
- Usually there is an associated head injury.

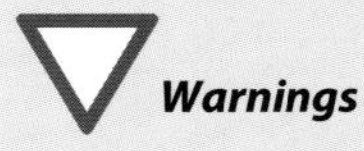

Warnings

- Priority in treatment is cardio-pulmonary stabilization.
- CT scan is contra-indicated in an unstable patient.

Controversy

- Abdominal CT scan:
  - If patients are stable but major solid organ injury suspected.
  - If a hollow viscus injury is suspected (warranting emergency surgery).
  - When accompanying head injury.
- Abdominal radiograph is unreliable in 50%.

Urgency

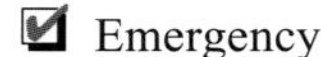

☑ Emergency
☐ Urgent
☐ Elective

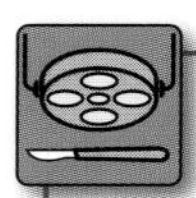

What the Surgeon Needs to Know

- Is there need for emergency laparotomy?
- Where is the major organ injury?

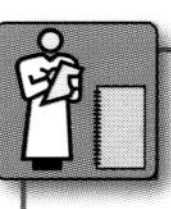

Clinical Differential Diagnosis

- Referred pain from the chest (rib fractures, hemo/pneumothorax).
- Referred pain from a pelvis injury (fracture).
- Abdominal wall contusion.
- Transitional zone pain in paraplegia.

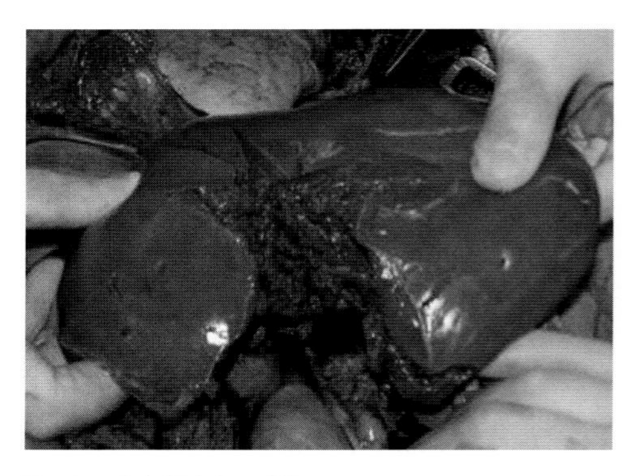

Ruptured right lobe of liver

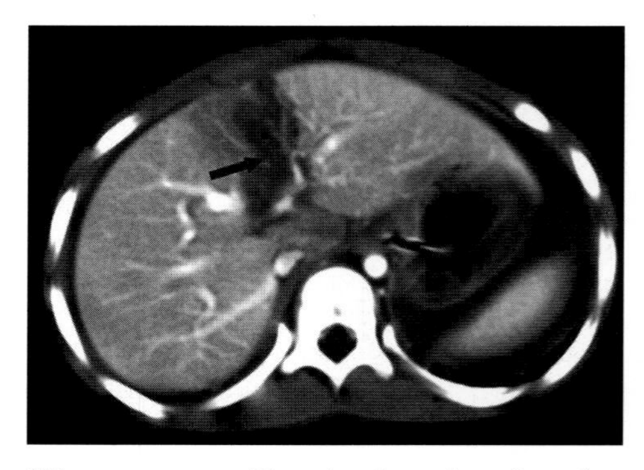

CT post-contrast – There is a large, hypodense laceration of the liver (*arrow*) extending towards the confluence of the left and right portal veins

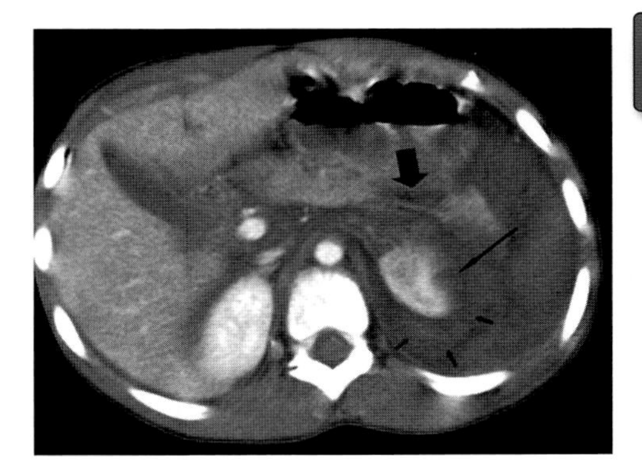

CT post-contrast – CT demonstrates a fractured pancreas (*thick arrow*), left perinephric hematoma (*small arrows*) with an associated renal contusion (*long arrow*) and haemoperitoneum

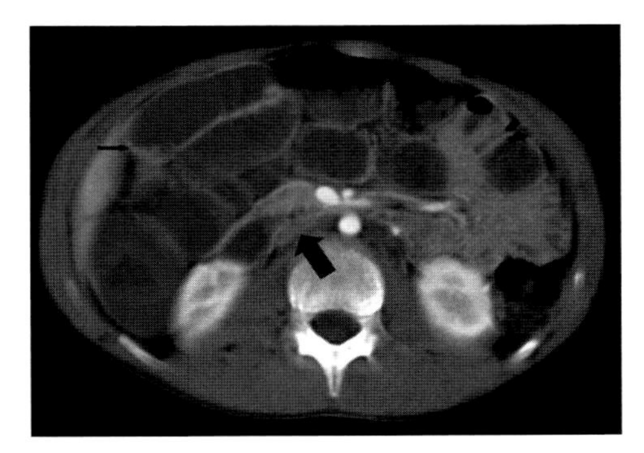

CT post-contrast – There is dilatation and intense enhancement (*thin arrow*) of the small bowel wall, consistent with shock bowel. Note the small IVC (*thick arrow*)

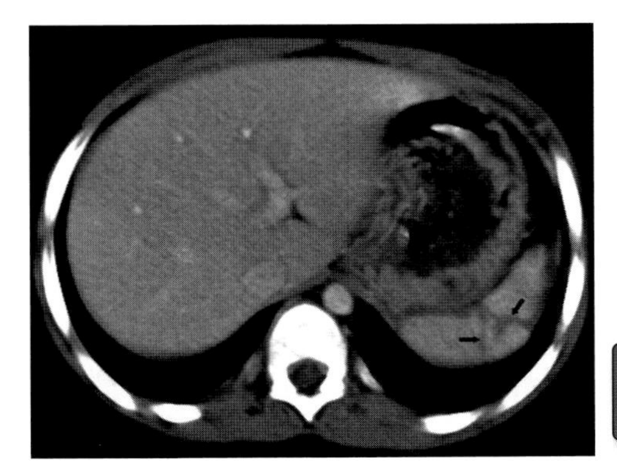

CT post-contrast – There are multiple hypodense lacerations (*arrows*) of the spleen (splenic fracture)

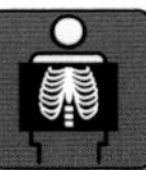

Imaging Options

- Primary: CT
- Alternative: US (recommended only as triage tool to detect free fluid)
- Follow-on: Cystogram (high pressure)

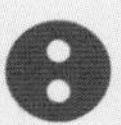

Imaging Findings

CT

- Intraperitoneal free fluid: Around liver or spleen, Morrison's pouch, in pelvis
- Low density lesions in solid organs: Contusions
- High density within contusions: Active haemorrhage
- Linear low densities in solid organs: Lacerations
- Edematous, enhancing bowel wall: Shock bowel
- Thick bowel wall: Haematoma
- Free air: Perforation

Tips

- Unstable patients go to theatre without CT.
- Oral contrast not necessary (causes delay and patient should be NPO in case of surgery).
- US gives false sense of security as it can miss organ injury and renal vascular injury.
- Use lung windows in the abdomen to detect free air.
- Objective of CT: Identify organ injury in case of urgent surgery later; exclude renal vascular injury, identify missed free intraperitoneal air, detect free fluid

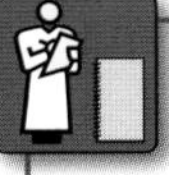

Radiological Differential Diagnosis

- Non-accidental injury

Trauma Chest

Surgeon: A. B. van As
Radiologist: A. Maydell

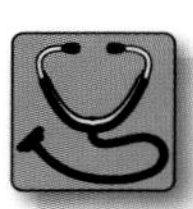

Clinical Insights

- The most common cause is blunt trauma.
- The rib cage is mostly cartilaginous and can be compressed significantly without fractures.
- The majority of injuries are pulmonary contusion, hemothorax and pneumothorax.

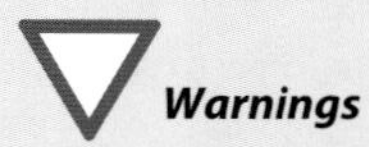

Warnings

- Children may have extensive myocardial or pulmonary contusions without obvious rib fractures.
- Children are easily "over"-ventilated and susceptible for iatrogenic baro-trauma, pneumothorax and placement of the ET tube in a main bronchus.

Controversy

- Widened mediastinum may indicate major vessel injury; however, ruptured aorta is extremely rare in children under 12 years.

Urgency

- [x] Emergency
- [ ] Urgent
- [ ] Elective

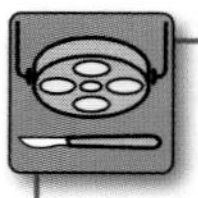

What the Surgeon Needs to Know

- Does the child require chest drains?
- Does the child require thoracotomy?
- Is there significant coexisting abdominal pathology?

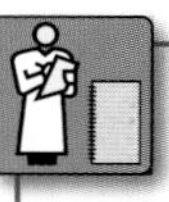

Clinical Differential Diagnosis

- Pre-existing pulmonary disease: TB, HIV/AIDS, etc.

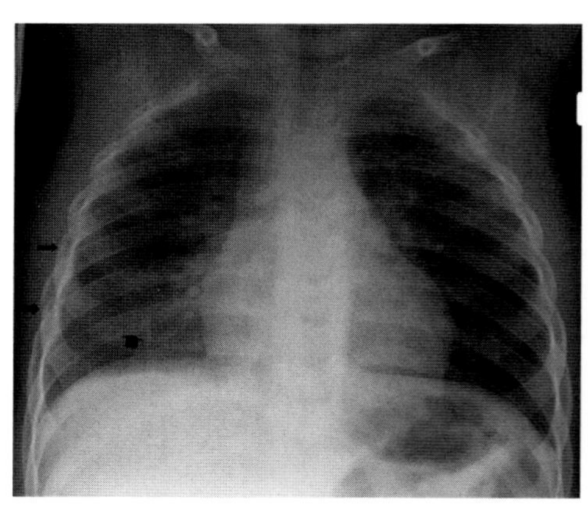

CXR – Demonstrates right-sided fractures involving ribs 5 and 6 laterally (*small arrows*) with minimal pleural thickening, suggestion of an underlying contusion (*thick arrow*) and no visible pneumothorax

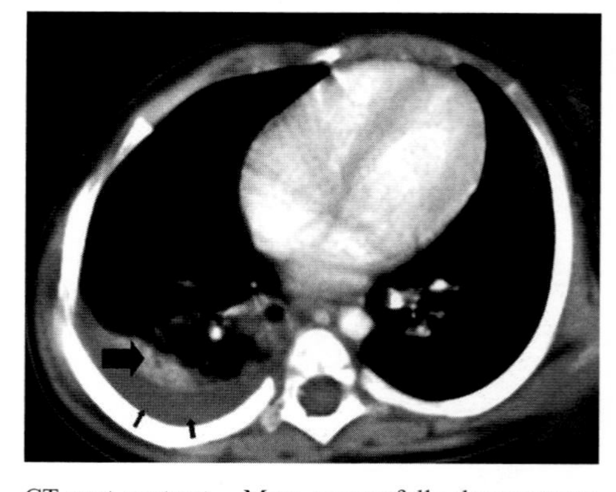

CT post-contrast – More successfully demonstrates the lung contusion (*thick arrow*) and haemothorax (*small arrows*) not well-appreciated on the CXR in the previous figure

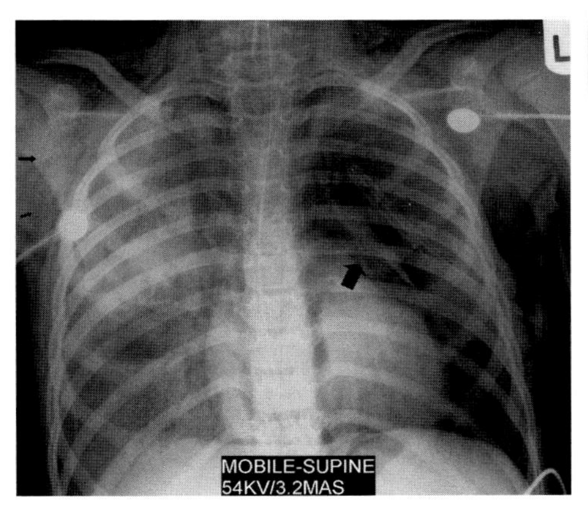

CXR – Demonstrates extensive right-sided lung contusion and it is difficult to exclude an associated haemothorax in the supine position. There are bilateral pneumothoraces lying medially predominantly (*thick arrow*), with an intercostal drain on the left. An ET tube and nasogastric tube are also in situ. There is extensive surgical emphysema (*small arrows*)

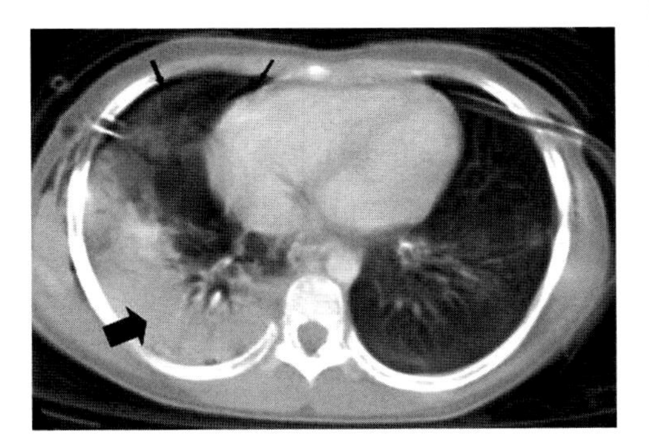

CT lung window – Demonstrates bilaterally sited intercostal drains with extensive right-sided lung contusion (*thick arrow*). The pneumothoraces are almost completely drained but the residual air lies anterior and medially (*small arrows*) in the supine patient

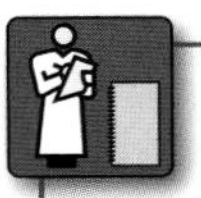

Radiological Differential Diagnosis

- Non-accidental injury

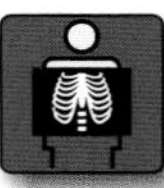

Imaging Options

- Primary: CXR
- Follow-on: CT
- Back-up: US, UGI, angiography, MRI

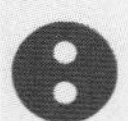

Imaging Findings

CXR

- Haemo/pneumothorax
- Pulmonary contusion
- Rib fractures (new/old)
- Wide mediastinum
- Diaphragmatic rupture
- Herniation of abdominal contents

CT

- Best option for accurate assessment of contusions

US

- Haemothorax, pericardial effusion, subcapsular haematoma

Angiography

- Vascular injury

MRI

- Spinal cord involvement

Tips

- CXR is usually sufficient to follow course of blunt trauma.
- Only stable patients must be accepted for CT.
- Pulmonary contusion, pneumothorax and rib fractures are common. Aortic injury uncommon.
- Over half of rib fractures in children younger than 3 years may be due to child abuse – Look for evidence of previous trauma.

Tuberculosis of the Abdomen

Surgeon: C. Davies
Radiologist: H. Douis

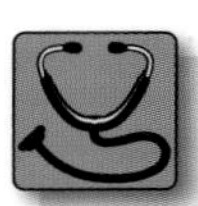

Clinical Insights

- TB of the abdomen is not an uncommon manifestation of the disease in endemic areas.
- When present, it may involve:
  - Bowel – Causing failure to thrive, bowel obstruction and fistulae
  - Peritoneum – Giving rise to the classic millet seed appearance of the peritoneum and ascites
  - Mesenteric and retroperitoneal lymph nodes – Important to differentiate from lymphoma
  - Solid organs – Mimicking pyogenic abscess, primary and metastatic malignancy

Warnings

- Patients with peritoneal TB often present with an acute abdomen
- HIV, TB and lymphoma often co-exist
- Diagnosis is made by minimal peritoneal or nodal biopsy, and any surgical manipulation of the bowel will result in perforation and fistulae

Controversy

- Nutritional support and TB therapy may resolve the problem without complications

Urgency

- ❑ Emergency
- ❑ Urgent
- ☑ Elective

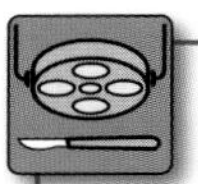

What the Surgeon Needs to Know

- What is the site of involvement?
- Are there any complications evident (free air, obstruction)?
- Are extra-abdominal sites involved (lungs)?

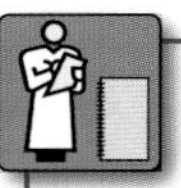

Clinical Differential Diagnosis

- Inflammatory bowel disease
- Infective enteritis
- Metastatic disease
- Lymphoma
- Pyogenic abscess
- Solid organ neoplasia

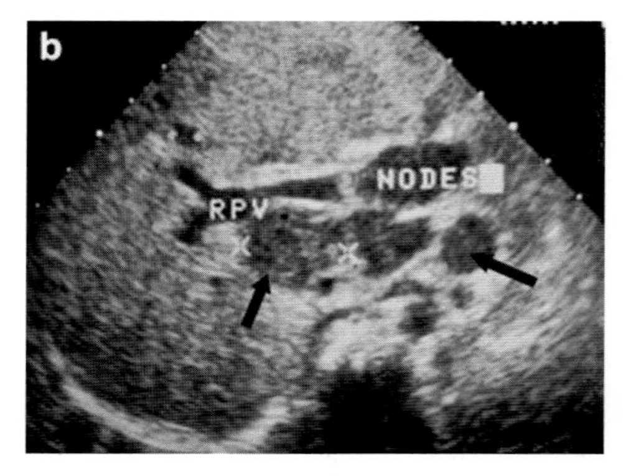

US transverse upper abdomen – Demonstrates lymphadenopathy predominantly involving the para-aortic group (*arrows*) in keeping with abdominal TB

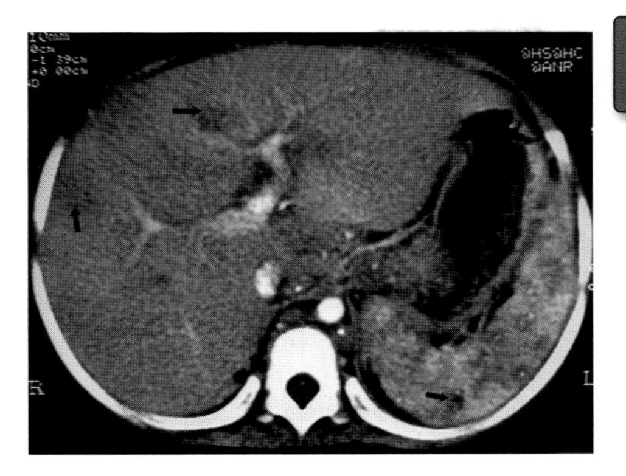

CT post-contrast – Demonstrates low density lesions in the liver and spleen (*arrows*) as well as calcified para-aortic lymphadenopathy of abdominal TB

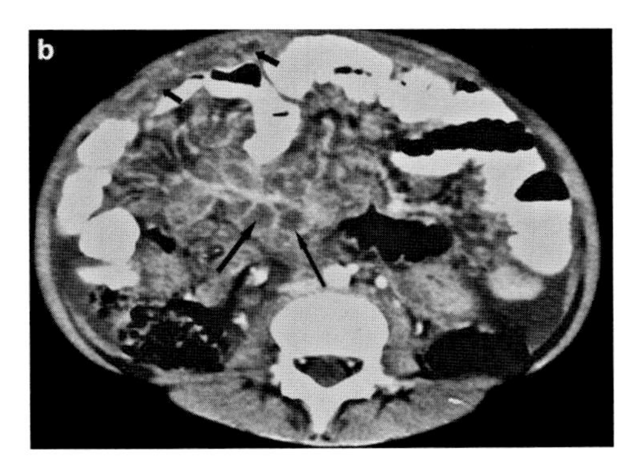

CT post-contrast – Omental cakes are seen immediately deep to the anterior abdominal wall (*short arrows*). There is also mesenteric lymphadenopathy (*long arrows*) splaying the vessesls and ascites in the para-colic gutters

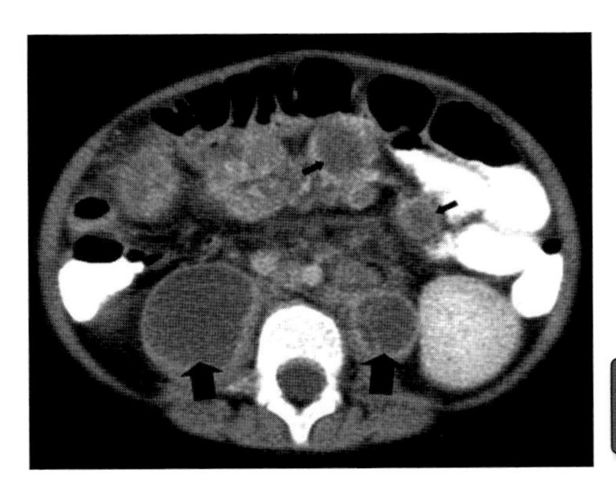

CT post-contrast – Paravertebral psoas abscesses (*thick arrows*) and low density ring-enhancing lympadenopathy (*small arrows*) are characteristic features of TB

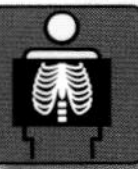

Imaging Options

- Primary: US
- Follow-on: CT/CXR/contrast enema/small bowel study
- Alternative: MRI

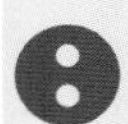

Imaging Findings

US

- Mesenteric thickening > 15 mm
- Calcified lymph nodes
- Dilated bowel loops
- Ascites
- Omental mass
- Focal lesions in liver and spleen

CT

- Peritoneal thickening/omental cakes
- Lymphadenopathy (low density and rim enhancement)
- Solid organ lesions (liver and spleen)
- Ascites (high density)
- Bowel wall thickening
- Inflammatory masses in omentum or ileocaecal region

Small Bowel Study/Contrast Enema

- Thickening of bowel loops
- Narrowed thick-walled caecum and terminal ileum

Tips

- Forty percent have a positive chest radiograph.
- Calcified or ring enhancing lymph nodes in abdomen or chest are best clues.
- Psoas TB abscesses and TB spondylitis may also be seen on AXR, US and CT.

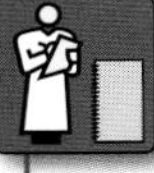

Radiological Differential Diagnosis

- Inflammatory bowel disease
- Malignancy, e.g. lymphoma
- Other infection

Urachal Abnormality (Patent Urachus/Urachal Cyst/Sinus/Diverticulum)

Surgeon: J. Loveland
Radiologist: T. Kilborn

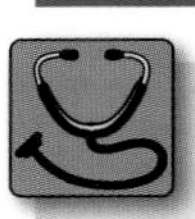

Clinical Insights

- The urachus is a connection between the foetal bladder and the amnion. It is normally obliterated in foetal life.
- Embraces a spectrum of anomalies originating from varying degrees of patency of the urachus:
  - Urachal diverticulum of the bladder
  - Urachal cyst
  - Urachal sinus
  - Patent urachus

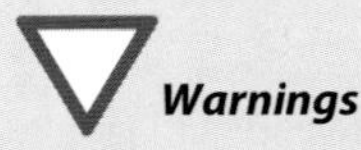

Warnings

- Where complete urachal patency exists, the bladder may prolapse through the umbilicus onto the abdominal wall.
- Patent urachus may be associated with bladder outlet obstruction.

Controversy

- Although recently described, laparoscopic repair is of uncertain benefit

Urgency

- ❑ Emergency
- ❑ Urgent
- ☑ Elective

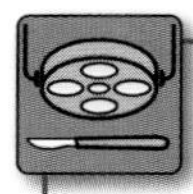

What the Surgeon Needs to Know

- What is the extent of the lesion?
- Where is the lesion in relation to surgical landmarks?
- Is this a vitello-intestinal duct lesion?
- Anatomy of distal urinary tract

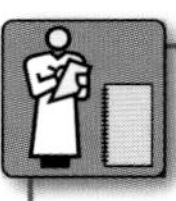

Clinical Differential Diagnosis

- Vitello-intestinal duct remnant
- Umbilical polyp/granuloma
- Meckel's diverticulitis
- Cutaneous infection/abscess

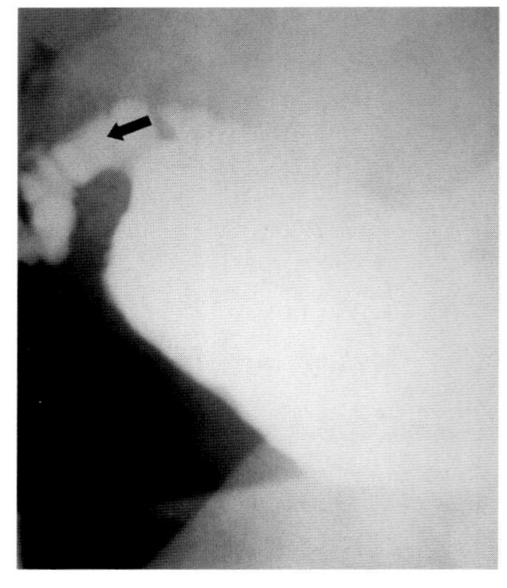

MCUG lateral – Showing contrast outlining a patent urachus (*arrow*) (communicates with the skin surface)

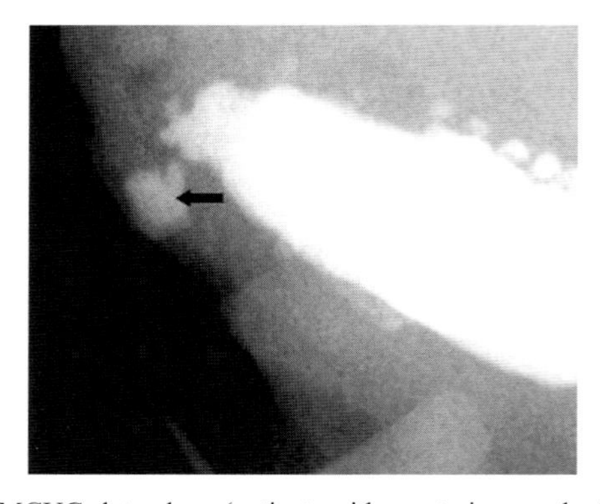

MCUG lateral – (patient with posterior urethral valve) showing urachal diverticulum (*arrow*) (does not communicate with the skin)

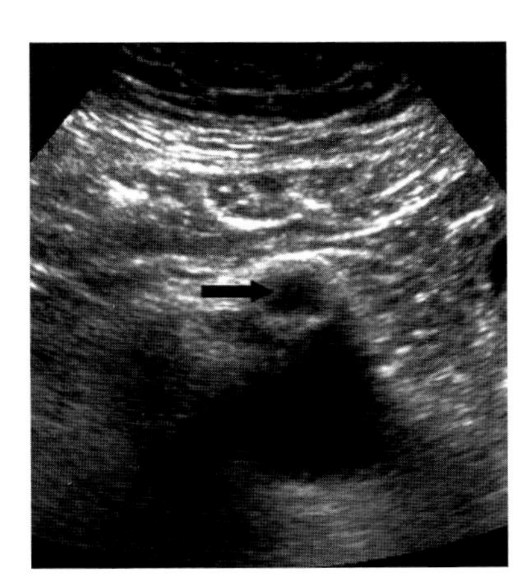

US – Showing a urachal cyst (*arrow*) anterior to apex of bladder deep to the umbilicus (does not communicate with the skin or the bladder)

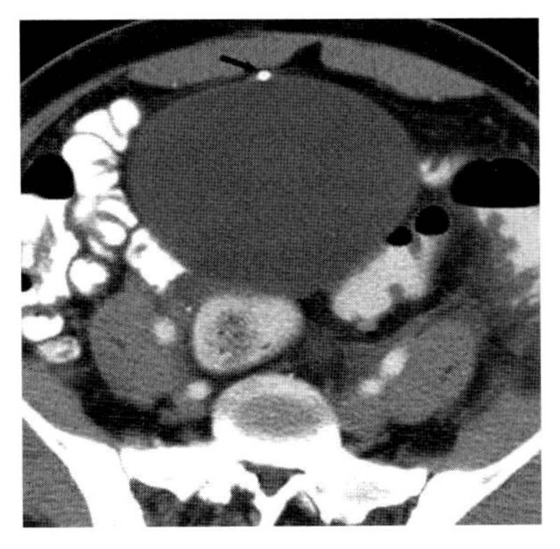

CT – Shows a calculus complicating a urachal diverticulum (*arrow*)

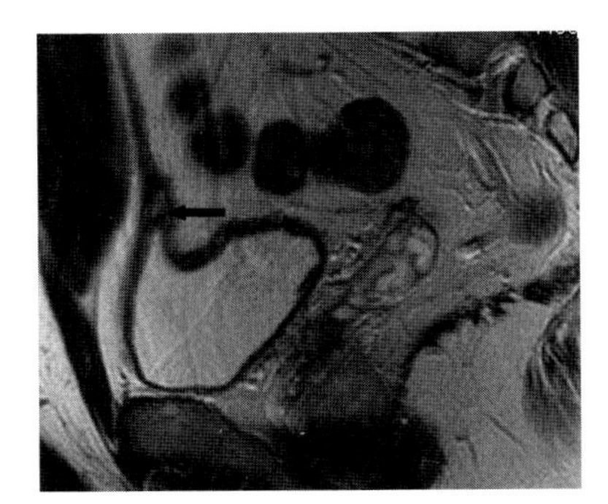

MRI T2 sagital – Shows a urachal diverticulum (*arrow*) at the bladder apex extending to but not communicating with the umbilicus

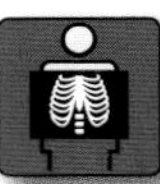

Imaging Options

- Primary: Fluoroscopy (MCUG/sinogram)
- Back-up: US
- Follow on: CT/MRI

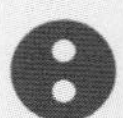

Imaging Findings

MCUG

- Patent urachus – Contrast extends from the apex of the bladder to umbilicus.
- Urachal diverticulum – Diverticulum at the bladder apex without connection to the abdominal wall.

Sinogram

- Urachal sinus – Contrast outlines a blind-ending tract at the umbilicus.

US

- Urachal cyst – An anechoic/hypoechoic cyst below the umbilicus. High resolution scanning may see the urachal tract towards the bladder.

CT

- Usually reserved for infected urachal cysts.
- Infected cysts are peripherally enhancing and lie just below the umbilicus.

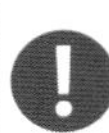

Tips

- A solid mass antero-superior to bladder dome with heterogeneous enhancement or calcifications – Consider complication of carcinoma (adolescents)

Varicocoele

Surgeon: A. Alexander
Radiologist: H. Lameen

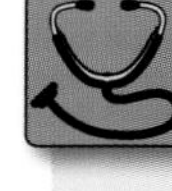

Clinical Insights

- Affects 15% of men usually in the left hemiscrotum (may be bilateral).
- Classically detected in the peri-pubertal period.
- Three grades:
  - Grade 1: Mass less than 1 cm
  - Grade 2: Mass 1–2 cm
  - Grade 3: Mass >2 cm
- Associated with compression of the left renal vein by the superior mesenteric artery (nut-cracker phenomenon).
- Associated with male infertility, particularly secondary infertility. This is the principle reason for surgical correction.
- Treated by ligation or laparoscopic clipping of the gonadal veins (arterial and lymphatic ligation included in some procedures).

Controversy

- Indications for surgery are not uniformly agreed upon but include:
  - Persistent testicular volume differential > 10%
  - Altered sperm counts, motility or morphology
  - Discomfort/pain

Urgency

- ❑ Emergency
- ❑ Urgent
- ☑ Elective

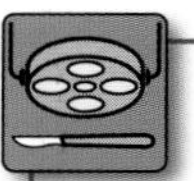

What the Surgeon Needs to Know

- Grade of varicocoele
- Enlargement on valsalva
- Are the contralateral vessels normal?
- Is the "nut-cracker phenomenon" present?

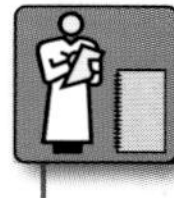

Clinical Differential Diagnosis

- Paratesticular mass
- Lymphatic malformations
- Hydrocoele

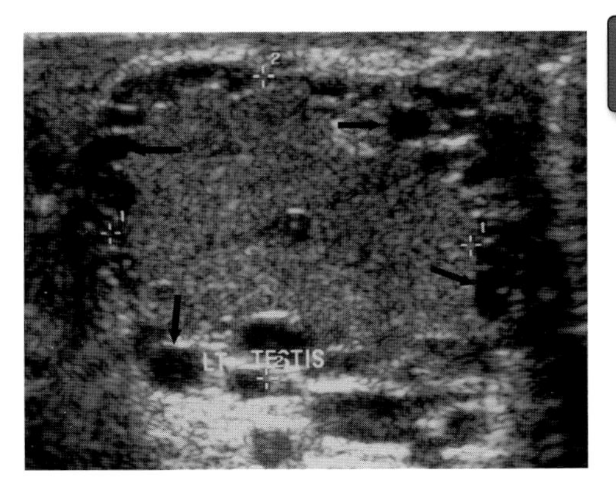

US scrotum – Demonstrates the serpigenous anechoic structures surrounding the testis (*arrows*)

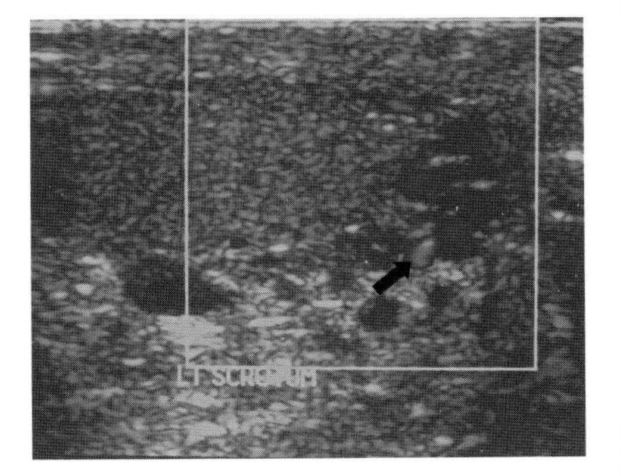

US colour Doppler of the scrotum – May demonstrate flow (*arrow*) within these structures indicating that they are vascular (venous) as seen in this child

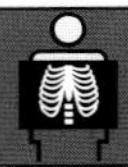

Imaging Options

- Primary: US

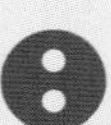

Imaging Findings

US

- Tortuous anechoic serpigenous structures adjacent to upper pole of the testis
- Doppler may show flow
- Increase in size in the erect position or valsalva
- If chronic may see phleboliths

Tips

- Standing position increases the diagnostic accuracy of the US
- Majority are left-sided but can be right or bilateral
- US of the abdomen could exclude retroperitoneal mass as a secondary cause

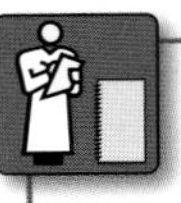

Radiological Differential Diagnosis

- Indirect inguinal hernia
- Epididymitis
- Paratesticular tumour

Venous Malformations (Including Klippel Trenaunay Syndrome)

Surgeon: A. Potgieter
Radiologist: T. Kilborn

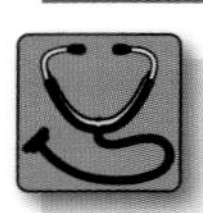

Clinical Insights

- Are composed of thin-walled, dilated, sponge-like channels.
- They are congenital, grow commensurately with the child, but may only manifest later in the childhood.
- In general, they are blueish, soft, compressible low-flow anomalies.
- They expand with dependency or after a valsalva manoeuvre.
- Principally occur in skin and subcutaneous tissue, but may involve deeper tissues.
- Phlebothrombosis is common leading to distention, firmness and pain.

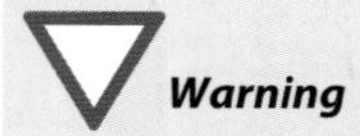

Warning

- Important to distinguish hemangioma (a benign neoplasm) from a vascular malformation (including venous malformations)

Controversy

- Treatment options most appropriate

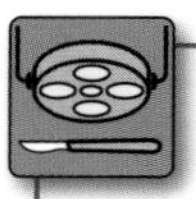

What the Surgeon Needs to Know

- The nature and extent of the lesion
- The structures involved
- Flow characteristics

Urgency

- ❑ Emergency
- ❑ Urgent
- ☑ Elective

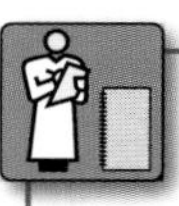

Clinical Differential Diagnosis

- Other vascular malformations:
  - Capillary
  - Lymphatic

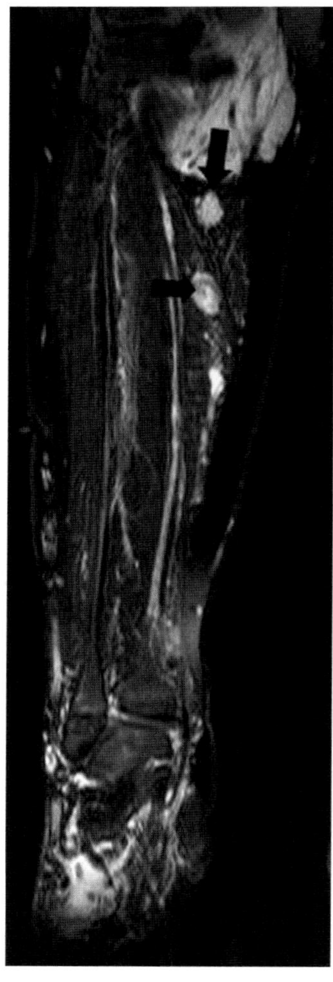

MRI coronal T2 fat saturation – Shows multiple linear and serpentine areas of high signal representing dilated veins with slow flow. This is especially evident medial to the knee (*arrows*)

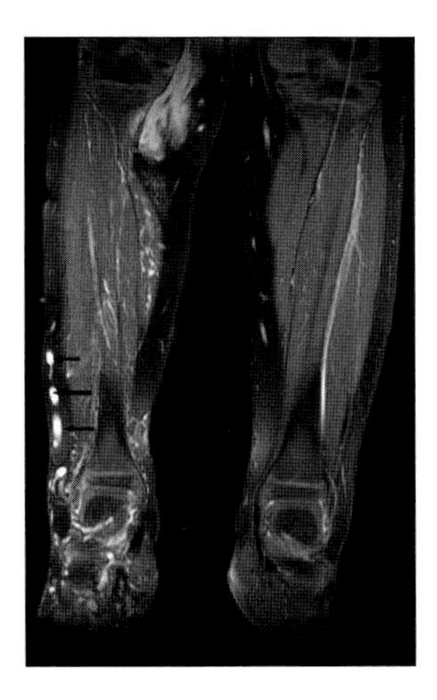

MRI gadolinium enhanced coronal T1 with fat saturation – In the same child as in the previous figure. Note the enhancement of an enlarged vascular channel (*arrows*) compared with the normal left leg

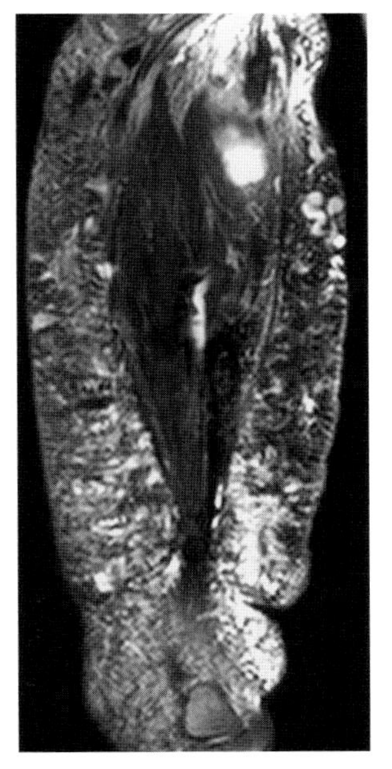

MRI coronal fat saturated T2 – Of the lower leg showing a lymphatico-venous malformation in Klippel Trenaunay syndrome. Note the marked thickening of the subcutaneous soft tissues and the dilated, tortuous vascular channels

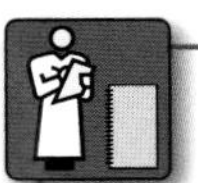

Radiological Differential Diagnosis

- High flow malformation (show flow voids on T2)
- Lymphatic malformation
- Sarcoma (if features do not conform fully to malformation, get a biopsy)

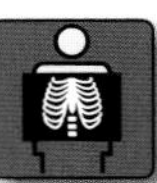

Imaging Options

- Primary: MRI with contrast
- Back-up: US
- Alternative: X-ray and CT

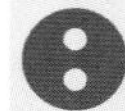

Imaging Findings

MRI

- Best modality to display the extent, showing increased thickness of the soft tissues and prominent subcutaneous venous channels.
- Intermediate signal on T1 (greater than muscle), and high signal on T2.
- MR venography useful to demonstrate dilated and anomalous veins.
- Gradient echo sequences show slow flow vessels best.
- T1 post-gadolinium can identify vessels with slow flow and enhancing septae of lymphaticovenous malformations.

US

- Limited value in diagnosis
- Can confirm the venous nature of the malformation but cannot show extent
- Used to direct percutaneous sclerosant therapy

X-Ray/CT

- Phleboliths are unique to low flow venous malformations

Tips

- Klippel Trenaunay Syndrome (KTW) is a mixed capillary, lymphaticovenous malformation with overgrowth of the affected limb.
- MRI in KTW shows varicosities of superficial veins and persistence of valve – less embryonic and deep venous channels.
- X-Ray will show phleboliths, overgrowth of the affected limb and cortical thickening of the adjacent bone.

Vesicoureteric Reflux (VUR)

Surgeon: J. Lazarus
Radiologist: A.M. du Plessis

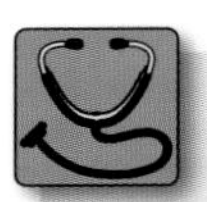

Clinical Insights

- Describes the retrograde flow of urine from the bladder to the ureter.
- An MCUG or "contrast" ultrasound (children <2 years) and indirect radionuclear cystogram (>2 years) establishes the diagnosis and its severity.
- Annual ultrasound examinations are indicated until VUR has resolved.

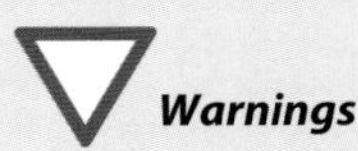

Warnings

- Some cases may result in chronic pyelonephritis, hypertension and chronic renal failure.
- Fifty percent of children with a UTI have VUR.

Controversies

- Investigation algorithms and treatment plans are evolving.
- Presently antibiotic prophylaxis is initially instituted with surgery reserved for specific indications:
  - Grade
  - Frequency and severity of breakthrough infections
  - Secondary VUR

Urgency

❑ Emergency
❑ Urgent
☑ Elective

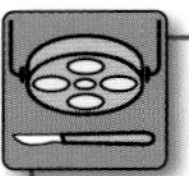

What the Surgeon Needs to Know

- Presence and grade of reflux
- Impact on the renal unit:
  - Size and interval growth
  - Cortico-medullary differentiation
  - Scarring
  - Dysplasia

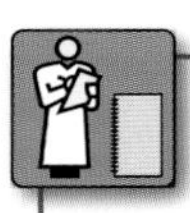

Clinical Differential Diagnosis

- Hydronephrosis and/or hydroureter of any other cause
- Secondary reflux (posterior urethral valves, neuropathic bladder, etc.)

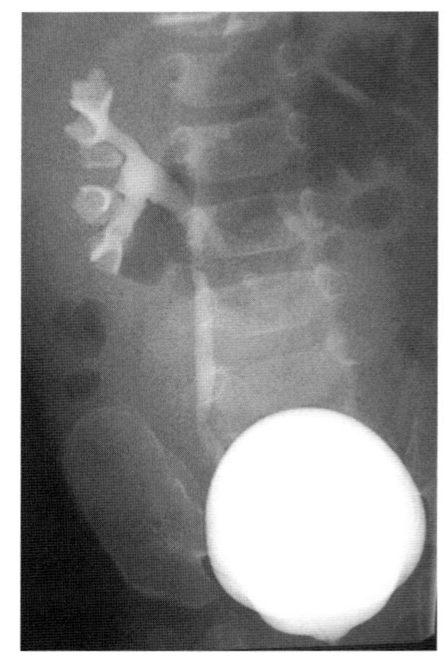

MCUG – VUR is demonstrated in a normal calibre ureter and in calyces that are not dilated on the right

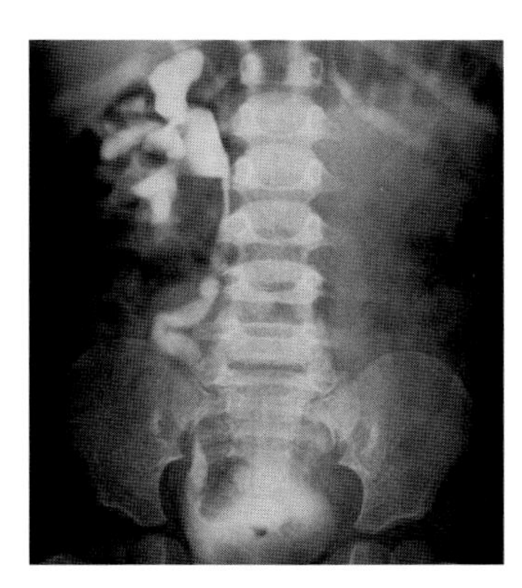

MCUG – VUR is demonstrated with dilated calyces but normal caliber ureter on the right

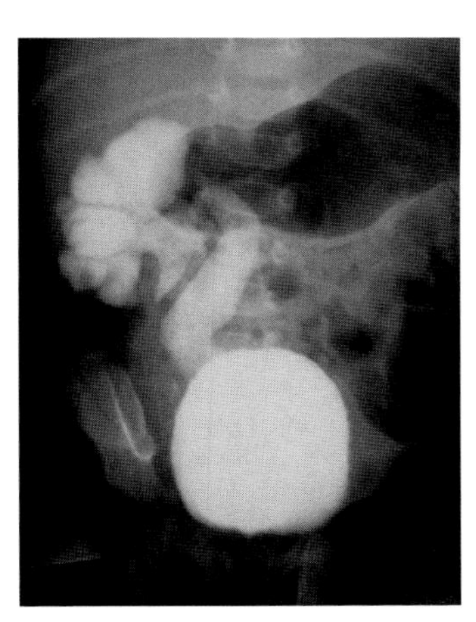

MCUG – VUR is demonstrated with dilated calyces and ureter on the right

Tips

- MCUG done with water-soluble contrast diluted 1:1 with sterile water.
- MCUG: Examination of choice for excluding posterior urethral valve in boys.
- MAG 3: Screening for females and follow-up of both sexes. (Less radiation but does not demonstrate urethra)
- Grading systems vary – Its more useful to describe the level of relux (into urethra only or into kidney) and any dilation (calyces and urethra).

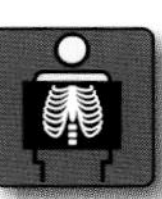

Imaging Options

- Primary: US (indicated with antenatal detection of abnormalities)
  MCUG
  Cysto sonography
- Alternative: Nuc Med (MAG 3)

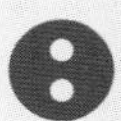

Imaging Findings

US

- Poor in detecting/predicting reflux
- When normal does not exclude reflux and when caliectasis does not indicate reflux
- Used to detect dilatation of urinary tract and anomalies

Cystosonography

- Major advantage is that there is no radiation involved
- Requires catheterisation and continual scanning to identify contrast in ureter and collecting system
- Does not assess urethra

MCUG

- Contrast seen flowing retrograde from bladder into ureter and renal collecting system
- Graded according to degree of dilation
- Assess urethra for PUV

Nuc Med (Mag 3)

- Less radiation than MCUG
- Radioactive tracer extends retrograde from bladder
- Can be performed "direct" by bladder catheterisation or "indirect" by IVI injection (indirect requires toilet training)

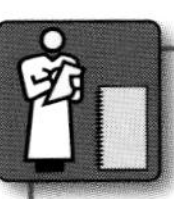

Imaging Differential Diagnosis

- MCUG mimics of uereteric reflux – Normal bowel surrounded by air or ileopectineal line
- Radio opaque stones – Watch for drainage post-void

Wilm's Tumour (Nephroblastoma)

Surgeon: S. Moore
Radiologist: N. Wieselthaler

Clinical Insights

- Embryonal neoplasm of kidney in childhood
- Clinical features:
  - Most common cause of a renal mass in children
  - Occurs mostly around 3–4 years
  - Tumour silent for a long time, presenting as an asymptomatic mass
  - Hypertension or haematuria occur in 20%
  - May bleed into tumour and "rupture" after minor trauma
  - Pulmonary metastases occur in 5–15%
  - 5–10% bilateral tumours

Warning

- Associated anomalies seen in 15%:
  - Beckwith-Weidemann syndrome
  - Hemihypertrophy
  - WAGR
  - Denys-Drash syndromes

Controversy

- Errors in diagnosis 5% (cystic Wilm's and xanthogranulomatous pyelonephritis)

Urgency

- ❑ Emergency
- ❑ Urgent
- ☑ Elective

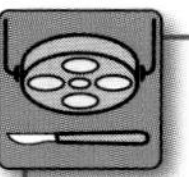

What the Surgeon Needs to Know

- Extent of disease – Local stage
- Renal vein, IVC or intracardiac tumour thrombus
- Bilateral kidney involvement
- Metastatic spread

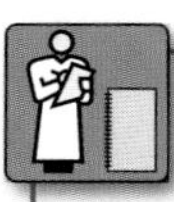

Clinical Differential Diagnosis

- Neuroblastoma
- Hydronephrotic kidney
- Multicystic kidney
- Nephroblastomatosis
- Other renal and retroperitoneal tumours (e.g. clear cell sarcoma)
- Mesoblastic nephroma

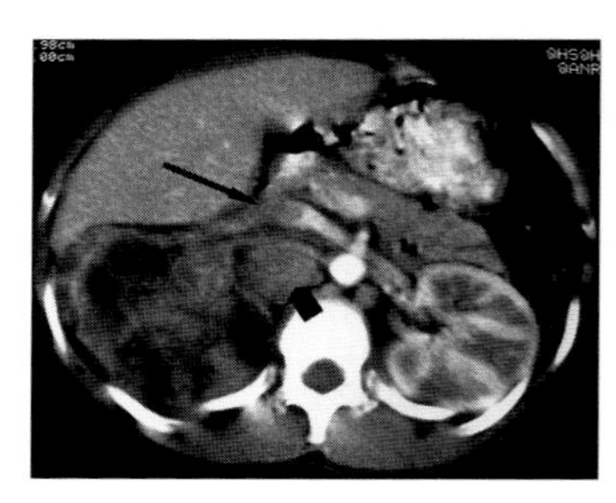

CT axial CT post-contrast – Right Wilm's tumour with thrombus in right renal vein extending into IVC (*long arrow*) and para-aortic adenopathy (*short arrow*)

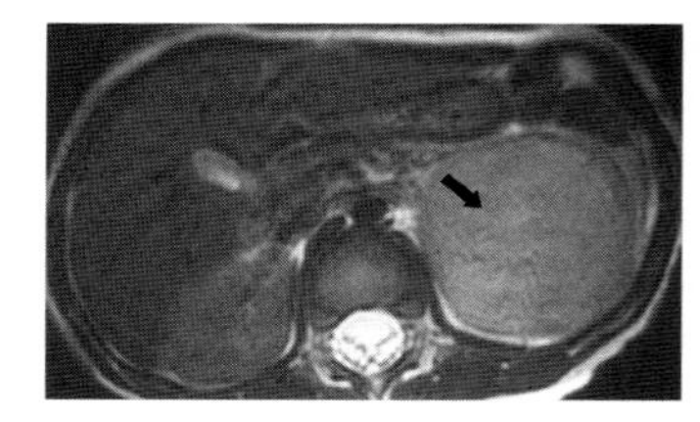

MRI STIR – Shows a relatively high intensity mass in the left kidney (*arrow*) consistent with a Wilm's tumour

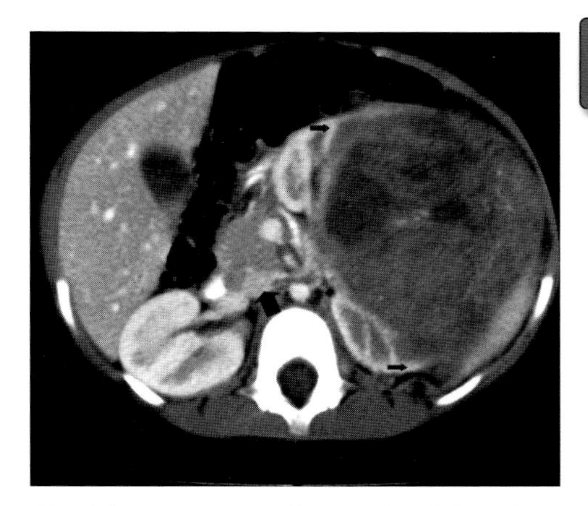

CT axial post-contrast – Left predominantly hypodense Wilm's tumour with classic "claw-sign" (*small arrows*) and patent left renal vein (*thick arrow*)

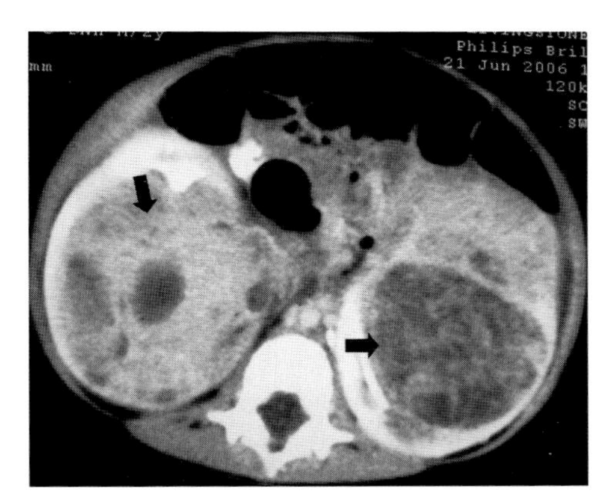

CT axial post-contrast – Bilateral renal Wilm's tumours (*arrows*)

Tips

- Look for "claw sign" for renal origin
- 10% bilateral, 10% calcify
- Displaces adjacent organs and vessels, not encases
- 15% have associated congenital abnormality
- CT must include chest for lung metastases
- IVC tumour thrombus expands the vessel – compressed vessels are unlikely to contain thrombus

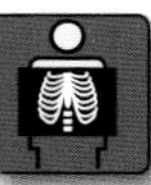

Imaging Options

- Primary: US, CT or MRI

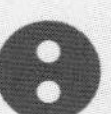

Imaging Findings

US

- Inhomogeneous mass with necrosis
- Doppler for differentiating tumour thrombus from venous compression

CT

- Large heterogeneous mass arising from kidney
- Poorly enhancing, ±necrosis, haemorrhage, cysts
- May extend into renal vein and IVC
- Local extension to nodes and perirenal fat
- Mets to lung (liver 20%)

MRI

- T1 hypointense, T2 mixed/hyperintense

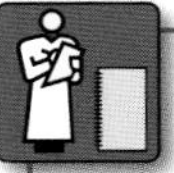

Radiological Differential Diagnosis

- Mesoblastic nephroma – solid/homogenous/infants
- Rhabdoid tumour – <1 year
- Clear cell sarcoma
- Neuroblastoma – More calcified, suprarenal, encases vessels
- Leukaemia/lymphoma ("tigroid" pattern of enhancement)
- Multilocular cystic nephroma – Indistinguishable from cystic Wilm's tumour
- Renal cell carcinoma (older children)

Index

Printing and Binding: Stürtz GmbH, Würzburg